Disorders of the Lumbar Spine

Disorders of the LUMBAR SPINE

ARTHUR J. HELFET,
B.Sc. (Cape Town), M.D., M.Ch.Orth. (Liverpool),
F.R.C.S. (England), F.A.C.S.

Clinical Professor, late Chairman, Department of Orthopaedic Surgery, Albert Einstein College of Medicine, New York; Formerly Consulting Orthopaedic Surgeon, Hospital for Joint Diseases, New York; formerly Senior Visiting Orthopaedic Surgeon and Lecturer in Orthopaedic Surgery, University of Cape Town and Groote Schuur Hospital, Cape Town, R.S.A.; Hunterian Professor, Royal College of Surgeons

and

DAVID M. GRUEBEL LEE,
M.B.B.Ch. (Witwatersrand), F.R.C.S. (England),
F.R.C.S. (Edinburgh)

Chairman, Department of Orthopaedic and Emergency Surgery, Frimley Park Hospital; Consultant Orthopaedic Surgeon, West Surrey/N.E. Hampshire Health District of Surrey Area Authority Group of Hospitals; Consultant Orthopaedic Surgeon, Rowley Bristow Orthopaedic Centre, Pyrford Hospital, Byfleet, Surrey, England

With 14 Guest Authors

J. B. Lippincott Company
Philadelphia   Toronto

ISBN 0-397-50381-4
Library of Congress Catalog Card Number 77-16571
Printed in the United States of America
1   3   5   4   2

Library of Congress Cataloging in Publication Data

Helfet, Arthur J
  Disorders of the lumbar spine

  Bibliography: p.
  Includes index.
   1. Vertebra, Lumbar—Diseases.   2. Backache.
I. Lee, David M. Gruebel, joint author.
II. Title
RD768.H44   616.7′3   77-16571
ISBN 0-397-50381-4

Guest Authors

Louis Berman, M.B., B.Ch., F.R.C.P. (E.)
Consultant Physician and Rheumatologist
Johannesburg General Hospital and University
 of Witwatersrand Medical School
Johannesburg, R.S.A.

Carl W. Coplans, M.R.C.S. (Eng.), L.R.C.P.
 (Lon.), D.Phys.Med. (R.C.S.&P.)
Senior Lecturer in Physical Medicine
University of Cape Town;
Senior Specialist in Physical Medicine
Department of Physical Medicine and
 Rehabilitation
Groote Schuur Hospital; and
Head, Department of Physical Medicine
Somerset Hospital
Cape Town, R.S.A.

Michael Devas, M.Ch., F.R.C.S.
Consultant Orthopaedic Surgeon
Hastings, England

Pieter D. de Villiers, M.B., Ch.B. (Cape Town),
 D.M.R.D. (Eng.), F.F.R. (Eng.)
Radiologist, Eugene Marais Hospital;
Formerly Professor of Radiology
University of Pretoria and
Head, Department of Radiology
H. F. Verwoerd Hospital
Pretoria, R.S.A.

George F. Dommisse, M.B., Ch.B. (UCT), M.D.
 (Pret.), Ch.M. (UCT), F.R.C.S. (Edin.)
Associate Professor
Department of Orthopaedics
University of Pretoria;
Member of the Faculty of Orthopaedics
College of Medicine of South Africa;
Vice-Head, Orthopaedic Department

H. F. Verwoerd Hospital
Transvaal Provincial Hospital Services
Pretoria, R.S.A.
Honorary Member
Scoliosis Research Society of North America
Founder Member
International Society for the Study of the
 Lumbar Spine

R. P. Gräbe, M.B., Ch.B. (Pretoria), M. Med.
 (Orth.) (Pretoria).
Professor and Head, Department of
 Orthopaedics, Kalafong Hospital,
University of Pretoria
 Pretoria, R.S.A.

J. G. Hannington-Kiff, B.Sc. (Hons), M.B., B.S.,
 M.R.C.S., L.R.C.P., F.F.A.R.C.S.
Director, Pain Clinic and Department of
 Clinical Investigation,
Frimley Park Hospital;
Consultant Anaesthetist, South West Thames
 Regional Health Authority;
Clinical Tutor, British Postgraduate Medical
 Federation, University of London

P. Kinnard, M.D.
Senior Resident in Orthopaedic Surgery
University of Saskatchewan College of
 Medicine
Saskatoon, Saskatchewan

W. H. Kirkaldy-Willis, M.A., M.D. (Cantab.),
 F.R.C.S. (E.), F.R.C.S. (C.), F.A.C.S.
Professor of Orthopaedic Surgery
University of Saskatchewan College of
 Medicine
Saskatoon, Saskatchewan

R. W. MacKay, M.D., F.R.C.P. (C.)
Assistant Professor of Pathology
University of Saskatchewan College of
  Medicine
Saskatoon, Saskatchewan

John Reilly, M.B., Ch.B.
Resident, Orthopaedic Surgery
University of Saskatchewan College of
  Medicine
Saskatoon, Saskatchewan

Louis Solomon, M.D., F.R.C.S.
Professor of Orthopaedic Surgery
University of the Witwatersrand Medical
  School and

Chief Orthopaedic Surgeon
Johannesburg General Hospital
Johannesburg, R.S.A.

John H. Wedge, M.D., F.R.C.S. (C.)
Assistant Professor of Orthopaedic Surgery
University of Saskatchewan College of
  Medicine
Saskatoon, Saskatchewan

K. Yong-Hing, M.D., Ch.B., F.R.C.S. (Glasgow)
Department of Orthopaedic Surgery
University of Saskatchewan College of
  Medicine
Saskatoon, Saskatchewan

Preface

*Man in sooth is a marvellous, vain, fickle and
unstable subject.*

Michel de Montaigne

The pattern of behavior of the normal back and the nature of the events and incidents which lead to derangement and misbehavior have intrigued the practitioner since primitive times.

The vast increase in knowledge and in the elegant aids to diagnosis and treatment in this golden age of science should ease our anxieties, but, alas, the vicissitudes of living in a world of increasing violence and mechanical complexity aggravate rather than solve the problems of man's back and its aches. Population explodes, transport is faster and less safe, both industry and the household present hazards, and even sport becomes relentless and ruthless. Pain in the back is a malady likely to be with us for a very long time.

Our concerns, then, must be to prevent accidents, to protect the patient from hurt and illness, and to heal and to readjust the injured, both physically and mentally. All disease is heir to the tyranny of pain, against which the genius of modern research is in constant rebellion.

For many centuries the medicine men of the East were aware of, and used, the influence of the psyche. Western medicine, on the other hand, is comparatively recent in its study of the role of the mind and emotions on the physical manifestations of disorder. Significant, therefore, is the increasing use in the West of Eastern techniques. The interrelationships of the systems are now better understood by both disciplines.

Through all these changes the traditional image of the "physician" has been one of compassion and clinical skill, all-observant and considerate of the patient. Indeed, amidst all the advances of treatment, these qualities, demonstrated nowhere more keenly than in the management of backache, remain essential.

The interest and advantage of 40 years of study of man's back and its ills have encouraged the authors to write this book for the clinician, be it physician or surgeon, who treats a *patient* as well as a disorder of the lumbar spine.

Arthur J. Helfet

Contents

Disorders of the Lumbar Spine

1 Introduction

The commonplace of schoolbooks of
tomorrow is the adventure of today.
Jacob Bronowski

"Backbone" conjures up a picture of resolution and gallantry in nation, army, or man. The "spineless" are without courage or will. Such images have influenced our idea of the functions of the vertebral column. How else do we explain the mystique surrounding the manipulator's click or the dread of any surgical procedure on the backbone? The purpose of this book is to dispel these fancies not only by relating backache to the whole patient but also by establishing understanding and precise diagnosis.

When, during the earlier years of this century, it was realized that the prolapsed intervertebral disc could give rise to the symptoms of sciatica, a logical focus for the study of the mechanical features of backache was established. But backache may also be a symptom of vascular or renal disease, a manifestation of psychosomatic stress, a cloak for an unresolved personality conflict or underlying insecurity. One must always remember in the management of patients with backache, that the patient must be considered and not only the mechanical disorder.

This book discusses aspects of medical and surgical practice, of orthopaedics and physical medicine, of neurology and neurosurgery, of rheumatology and acupuncture, of radiology and physiotherapy, including the art of manipulation. As definition improves it is possible to distinguish clinically disabilities produced by derangements of the spine from those due to injury or strain of muscles and ligaments, with or without adjacent nerve involvement, and to recognize when back pain is of extraspinal origin. Treatment may thus be more reasonable and more precisely directed. The practice of rule of thumb trial of antiinflammatory medication, corsets and physiotherapy to initiate conservative treatment, and routine myelogram and laminectomy when it fails, is often unsatisfactory and time-wasting for patient and physician.

At the same time it is important to realize the limited role played by surgical intervention. P. H. Newman reports that of each 100 patients who consult their general practitioner, 10 are referred to hospital and less than 1 per cent are treated by operation. From the author's records (A.J.H.) over a 10-year period, 1260 patients were referred as "discs" for treatment. They included 63 disabled by spondylolisthesis or spondylosis. Using strict criteria, a clinical diagnosis of derangement of a lumbar disc was made in 684. In all, including those in whom instability was the prime indication, operation was necessary in 138, or 8 per cent of the total of 1260. Of these, 11 required reoperation during the next 5 years, usu-

1

ally fusion or, for some whose original procedure was for spondylolisthesis, refusion.

Since prolonged disability caused by a deranged disc affects associated joints and muscles, the treatment of low backache and sciatica due primarily to the affected disc is not merely its surgical removal. The associated strain or backache must be treated as well. Reablement and rehabilitation are essential and must be complete.

Clinical examination and management of derangement and instabilities of intervertebral joints and their discs are the main subjects of this book, with some emphasis on the phenomenon of anatomical instability, which the authors consider responsible for most back pain and disability of mechanical origin.

The text is complemented by a number of distinguished contributions. *Professor Kirkaldy-Willis, John Wedge* and *their colleagues* at the University of Saskatchewan demonstrate and explain the anatomical changes that are basic to the clinical syndromes of back pain and their treatment. There is also their thoughtful interpretation of the increasing significance of "spinal stenosis."

Investigation by the modern range of roentgenographic and neuroroentgenographic techniques is superbly illustrated and interpreted by *Dr. Pieter de Villiers,* who maintains, "Mistakes are less often due to faulty interpretation than to inadequate radiography."

Professor Louis Solomon and *Dr. Berman* discusses the pathological and clinical features of rheumatoid arthritis of the spine and the ankylosing spondyloarthropathies. The distinctions between these disorders are defined and a rational approach to treatment is outlined.

Dr. John Hannington-Kiff writes a refreshingly original description of the medical management of pain and inflammation based on his pharmacologic and biophysiologic research.

Dr. C. W. Coplans describes the physical and injection treatment of backache and defines the indications and methods of orthodox orthopaedic manipulation designed to restore the normal pattern of movement rather than to reduce unproven and ill-defined subluxations. Manipulation is valuable, but it can be useless or harmful when inappropriate.

Professors George Dommisse and *R. P. Gräbe* present the results of recent research into the "failed operation" and advocate the remedies, including the refined techniques of microsurgery. A spinal surgeon, rather than an orthopaedic or a neurosurgeon, is the appropriate leader of the team.

Mr. Michael Devas describes his own views after recently undergoing laminectomy for a prolapsed lumbar disc. It is not often that a distinguished orthopaedic surgeon has given us the benefit of his experiences on the "receiving end" of surgery.

Thanks are due to those whose help was ready and unstinted; especially to Lydia Gruebel Lee, who edited with skill and patience, and to J. Stuart Freeman, Jr., and Suzanne Boyd, who, in the Lippincott tradition, have encouraged and facilitated progress and production of this book.

2 Clinical Problems of the Lumbar Spine

A number of clinical syndromes that cause pain in the back will be discussed before the anatomical features of mechanical breakdown of the spinal column in the lumbar region are given. Patients suffering from lumbar pain and disability can be grouped for ease of diagnosis and treatment.

CHILDHOOD INSTABILITY

Pain in the back is rare in children before adolescence, but when it does occur it is sudden and severe. It is more common in the thoracic or thoracolumbar spine, but it may also affect the lumbar region. A trivial, rotational movement will provoke an attack of screaming. Even breathing is difficult. Medical advice is therefore sought at an early stage. The child fears examination, adopts a stiff posture, and tries to rest the back. Muscle spasm, both voluntary and reflex, is present.

There is no bony tenderness, although palpation of the erector spinae muscles causes pain. Any attempt at straight-leg raising may increase the child's symptoms, as may rotation of the legs and pelvis. The pain is localized precisely, but signs of root compression are absent.

The syndrome bears all the features of intervertebral instability, but it is uncertain whether the pain arises in the zygapophyseal joints or the disc itself. When the patient is sedated and put to bed, symptoms subside, suddenly or within a few days. This suggests a mechanical lesion occurring in normal tissues. Attacks may be frequent enough to warrant the wearing of a polythene brace for a time.

The child may have only one attack or repeated episodes over a few months or years, but the condition usually disappears with further growth. Roentgenographs show nothing abnormal, and the only significant feature is that the children usually have congenital ligamentous laxity.

THE ADOLESCENT LOCKED BACK

Adolescent backache is uncommon, but it is often resistant to treatment. The parents are likely to be concerned and to press for active treatment and a firm prognosis, since the young person's education and athletic abilities are threatened. It is often the best sportsmen who are vulnerable to such attacks. Adolescents who suffer from Scheuermann's epiphysitis or osteochondritis are especially at risk.

This condition causes pain in the thoracolumbar spine in a young person

3

during the final growth spurt. Slight spinal deformity of the kyphotic type, with a thoracic hump, craning neck, and straight (i.e., kyphotic) lumbar spine is characteristic. The greatest spinal deformity is at the thoracolumbar junction, where the meeting of thoracic and lumbar segments results in an almost angular kyphos, with poor posture and muscle spasm. It is difficult to know whether the tight hamstring muscles are a cause or a result of the condition.

The diagnosis is confirmed by roentgenography. Typical features include irregular ossification of the vertebral end-plates, narrowing of thoracic disc spaces, Schmorl's nodes in the thoracic and thoracolumbar region, and an increased anteroposterior diameter of the vertebral bodies of the kyphotic thoracolumbar segment with anterior wedging. The latter is considered pathognomonic.

Abnormality of the lumbar disc spaces is unusual, except in a variation of the condition without significant thoracolumbar kyphosis. In this case the thoracic curve is compensated by an extreme lumbar lordosis with abnormal compression on the mid-lumbar discs forcing them forward and downward. Since the strength of the abnormal vertebral end-plate is not equal to the compressive force, damage occurs to its anterosuperior portion, which may break. It ossifies separately, or remains unossified, to give the typical roentgenographic feature known as the Butler lesion.[2]

The mere absence of roentgenographic changes does not preclude damage to the lumbar discs. Acute locking of the lumbar spine may occur without it. Even after fusion of the end-plate epiphysis, the back can suffer sudden, mechanical locking.

Locking in an adolescent's back is probably discogenic. It is accompanied by loss of straight-leg raising, often bilaterally, and by pain in the legs. Nerve root signs are infrequent, but when present indicate that the condition will not resolve easily.

Such recalcitrance is an indication of the strength of healthy tissue in the adolescent back. It takes a great deal of pressure to displace nuclear material. It cannot be squeezed like toothpaste; instead, large lumps are displaced to impinge against a strong, annular ligament. Such intervertebral prolapse is particularly difficult to reduce. Unlike degenerate material, nuclear tissue does not shrivel.

The stretched annulus causes reflex spasm, with muscle pain and tilting. Rupture of the annulus follows great provocation only, and the nerve roots are seldom stretched. Recovery does occur spontaneously but is often protracted. Occasionally, a patient is left with severe disability, so that operation becomes essential.

TRAUMATIC DISC PROLAPSE

Traumatic prolapse is found in young adults; more commonly they are male and are usually employed in heavy work, often involving the lifting of weights. Furniture movers, dockers, miners, truck drivers (who have to load their own trucks), and medical and nursing workers, are particularly vulnerable.

The patient develops acute pain in the back immediately after lifting a weight in a heedless way or unexpectedly bearing a heavy load, as for example, when the worker slips or his helpers release their grip prematurely. The sudden force is taken by the flexed and rotated spine. He develops an immediate, mid-line lumbar pain severe enough to stop him in his tracks. He is afraid to move and feels his back locked by the pain.

This may extend into the leg at the same time or shortly thereafter, in the sciatic distribution. There may be loss of nerve root function. The pain is severe enough to drive the sufferer to his bed in the first attack. Recumbency relieves his symptoms.

THE "YOUNG EXECUTIVE SYNDROME"

Of all types of severe back pain, that occurring in healthy adults between the ages of 35 and 45 is most common. It may be increasing in the urban population.

Patients with this syndrome tend to share personality traits and circumstances. They are often at the upper levels of executive responsibility but are seldom at the top of the ladder of command. They are more likely to have the position of "first lieutenant" and consequently are subject to the pressures of a subordinate role. Many have been recently promoted and feel that they have to prove themselves. They are hard-working, conscientious, and ambitious, but harbor secret fears about the ability to cope.

Women who feel restricted because they are not engaged in a business or professional career, or who may resent having to run a home and cope with the children while their husbands commute to the city or take sudden, overseas business trips, develop the syndrome.

The injury is often unexpectedly trivial: a briefcase lifted with rotated back, bending to pick up the morning paper, even a sneeze can precipitate the attack. The result is the same as in traumatic prolapse: sudden lumbar pain is followed by sciatica.

The story appears straightforward, but further questioning reveals that the patient may have had backache for months, often fluctuating in severity but not directly associated with trauma. It has seldom prevented him from doing anything. On the contrary, the extent and nature of the patient's physical activity during this period is surprising. Again and again one hears stories from those who, apparently fully employed in a challenging job, lay patios in their spare time, build house extensions, redecorate homes, or cope alone with infirm relatives. This illogical pressure of activity characterizes the syndrome.

From this pinnacle the patient is precipitated into profound incapacity. There is a precise logic in this physical breakdown. The businessman's incessant work has been a sign of this conflict. The question of whether he could cope has been answered in the negative. Insecurity manifests itself in psychosomatic distress and useless, even punishing, activity. The syndrome is one of "a storm in the midst of a calm."

Collapse is therapeutic, since it allows the patient to rest, and gives a socially acceptable reason for doing so. Even the strongest among us need such support. The only time the late President Kennedy appeared in public using crutches to rest his constantly painful back was on his return from his first meeting with Khrushchev in Vienna.

It must be emphasized that the prolapse is real and is as likely to lead to operation as any other. Unless the underlying stress is relieved, surgery is even more likely.

Not all attacks of lumbar pain at this age are predominantly psychosomatic. There may be a mechanical fault, either developmental or acquired. The patient may have developed the psychological overlay because of long-standing back pain and incapacity.

Patients of other ages with disc prolapse are less likely to have a psychological stimulus. The young develop other psychosomatic conditions due to the stress of growing, while the aging suffer from the realization of failing abilities; but the target organ is not the lumbar spine.

It seems that in the middle years, the disc material of the lower lumbar spine is vulnerable to psychological stress. It is known that nuclear material in this region has undergone sufficient chemical change to differ from the young man's disc, both macroscopically and biochemically.[4] It has lost elasticity and become "degenerate."

Presumably it is prone to swelling,

since prolapsed nuclear material in this age-group is often found at operation to be under great tension. Pathological increase in intervertebral pressure will cause pain by stretching the intact annulus and will allow disruption of the ligaments, with disc prolapse, by comparatively insignificant injury. It is thought that psychological stress may be one cause of such disc swelling, but the mechanism is not understood.

It is not only the lower·lumbar spine that is vulnerable at this age. Similar symptoms may develop in the lower cervical spine, before, during, or after an attack of back pain. The discs in this region deteriorate at the same time.

DISC PROLAPSE IN THE MIDDLE-AGED

Middle-aged people also suffer lumbar disc prolapses. Except for a difference in emphasis, the essential features are similar. Psychological stress is not usually as evident as in younger patients, and the force required to precipitate the injury is less. More advanced degeneration means a softer disc to displace.

The history may reveal one attack or a series of episodes over a number of years, after which the attacks cease spontaneously. They are not usually as severe or incapacitating as in younger men and are less likely to require surgery.

The term "middle-aged" may apply to the disc and not to the patient himself. The disc has often reached the stage of collapse in which narrowing of the intervertebral space, sclerosis of surrounding, weight-bearing bone, and osteophytic lipping are roentgenographically visible: yet the disc with local roentgenographic changes is not necessarily the focus of the patient's symptoms. An apparently normal disc above or below may be the site of prolapse and may well behave like that in the young patient.

CLAUDICATION OF THE CAUDA EQUINA

Claudication of the cauda equina has been understood and diagnosed only recently. The term is appropriate, provided it is used to describe a symptom characterized by pain in the back and leg severe enough to cause a limp. *Claudication* is an allusion to the limp developed by the Roman Emperor, Claudius.

As in other forms of claudication, the symptom is intermittent, increasing with activity and relieved by rest. Usage has added a suggestion of vascular insufficiency to the term.

Some patients with mechanical disease of the spine, especially in late middle or old age, have pain in the legs and back on effort. They describe a precise effort tolerance before the symptoms begin. If walking is continued, the pain increases until the legs become weak, and further effort may produce sensory disturbance. In many cases the pain subsides and strength returns to the limbs if the patient stops walking: in others, the patient may have to sit or lean against something for a while before continuing. The period of rest may be brief or as long as a quarter of an hour. It seldom lasts longer. Patients with this condition are comfortable when sitting or lying down, but are unable to cope with the increasing oxygen demands of exercise.

Discomfort and pain are hardly ever limited to one segment of the spine but extend distally as far as the sacrum. Some cases gradually deteriorate; the patient complains of decreasing effort-tolerance and increasing weakness that makes him almost chair-bound. This is not invariable; as with intermittent claudication due to peripheral arterial obstruction, the condition may stabilize and the sufferer accommodate to his disability. The pattern of symptoms in the elderly, usually due to femoral arterial block, is familiar to vascular surgeons. It may also follow profunda femoris block or even the Leriche syndrome (aortic bifurcation obstruction).

Because of the number of small-caliber spinal vessels, it is difficult to demonstrate the block by arteriography. There is no reason to doubt that mild compression leads to intermittent claudication. Severe compression of end-vessels results in major damage to the spinal cord with necrosis of neurones followed by transverse myelitis.

The following cases, seen by one of the authors, are illustrative:

CASE 2-1. A 20-year-old policeman suffered acute, traumatic, central L5–S1 prolapse when he fell on duty and landed on his buttocks. Emergency laminectomy and complete disc removal resulted in full recovery, but 3 weeks later, after his discharge from the ward, he developed permanent perineal sensory loss, with a paralyzed bladder and patulous anus. Myelography failed to reveal a block, or even any indentation, of the Myodil column. There was no sign of infection, hematoma, or recurrent prolapse. In the end, neurosurgical opinion was that irrecoverable, avascular necrosis of the cauda equina had occurred.

CASE 2-2. A 63-year-old foreman mechanic developed typical features of claudication of the cauda equina. In hospital he was able to walk only 40 feet before having to rest. Attempts by the physiotherapists to make him walk further led to weakness of the legs, until he could no longer stand. Myelography showed L5–S1 lateral disc prolapse, which, at operation, looked like a young man's prolapse in that the annulus was strong and the nuclear material tense, elastic, and gelatinous. Recovery was complete. It was not the disc but the blood vessels of the cauda equina that were middle-aged.

The lumbar spine is the region most commonly affected because of the frequency of obstructive, mechanical lesions in this area and perhaps because of the local distribution of blood vessels. Cauda equina syndrome is a result of spinal stenosis, described in Chapter 5.

Diagnosis depends upon the presence of an intact, peripheral arterial tree. Obliteration of a distal pulse should always be investigated immediately, but it should be borne in mind that obstruction at the aortic bifurcation does not cause the loss of distal pulses. There is always a significant delay in pulses in the legs compared with the arms. Aortic block or aneurysm can cause back pain and buttock claudication and should always be considered as a differential diagnosis.

Diagnosis is confirmed by myelography, which reveals one or more extradural swellings, diverting or obstructing the flow of contrast medium. The lesion, at this stage, is more frequently a transverse ridge of fibrosed material with osteophyte formation.[3] In some cases, blocks at several levels make treatment difficult.

Acute Central Disc Prolapse

Acute, severe central disc prolapse is uncommon, but when it does occur diagnosis is a matter of urgency, for, if delayed, the consequence could be permanent neurologic disability.

In most cases of disc herniation, extruded material comes to lie in a posterolateral position, producing unilateral signs and symptoms, but there is often some extension of the prolapse across the midline so that signs are present bilaterally. For practical reasons the term "acute central prolapse" should be reserved for cases of sudden onset, usually following trauma.

The patient develops bilateral signs and symptoms as well as loss of sacral sensation. Usually the loss of sensation is complete, extending from the perianal skin to the perineum; so that feeling is lost in the penis and scrotum in the male, and in the vulva in the female. The anal sphincter is patulous, while absent bladder sensation accompanies retention of urine.

Unless the cauda equina compression is relieved within a few hours, the paralysis of the bladder may be permanent. Even the delay of a few days may result in incomplete recovery, with the patient profoundly disabled by the loss of sphincter control.

Myelography shows a large and broad prolapse, compressing the dural sheath firmly enough to block the flow of cerebrospinal fluid. The patient should be prepared for immediate decompression and removal of the disc. Goldthwaite's original case was typical.

The author has seen the syndrome develop precipitately in healthy patients with unilateral disc prolapse; a sudden movement of flexion and rotation is followed by loss of sacral sensation. Usually there are prodromal symptoms of backache but it can occur without warning if the flexion injury is severe enough, for example following a fall onto the buttocks in which the lumbar spine is acutely flexed. A not inconsiderable number of patients develop the syndrome after incautious manipulation. Presumably a congenitally inadequate annulus, or one weakened by chronic inflammatory change, has ruptured.

Acute central prolapse is due only to maximal compression. In many cases there is some degree of cauda equina dysfunction, with bladder weakness ranging from minimal to severe. The volume of residual urine in the bladder, measured by urethral catheterization immediately after spontaneous micturition, is a precise indication of the degree of paralysis. Urgent decompression is necessary only in the presence of perineal anesthesia.

THE OSTEOPOROTIC BACK

Demineralization of the skeleton is so common in the later years of both men and women as to constitute, almost, the normal state of affairs. Urist reported an incidence of the condition in one woman in four and one man in five or six over the age of 70.

Albright postulated that osteoporosis was due to deficiency of the protein matrix in bone,[1] but more recent studies[5] have suggested that, as well as the loss of the protein structure on which apatite crystals are laid to constitute normal bone, patients have suffered a long period of calcium deficiency before the onset of the syndrome. It is probable that both calcium and collagen are lost in the condition.

Osteoporosis is a generalized state of skeletal tissues in which there is a reduction in the total amount of bone without a change in its chemical composition. Symptoms occur in those regions subjected to the greatest stress, such as the upper lumbar spine and the proximal half of the femur.

Clinically the disease is of insidious onset over years, with little to announce its presence to the patient except for aching in the bones and joints and the occasional sudden muscle cramp, the latter probably due to disordered calcium metabolism. These symptoms are so common in older patients that they seldom warrant attention either by the sufferer or the medical advisor.

Loss of calcium can be quantified by repeated roentgenographs of the spine in which a dried bone, such as a human phalanx, is incorporated so that a comparison can be made of bone density on the films taken at different times, usually by electronic measurement of light transmitted through the roentgenograph. Such techniques are difficult to calibrate and are usually confined to experimental procedures. Bone biopsy gives more certain measurement of the degree of osteoporosis.

The protein loss is mainly of collagen. Such loss occurs not only in the bones but in all tissues. Clinically it is most easily seen in subcutaneous tissues, especially on the dorsum of the hands, the skin of which is thin and atrophic. Subcutaneous veins are abnormally visible, giving a marbled appearance to the skin. There is abnormal capillary fragility, with petechiae or even larger collections of extravasated blood.

In time, the patient's spine begins to collapse, the increasing spinal curvature causing aching pain as the ligaments bear more weight. A decrease in stature due to thoracic kyphosis is observed. Pain in the lumbar or thoracolumbar region intensifies and becomes constant.

A few women appear to develop an acute version of the condition, with constant back pain and relatively rapid collapse of the spine. In some, the condition is severe enough to suggest a diagnosis of metastatic neoplasia or even hyperparathyroidism, but in these diseases the erythrocyte sedimentation rate is usually raised to levels appreciably higher than those found in osteoporosis.

Progressive thoracic kyphosis leads to crowding of the rib cage and consequent loss of chest expansion. Pulmonary disability adds to the patient's misery, as does the encroachment of the floating ribs on the iliac crest. Some patients' main complaint is of recurrent, sudden sharp pain in the hypochondrium. Careful questioning establishes the mechanical nature of this pain, which is due to the impingement of a twelfth rib against the iliac crest. Palpation confirms the diagnosis when the standing patient is asked to inhale: the tip of the lowest rib can be felt to click against the crest. Excision of the offending rib cures the pain.

Decreasing strength of the vertebral bodies may reveal an interesting fact of the physiology of the nucleus pulposus. The normal disc material behaves as a perfect elastic body, transmitting vertical compression forces horizontally, and so protects the vertebral and-plates from unacceptable force. Such a disc is normally under tension, while a "degenerative" disc has lost this property. In severe osteoporosis, this tension within the nucleus pulposus may be great enough to distort the weakened vertebral end-plate sufficiently to squash the body of the vertebra. The result is a characteristic fish-shaped appearance on a lateral roentgenograph. Collapse of the vertebral body may occur gradually, giving rise to an aching pain in the spine, but there may be sudden infraction of the body with resulting sudden pain that subsides gradually in 6 to 12 weeks.

Of all the causes of sudden, severe pain in the back of the osteoporotic patient, wedge fracture is the most common and the most significant. The fracture is pathological in that is is caused by trivial trauma, since the softened bone is unable to bear normal compression. The wedge fracture is always caused by a flexion movement of the spine. Most occur in the T12 or L1, because when an acute flexion force is applied to the spine, maximum compression is applied to the apex of the curve, just as an iron bar held at either end will break at the apex of the curve when an angulation force is applied to it. The fracture is stable, since the bone collapses but the posterior ligament complex does not rupture.

The degree of collapse depends upon the softness of the bone and on the force that has been applied. It varies from the minor wedge to very severe loss of height of the vertebral body.

The usual cause of fracture is a fall onto the buttocks, with flexion of the spine. One such case was that of a retired, 79-year-old doctor, who attempted to close one of those sliding sash windows still found in Victorian houses in the British Isles. He placed his hands on the window frame (as he had done previously on many occasions) and applied the weight of his body to the stiff mechanism. In his attempt to push the frame downwards, he felt something click in his upper lumbar spine and developed severe back pain.

This story of sudden pain is typical. There is associated spasm of surrounding muscles; the dispersing hematoma may even reach the surface and cause characteristic skin discoloration in the thin patient after a few weeks. An angular kyphos can be seen at the level of the fracture, and gentle percussion of the vertebral spines causes tenderness that is often severe in the early stages. Tenderness, abating gradually in 6 to 12 weeks, is an important sign of recent fracture. Lateral roentgenographs show the severity of the collapse, but even careful study of the films seldom reveals whether the fracture is new, because the roentgenograph, however good, does not show a break in continuity of trabeculae in the poorly-visualized bone of the osteoporotic patient.

Roentgenography cannot differentiate between new and old fractures. As a result, what the radiologist reports may well be a united fracture. The general practitioner, receiving such a report and failing to realize the significance of a recent trivial injury, concludes that the patient is suffering from disc prolapse. The palpating finger of the orthopaedic surgeon clarifies the situation, and a good prognosis can be given in most cases.

The patient is left with a kyphos and is liable to suffer repeated fractures at different levels. This leads to gradually increasing deformity.

SENILE COLLAPSE OF THE LUMBAR SPINE

With or without osteoporosis, time takes its inevitable toll of the human frame. Collapse of disc material comes to us all in the end, affecting mostly those regions of the spine subjected to the greatest force during normal activity. Despite genetic variation in the strength of disc material, most people in Europe and America have changes that would be roentgenographically evident in the lower cervical and the lumbosacral spine by their fifth decade.

In the normally-shaped spine, such changes occur in those areas in which the vertebral column is held in the extremes of its range of movement. A similar effect is present in any abnormal curve of the spine. Degenerative changes thus appear in the apex of the mid-thoracic kyphosis that follows adolescent Scheuermann's disease. Similar changes occur at the apex of the lateral curves of patients who have suffered adolescent or congenital rotational scoliosis. The adult who has walked with fixed flexion of the hips for many years, with resultant constant lumbar lordosis, is more likely to develop severe lower lumbar disc collapse than are those with normal hips.

In the end, senile kyphosis is the rule. Abnormal strain upon the intervertebral ligaments is its consequence, amounting in many patients to a disability. In some, lateral collapse of a mid-lumbar disc takes place. It can occur slowly or precipitately, with acute lumbar pain and spasm. Once begun, the angular collapse tends to accelerate because of the force of gravity. The increasing tilt causes deformity of the trunk with progressively poorer posture, which may cause joint strain in the lower limbs. The rate of development of deformity of the trunk, with accompanying pain and weakness, may be surprisingly quick.

Treatment, which consists of spinal bracing, may go a long way toward alleviating the condition. Attention should always be directed to muscle-strengthening exercises that are within the patient's mental and physical capabilities. An Occupational Therapy Department of a geriatric day hospital can be a great help in this regard.

REFERENCES

1. Albright, F.: [quoted in] "Therapeutic Insights II." Sandoz Australia, Pty., Ltd., 1975
2. Butler, R. W.: Long-term follow up of lumbar vertebral osteochondritis. J. Bone Joint Surg. *48B*:585, 1965.
3. Kirkaldy-Willis, W. H., Paine, K. W. E., Cauchoix, J., and McIvor, G. W. D.: Lumbar spinal stenosis. Clin. Orthop., *99*:30, 1974.
4. Mankin, H. J., and Orlic, P. A.: Effect of aging on protein synthesis in rabbit articular cartilage. J. Bone Surg. *47A*:1100, 1964.
5. Nordin, B. E. C.: the pathogenesis of osteoporosis. Lancet, *1*:1011, 1961.

Mechanical Causes of Lumbar Pain Other Than Disc Pathology

3

The clinical syndromes described in Chapter 2 are not the only causes of mechanical pain in the back. The intervertebral discs are by no means the only anatomical structures in the lumbar spine that give rise to pain. Muscles, ligaments, and the other synovial joints of, and surrounding, the central spinal column are vulnerable to the stresses of gravity and movement as well as the nucleus pulposus. They are also likely to suffer from strain, weakness, degeneration, and injury. A comprehensive classification of such lesions will not be attempted, but common causes of pain that simulate disc disease will be described.

FATIGUE AND SPINAL SAG

There is no exhaustive definition of the term "fatigue"; nor is the difference between fitness and unfitness in athletes easy to define. At the beginning of the season players tire easily and after training feel stiff and sore. This does not imply muscle strain. Following a strenuous game, a sportsman soon recovers when he has had a hot bath and adequate rest. Each day he is able to run further and play for longer periods without ill effect. It would seem that this is a physiological reaction to increasing activity.

On occasion, fatigue can be of more lasting significance. For example, after an operation on the knee the muscles waste. Overexercising or bearing weight before the muscles are strong enough to cope leads to effusion in the joint, followed by pain, tenderness, and the other signs of strain. A similar effect occurs after back operations. As long as the exercise program is within the limits of fatigue, reablement is effected without strain.

Some years ago, in an attempt to explain postoperative muscle weakness and wasting, it was postulated that there were two types of muscle fibers: the one controlling posture and the other for quick movement. Wasting of the latter, for example after disuse or operation, would leave a patient weak and fatigued after sudden activity such as sport, since he was trying to achieve repeated, quick movements with postural muscles. Recent histologic studies have shown that muscle fibers can indeed be divided into two groups by their staining properties, at least in children born with severe talipes equinovarus.[5] Other evidence suggests that a similar differentiation occurs in the muscles of patients after disuse.[3] The revival of the old theory would go a long way toward explaining pathological fatigue. It is certain that muscle wasting can occur within a short time of the onset of a condition that immobilizes a limb. A locked knee, a fractured long bone, or a prolapsed disc, all cause muscle wasting.

The daily fatigue of housework, agricultural or other hard labor leads to swelling and aching of the legs, but this disappears after a night's rest. In time, such overactivity causes persistent symptoms; a form of *chronic strain.*

Such recurring states of fatigue, if not interrupted by a program of alternate exercise and rest to maintain muscle tone, result in chronic lumbar backache. In time, the postural muscles fail, and the patient develops "spinal sag," with increasing lumbar lordosis, a round back, and drooping shoulders. Goldthwait described spinal sag and its effects in the following graphic way: "... the disturbance in rib and diaphragm movement, the bulging abdomen, the viscera dragging on the omentum, leading to shallow breathing, flatulence, and a tired existence."[4]

In the end, such faulty body mechanics lead to inflammatory swelling of the synovium of the zygapophyseal joints of the spine and to consequent osteoarthritic degeneration. At the same time, disc collapse occurs with spondylosis of the intervertebral joints.

The sagging posture leads to backache, but, especially in its early stages, this symptom may be relieved by postural exercises. There is a gradual restoration of normal muscle tone, helped, if necessary, by the temporary use of a Goldthwait brace. A system of exercise is described in Chapter 10. Care must be taken not to allow the patient to overexercise, for when he is run down and tired from overwork, vigorous exercise to "get fit" is not an antidote, unless it is blended judiciously with rest. Overexertion increases the strain on tired muscles.

In adolescence, fatigue commonly follows the spinal sag that results from the bone collapse characteristic of Scheuermann's osteochondritis. Postural exercises are as important in this condition as in the sag that occurs in later life.

ABDOMINAL WALL COLLAPSE

The security and comfort of the back depend not only on the lumbar muscles and ligaments but also on the strength of the abdominal wall and prevertebral muscles. In all cases of chronic pain in multiparous women, the abdomen should be palpated to determine if divarication of the rectus abdominis muscle is present. Such divarication is a good indication of the extent of pathological stretching of the abdominal muscles.

The clinical test for the diagnosis of rectus divarication is to ask the patient to lie supine and then to raise the head from the pillow. The examining hand can easily feel the gap between the contracted pillars of the rectus, and the fingers will sink into the soft abdominal wall.* The width of the gap may vary from 1 cm. to a hand's breadth.

Whatever the cause of the sagging abdominal wall, visceroptosis follows, and it leads to strain on the lumbosacral ligament. This in turn produces stretching of the anterior common ligament, which becomes thickened and even ossified. Eventually this physiological attempt to buttress the lumbar spine fails, and severe lumbar lordosis develops. In the end the patient has chronic lumbar pain which, although not severe, is difficult to overcome.

Physiotherapy, in the form of heat, massage, diathermy, or the like, can be of no help in this condition. A spinal brace is also useless, since, to support the lordotic lumbar spine in the vertical position, its curve must be greater than that of the lordosis. However, a modern elastic corset of two- or three-way stretch material available in any store, will support the abdominal wall and overcome the lordosis.

To prevent abdominal collapse care should be taken during the antenatal period to prevent obesity, and abdominal strengthening exercises should be per-

---

* Guy Beauchamp: Personal communication.

formed, especially isometric contraction of the muscles. These, together with deep breathing exercises, prevent excessive stretching of the muscle sheets by the enlarging uterus. In a similar way adequate postpartum exercises aid the restoration of the abdominal wall; especially important if the woman intends to become pregnant again.

Intractable divarication of the rectus is best treated by surgical repair when childbearing is finished. Until such time, obesity should be prevented. Thereafter exercises to flatten the lumbar curve must be performed, together with isometric exercises for the abdominal wall. Back extension exercises are obviously contraindicated.

ACUTE AND CHRONIC STRAINS OF MUSCLES AND LIGAMENTS

Acute Strains

After lifting a heavy weight or making a sudden twisting movement the patient experiences immediate pain, which may stop him in his tracks. The episode may be transitory. Usually it is followed by a pain-free interval, after which the patient develops stiffness that limits his mobility. The stiffness subsides gradually over a few days. In the athlete, the pain of a sprained ligament in an ankle, knee, or in the back is typically mild while the injured part is warm from the game, but the pain strikes him with greater severity in the changing room or after a night's rest.

This clinical syndrome differs from complete rupture of a ligament or muscle when, after a brief sensation of snapping accompanied by a stab of pain at the time of the injury, loss of function is the predominant symptom and pain may be minimal. Later, the joint tends to give way under stress.

Chronic Strains

Burrows and Coltart defined the adhesions that form in chronic strain as "scar tissue which interferes with the normal free play between the parts of the motor system." The lesion occurs at the junction of tissues of differing elasticity, for example where muscle fibers or ligaments are attached to bone or tendon. Disruption of such fibers with hemorrhage is followed by reactionary swelling. The extent of the process depends upon the severity of the strain.

The exudate that forms is organized by tissue repair to form fine fibrous adhesions, which are probably responsible for pain on movement as they are subjected to tension. Manipulation is a successful form of treatment if it results in the snapping of these adhesions.

The diagnosis of chronic strain is made when a patient with a history of previous injury has a palpable swelling in the muscle or ligament with finger-point tenderness. If the rupture has been a complete one, a gap will be felt, accompanied by a greater degree of swelling than is the case in partial rupture, but the patient has less pain or tenderness.

FRACTURES OF THE LUMBAR TRANSVERSE PROCESSES

Any twisting movement of the spine, especially if caused by sudden powerful but uncontrolled muscle contraction, can fracture one or several of the lumbar transverse processes. This is probably the most common avulsion fracture in the body, and in its most severe form may involve all the lumbar transverse processes on one side of the spine.[1]

Painful at first, transverse process fractures rarely cause prolonged disability. The pain is best treated by the injection of a local anesthetic agent into the site of the hematoma and swelling and by the immediate administration of proteolytic enzymes and antiinflammatory medication by mouth. Since the fractures are really muscle injuries, accompanied by no instability, activity is preferable to rest. Immobilization is not indicated. In many cases the avulsed tip of the transverse process is separated so widely from the rest of the bone that it fails to unite. It is of no significance, and the patient makes a full recovery from the injury.

SLIPPED LUMBAR EPIPHYSEAL END-PLATE

From birth the endochondral bone of the lumbar spine is covered by a plate of epiphyseal cartilage on the upper and lower surfaces of each vertebra (Fig. 3-1). A ring of secondary centers of ossification appears within this end-plate at about the age of 14 (Fig. 3-2), and it fuses to the primary bone by the age of 20 (Fig. 3-3). Damage can occur to the end-plate in young people if it has been subjected to severe injury or if it is softened by a pathological condition (Fig. 3-4, 3-5).

Adolescent Vertebral Epiphysitis

Adolescent vertebral epiphysitis (vertebral osteochronditis, Scheuermann's syndrome) was described in Chapter 2. It leads to epiphyseal end-plate damage in the lower thoracic spine, when intervertebral disruption of the end-plate by the nucleus pulposus results in the typical lesion seen in the lateral roentgenograph, the Schmorl's node (Fig. 3-6). This relatively common lesion may even be seen in the lumbar spine if it is straight (that is,

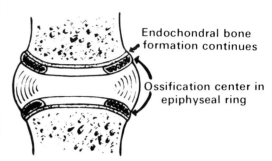

AT ADOLESCENCE

Endochondral bone formation continues

Ossification center in epiphyseal ring

FIG. 3-2. Diagram of the development of the vertebral cartilage end-plates in an adolescent.

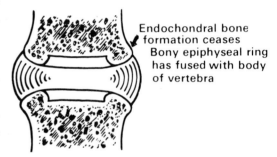

FULLY GROWN

Endochondral bone formation ceases
Bony epiphyseal ring has fused with body of vertebra

FIG. 3-3. Diagram of the development of the vertebral cartilage end-plates in a fully grown child.

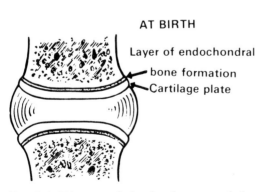

AT BIRTH

Layer of endochondral bone formation
Cartilage plate

FIG. 3-1. Diagram of the development of the vertebral cartilage end-plates in a child at birth. (see Figs. 3-2, 3-3).

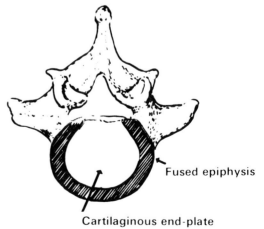

Fused epiphysis

Cartilaginous end-plate

FIG. 3-4. The adult end-plate.

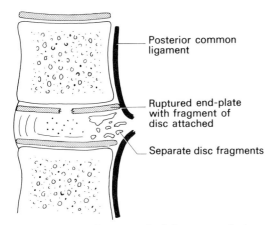

FIG. 3-5. How the normal adolescent end-plate is damaged as a result of severe injury.

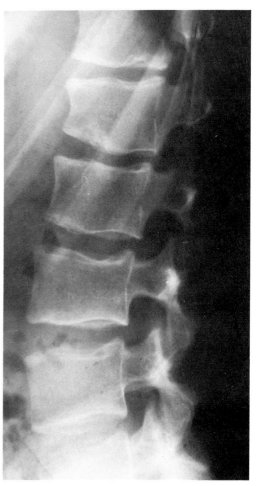

FIG. 3-6. A roentgenograph of the thoracolumbar spine shows many of the features that follow vertebral osteochondritis. In the highest visible disc a posteriorly placed Schmorl's node is present. At the next level, disruption of the inferior end-plate of the vertebral body has occurred anteriorly, following anterior prolapse of the disc during growth. The lumbar spine is kyphotic. In contradistinction to traumatic rupture this lesion occurs with minimal injury. Note the lack of ossification of the separated fragment.

kyphotic). However the normally lordotic lumbar spine, when subjected to compression, transmits the force forward and downward. If the end-plate cartilage has been softened by epiphysitis, its anterior border can be injured, or even disrupted, leaving a fragment of cartilage to ossify separately. This lesion was described by Butler who commented on its benign nature and the rarity of symptoms.[2] It may be seen in patients suffering from Scheuermann's syndrome, but is commonly seen as a chance finding in lateral roentgenographs of the lumbar spine taken in later life. The patient is then often suffering from other disc pathology, often at a lower level. Unless recognized for what it is, it may be misdiagnosed as some sinister condition such as tuberculous spinal disease, which it does not resemble roentgenographically. Sclerosis of the surrounding vertebral body makes differentiation easy in most cases.

Traumatic Slipped Epiphysis

A similar injury to the anterior part of the end-plate can occur in the normal adolescent spine. It is rare. In nearly four decades of orthopaedic practice, the author (A.J.H.) has demonstrated the lesion in only three patients at operation. A presumptive diagnosis was made in four others. It was interesting to find that some instances of persistent back pain and sciatica in adolescents were due to the protruding edge of the slipped part of the cartilaginous end-plate.

All the patients with this condition were tall, well-built young men, between the ages of 15 and 18, with long backs. Each had been subjected to traumatic stress which was excessive for his immature skeletal development. Three were injured while playing rugby for the University First Team. A fourth, also a university student, was at home on the farm for the vacation and had helped unload 200-lb. bags of wheat from a wagon. Toward the end of the day, when he had become overtired, his back had collapsed and locked. The pain and disability of a fifth patient, aged 15 years, originated the first time he attended a weight-lifting class. Another young man had slipped and fallen badly before the onset of his symptoms.

The acute phase of the condition is characterized by great pain, with clinical signs similar to those of disc prolapse, but at an upper lumbar level. Roentgenographs show no abnormality other than immobility due to muscle spasm, for the cartilage end-plate is not radiopaque.

After 2 or 3 weeks' with no improvement, the space was explored in two patients. In each case a prolapse of ragged pieces of disc material was found with fragments attached to the under-surface of the posteriorly displaced upper cartilaginous end-plate. The disc fragments were excised, and the protruding edge of the end-plate was snipped off.

CASE 3-1. A boy of 15 was injured in November, 1959. When examined 4 months later he was still in bed, unable to bend his back. He complained of persistent pain which had increased in severity. At operation in March, 1960, 0.5 cm. of cartilaginous end-plate was found protruding beyond the lower border of L4, with ragged fragments of disc adherent to its lower surface. The disc itself was partially sequestered into the canal. The disc fragments were excised and the protrusion of the end-plate was nibbled off.

The specimen was sent for histological section, and the pathologist reported: "Sections show viable bone, hyaline cartilage, and fibrocartilage. Features are consistent with a biopsy from the cartilaginous end-plate. No evidence of malignancy was observed in these sections."

In all operated cases, convalescence was comfortable, with recovery of function and movement. The patients were soon fit for ordinary activities but were advised against participating in contact sports. None returned to playing rugby, but one patient was able to play golf, and another, tennis.

CASE 3-2 One of the patients mentioned above consulted me again 18 years later. He had recently felt pain in the upper lumbar spine while playing a game of tennis. He found that sudden turns in either direction caused sharper pain across the back.

Forced rotation of the thorax reproduced his pattern of pain, and tenderness was elicited over the interspinous ligaments and spaces at the T12–L1 and L1–L2 levels. Roentgenographs showed the anterior edge of the first lumbar vertebral to be underdeveloped (Fig. 3-7).

The patient's spine was manipulated gently under general anesthesia, after which he re-

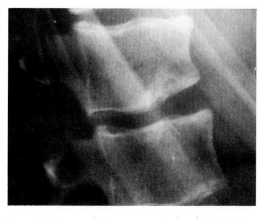

FIG. 3-7. Lateral roentgenograph of a 34-year-old man who has undergone operative removal of a ruptured vertebral end-plate at the age of 18. The deformed body of L1 can be seen with early retrospondylolisthesis.

gained a full range of motion. Spinal bracing and a program of exercise resulted in normal muscle tone and comfortable movement for a few months, during which he worked long hours as a hotel manager. In the end, his discomfort returned, but it has been controlled by the patient's acceptance of a lighter job with shorter hours.

Not infrequently roentgenographs of adult lumbar spines show stunting of the lumbar vertebral margins similar to those shown above. We must presume that epiphyseal injuries during the final growth spurt are more common than has been suspected, and that, at least in some cases, vertebral "epiphysitis" is actually the result of individual trauma to a joint.

"SACROILIAC STRAIN"

Some orthopaedic surgeons deny that the sacroiliac joints ever give rise to mechanical symptoms and maintain that it is only disease of the joints (such as ankylosing spondylitis or even, infrequently, tuberculosis) that causes pain. It is certainly true that in many cases pain in the region of the sacroiliac joints is actually referred from the lumbar spine, yet the many roentgenographic examples of osteophyte formation and sclerosis of the surrounding bone that can be seen, even in relatively young patients, suggest at least the possibility of symptoms arising in these joints.

The argument that the sacroiliac joints have no function since they are capable of very little movement is similarly without merit. There is no evolutionary evidence, from other species, of a tendency toward fusion of these joints, despite the increasing portion of the body weight that they bear constantly, in those animals that seldom rest the trunk on the ground. It is probably that their main function is as shock absorbers, to prevent reactive forces from the limbs reaching the spinal column. The joints consist of a large posterior sacroiliac ligament and a synovial joint, the opposing cartilaginous surfaces being complex in shape but congruous to each other, with raised areas and depressions.

By the fifth decade—and, in some individuals, considerably earlier—oblique roentgenographs of the joints reveal the changes we associate with osteoarthritis: inferior osteophytic lipping, which may be severe enough to be described as "parrot-beaking," irregularity of the joint line, and surrounding bony sclerosis. These changes are often symmetrical and in many patients cause no symptoms. In other cases the patient develops pain in one joint, despite the apparent similarity of the two sides on roentgenographs.

In such cases there is often a history of a wrenching injury to the joint. Often the story is very much like that of sudden disc prolapse, the patient describing the onset of pain on bending forward and twisting. He finds himself stuck suddenly in a doubled-up position, unable to straighten his back to any extent. The feeling of instability when he attempts to do so prevents him walking for some hours, after which it gradually wears off or even, in some cases, returns suddenly to normal. Even then he may have difficulty in bearing weight on the affected leg, and may feel that the joint is "out of place."

Whether subluxation really occurs has for many years remained an open question between orthopaedic surgeons and osteopaths. Roentgenographs fail to show convincing signs of subluxation, and the complex shape of the joint does not suggest that such an incongruous movement of its parts would occur easily. Yet the occasional story of a sudden unlocking of a joint indicates a mechanical origin to the symptoms, just as it does in the knee or shoulder joint.

In the majority of patients, although the cause of the first episode of pain is mechanical in nature, the pain persists long after the locking subsides. It fluctuates in intensity, exacerbated by weight bearing and relieved by rest, but is seldom absent for long. It may continue for months or even years and may then subside, only to return years later when the patient experiences another traumatic episode. Subsequently, trigger movements may become increasingly trivial.

The pain is aching in nature, increased by weight bearing, and extends from the region of the sacroiliac joint posteriorly down the outer side of the leg to the lateral aspect of the knee. Occasionally it extends below the knee. It is easy to attribute it mistakenly to sciatica or even hip pathology. There is always tenderness localized to the sacroiliac joint posteriorly, and pressure in this region may reproduce the pain down the leg. In some cases thickening of the soft tissues at the back of the sacroiliac joint is palpable. Straight-leg raising and femoral nerve stretch are normal, so that nerve root compression can be ruled out. The pain can be reproduced by straining the sacroiliac joint. This can be performed by the application of the weight of the examiner to the iliac crests when the patient is lying supine on a hard bed. In this way the sacroiliac ligaments are stretched as the joint is opened up. The patient is then asked to lie in a lateral position and the examiner leans both arms, with elbows extended, on the superior iliac crest, thus pressing the joints together to test the synovial part of the joints. Either or both tests may cause pain.

The joints can also be stressed if the patient is made to lie supine on a hard bed and each leg in turn is used as a lever to rotate the pelvis. The leg is held in the examiner's hands with the hip and the knee flexed to 90 degrees and is then fully rotated, externally and internally, while the patient's shoulders are held on the bed by an assistant. In this way, provided there is no pain or stiffness in the hip, rotational strain is put upon the sacroiliac joints. Pain may be elicited in the ipsi- or contralateral sacroiliac joint, during either internal or external rotation. Consideration of the movement and the side of the pain will reveal whether the affected joint has given rise to symptoms when it is stretched or compressed.

Finally, pain and tenderness of the symphysis pubis should be sought, and the joint carefully palpated to seek irregularities or osteophytes, distortion or step formation of either bone in relation to the other, and diastasis, especially in the pregnant woman.

It is not difficult to understand why a patient with symmetrical degeneration should have unilateral pain. Frequent observations of other degenerating joints, for example the hip, have shown that the inexorable process of articular wear is accompanied by fluctuating synovitis. It is the latter that causes the typical symptoms described above. The management of the patient is by treatment of the inflammation.

Certain groups of people are more likely to develop sacroiliac strain than the rest of the population. These may best be considered as those suffering from postpartum-, athletic- or congenital instability. It will be realized that there is often a combination of such causes. It should also be borne in mind that the two halves of the pelvis act in unison, and that therefore the instability is always of the pelvis as a whole. The two sacroiliac joints and the symphysis must always be considered together.

Postpartum Instability

In the last trimester of pregnancy many women experience pelvic instability, amounting in some cases to a temporary disability. At this time there is increasing ligamentous relaxation throughout the pregnant woman's body, but concentrated around the pelvis. It is thought to be an effect of the ovarian hormone, relaxin, the level of which is rising in preparation for parturition. Some women develop symphyseal diastasis in the last few weeks before delivery and may require admission to hospital as a result.

Repeated pregnancies seem to be a cause of sacroiliac instability, and it is not difficult to imagine that repeated ligamentous softening can lead to the initiation of degenerative changes within the joints as the recurrent abnormal weight bearing takes its toll. Some women, while still in their twenties, develop painful sacroiliac joints with widespread sclerotic changes in the iliac bones. The condition is often called "osteitis" of the iliac bones, the term suggesting an inflammatory or even infective lesion of the cortical bone, but there is no evidence to justify such a conclusion. Usually careful study of the roentgenographs suggests that the affected area of the iliac bone is that which is subject to abnormal weight bearing due to sacroiliac instability. The roentgenographic changes are not always permanent. In time, increasing degenerative changes within the joints themselves are associated with a gradual relief of pain. In these cases the sclerosis tends to subside. It is probable that in these patients, advancing capsular fibrosis, the inevitable accompaniment of degenerative change in a joint, stabilizes the joint and so reduces the stress on the ilium.

Instability in Athletes

Pain with stretching or laxity, instability, and recurrent subluxation of the sacroiliac joint, may follow acutely after a particularly violent injury of the pelvis. In athletes—such as long-distance runners, hurdlers, and jumpers—who put weight-bearing and "take-off" strain repeatedly on the same side of the pelvis, the onset may be gradual.

CASE 3-3 (Fig. 3-8). A typical example occurred in a 5,000-meter and cross-country national champion. He was assiduous in his training and ran long distances across rough country. Insidiously, toward the end of each run, discomfort followed by pain was felt in the right buttock. In time the pain became se-

vere and the distance he could run decreased. He could identify no specific injury. His running style was to hurdle or jump predominantly on the right foot.

Examination showed him to be a well-built young man of 25, fit and with a full range of movement of all joints, except the right sacroiliac. Weight bearing and passive pressure on the joint resulted in pain, which was also elicited by distraction of the pelvis; for when the patient lay on his back, heavy pressure on both superior iliac spines caused pain in the right sacroiliac joint and symphysis pubis. Similarly, when the patient lay prone and the pelvis was stabilized by the examiner's left hand, forced extension of the right leg reproduced the pain. Injection of a few milliliters of a local anesthetic agent into the interarticular ligaments of the joint gave instant, if temporary, relief. The spine moved freely. There was no tenderness of the lumbosacral joint or of the muscles of the back or pelvis.

Roentgenographs of the pelvis showed juxtaarticular sclerosis of the ilium. With full weight bearing on the right leg (and therefore with unilateral stress on the sacroiliac joint) the right side of the symphysis pubis rode up 3 mm. higher than the left.

In March, 1972, the joint was stabilized by transarticular bone graft. By the end of July fusion was sound. The patient started training again and in time could run 10 miles in 50 minutes.

In September, 1973, he felt pain in the left sacroiliac joint while running, with a sensation of instability on transferring weight to that side. The right side remained stable and symptom-free. The left settled with rest, but his competing days were over.

CASE 3-4. Two girl hurdlers developed similar symptoms, but without evidence of symphyseal displacement. They were advised to stop running for 6 months and thereafter recovered running comfort, but never fulfilled their early athletic promise.

CASE 3-5. Recently a man of 40 took up jogging to keep fit. He discovered a talent for distance running and within a year participated creditably in a marathon. He then developed low backache referred to the left buttock and thigh. Examination revealed sacroiliac strain with tenderness and pain on stress; both were

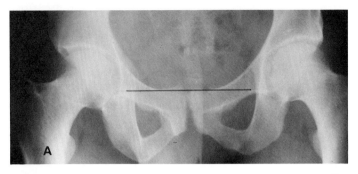

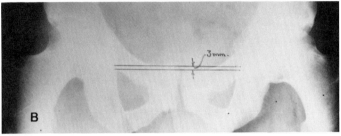

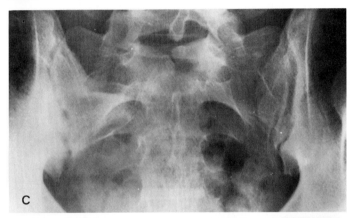

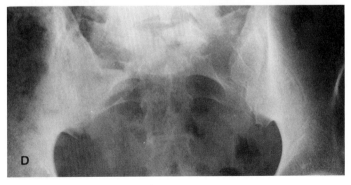

FIG. 3-8. *(A)* Roentgenogram of a patient lying supine. There is juxtaarticular sclerosis of the right sacroiliac joint, with irregularity of the joint margins. Similar appearances are present in the symphysis pubis. Only right hemipelvic instability can account for these features, but when the patient is not bearing weight, the symphysis pubis is in normal alignment. *(B)* When the patient stands on the right leg, the right pubis rides up 3 mm. *(C)* A close-up view shows accompanying congenital irregularity of the neural arches of L5 and S1. Note that the right sacroiliac joint has been fused by bone graft. *(D)* The roentgenograph shows sound fusion after transarticular graft.

relieved by the injection of a local anesthetic agent. Roentgenographs already showed juxtaarticular iliac sclerosis but without displacement on weight bearing. He was persuaded to give up long-distance running and has had no symptoms since.

Athletic instability has been described by Harris in professional football players who developed an added feature: avulsion stress fracture of the pubic bone adjacent to the symphysis pubis.[5b] A typical case involved a 36-year-old football player who developed pain in the back and the pubic symphysis severe enough to reduce his ability from that of a First to Third Division player. Inevitably he gave up professional sport in the end.

Congenital Pelvic Instability

Even without the stress of pregnancy or the severe rotational strains of professional sport, some patients develop pain in the back and symphysis pubis. They are usually young people who are fit and physically active. In such cases weight-bearing anteroposterior roentgenographs, with the patient standing on each leg in turn, reveal the characteristic subluxation of the symphysis pubis. A typical case was that of a 26-year-old salesman, who had had pain for 18 months. Until the diagnosis was established he had been thought to be suffering first from an obdurator hernia and then from a form of benign prostatitis, because of the site of his pain.

Symptoms are usually mitigated by reduced activity, with the intraarticular injection of local anesthetic agent and steroid in the severe case. Occasionally a pelvic band, to compress the iliac crests and support the pelvis, is helpful.

LUMBOILIAC PSEUDARTHROSIS AND TROPISM

There is a rare congenital abnormality of the transverse process of the fifth lumbar vertebra that gives rise to mechanical pain and locking of the back. Most congenital anomalies of pre- and postfixation of the lumbosacral region of the spine have little relevance to back symptoms, although, if they cause asynchronous movement, they play a part indirectly in the development of degenerative disease.

The abnormality that does matter, in some cases, is unilateral enlargement of a fifth lumbar transverse process, with a large vertical extension, so that it articulates with the iliac crest immediately above the sacral ala. The articulation may constitute a true synovial joint or there may be a pseudarthrosis above the sacroiliac joint. It may be vertical, a continuation of the sacroiliac joint, or even oblique or transverse. The anomaly of the transverse process is usually associated with a congenital abnormality of direction of the zygapophyseal joint between L5 and the sacrum *on the same side.* This latter abnormality has been called tropism.

Whether this combination of anomalies is always the cause of symptoms is unknown. That such unilateral tethering of L5 to relatively fixed sacrum and ilium can cause symptoms, is not in doubt. Two examples will be given:

CASE 3-6. A 33-year-old mother of two children had suffered recurrent locking of the back, always of sudden onset, with sharp pain localized to the sacroiliac joint. This always occurred when she rotated her extended lumbar spine to the opposite side. At first her symptoms were not severe. They gradually increased, and each period of locking was followed by several days' aching which prevented her doing her normal duties. The eventual disablement prevented her from joining her husband on their sailboat, and, finally, from getting in and out of a car. She was virtually confined to her home. All attempts at conservative therapy failed, but she was eventually cured by operation.

CASE 3-7. A woman of 29 presented with a similar story of locking of the back on rotation, although her pain was not as severe as that described in the above case. The attacks were less frequent, but the ache that followed each episode continued for months.

Roentgenographs revealed that her symptoms were not arising in the side of the congenital abnormality, but from the contralateral sacroiliac joint which, on the roentgenograph, looked normal, except for the possibility of early degenerative changes. Presumably, in her case, congenital tethering of the lumbar spine on one side had led to abnormal strain on the other.

The patient's condition was helped by the injection of a steroid and local anesthetic agent into the site of the tenderness, and muscle-strengthening exercises and the occasional use of an iliac band have prevented severe recurrence.

In those cases of lumbar transverse pseudarthrosis that do not respond to conservative treatment, especially if they casue severe disablement, operation is indicated. Excision of the abnormal transverse process cures the condition. The operation is difficult and can even be dangerous, since the extra process extends not only downward but forward, in some people reaching the brim of the pelvis. The unwary surgeon may find himself dissecting down a deep and gradually narrowing cavity that is not capable of expansion due to the presence of the iliac crest on the lateral side. He should remember that the ureter is not far away. Fortunately it is not necessary to excise the whole abnormal process. All that is required is the excision of the base of the transverse process. By this means the link between the body of the vertebra and the pesudarthrosis is broken, and mechanical symptoms can no longer occur. There remains the possibility that the tropism of the facets may later lead to lumbosacral instability, requiring local spinal fusion, but the author does not know of any case in which this has happened.

COCCYDYNIA

Of all the minor conditions presenting in the orthopaedic clinic, coccydynia is the one with most pitfalls for the inexperienced surgeon. The syndrome is characterized by pain, which may be severe, in the tip of the patient's tail. The pain is usually relieved when the patient stands and is exacerbated by sitting. It can be so severe that the patient has to carry a cushion or rubber ring to be able to sit for any length of time in comfort. The condition occurs more commonly in women than in men, usually in the fourth decade of life. It also occurs in girls in late adolescence.

There is often a history of trauma, the patient stating that the symptoms began after she struck the tip of her coccyx against some hard object. The blow may even have been severe enough to fracture the last segment of the sacrum, but the pain caused by local bruising usually settles, to be followed by a latent period without symptoms. A few weeks later the pain recurs, changed in character in that it is an aching or burning that spreads from the coccyx to the buttocks on either side.

There are several different types of coccydynia which can be differentiated by the clinician if he does not want a disgruntled patient returning repeatedly to his clinics. Diagnosis depends on taking a careful history and examining the coccyx itself carefully. This can only be done adequately by bimanual palpation, with one examining finger in the patient's rectum and the other on the perineum. Before this is performed, the lumbar spine must be examined fully, because lower lumbar central disc prolapse may cause no symptom other than mid-line pain referred to the tip of the coccyx, and may mimic coccydynia. In this case there is always immobility and usually spasm in the lumbar muscles and often a history of reduced bladder sensation and sphincter control. During rectal examination careful palpation of the pelvic organs must also be undertaken, to rule out rectal or gynecological causes.

CAUSES

The Immobile Coccyx

Injury to the sacrococcygeal joint, occurring during a difficult obstetrical delivery, may result in stiffness. The coccyx may even be dislocated. The resulting adhesions may cause pain during the sacrococcygeal movement that takes place on defecation and during subsequent deliveries.

Palpation reveals the stiffness of the joint on movement, and the pain is reproduced. Manipulation of the coccyx bimanually under general anesthesia may break down the adhesions, but if they are strong, or if the joint has been dislocated, operation offers the best chance of cure. Coccygectomy is unnecessary, since excision arthroplasty of the sacrococcygeal joint leaves a painless, mobile coccyx.

Congenital Prominence of the Sacral Tip

In this rare condition, which occurs equally in men and women, the patient, who is often thin, has a projecting bony prominence that is subject to trauma. It is easily visible at the base of the natal fold. Palpation shows it to be the tip of the sacrum (i.e., a narrow fifth sacral segment, and not the coccyx) that protrudes. The coccyx itself is mobile, nontender, and anteverted. The condition is best treated by excision of the bony prominence, provided the surgeon remembers that to do so he must open the spinal canal and detach the filum terminale.

Perineal Fasciitis

In the most common form of coccydynia, palpation reveals that the pain is not from the sacrococcygeal joint. Nor is the coccyx stiff. Instead, the muscles of the pelvic diaphragm are tender, or at least the fascial sheath overlying these muscles is the source of the patient's symptoms. In particular, the free edges of the anococcygeus muscle on either side are exquisitely tender. Movement of the coccyx reproduces the symptoms only when these muscles are stretched.

The syndrome is probably due to an inflammatory fasciitis, perhaps following some local injury to the sacrococcygeal joint followed by an extension of the inflammatory condition, similar to the spreading inflammatory condition in the shoulder. This would explain the latent period before symptoms recur as well as the severe aching or even burning nature of the pain. A frequent observation is that patients who develop this syndrome are tense people who transfer their psychological state to their muscles, which reveal a similar tension. They are literally "tight-arses." This may play a part in the potentiation of the condition, just as it may in hemorrhoids.

Treatment must be directed to the muscles of the pelvic diaphragm. Excision of the coccyx does not alter the symptoms, merely adding a tender scar to the patient's other discomforts. Most patients respond to anal dilatation under anesthesia, following which 40 mg. of intraarticular steroid and 2 ml. of a 2-percent solution of lignocaine is injected into each anococcygeal muscle. This is done with the patient in the lateral position, with the knees drawn up toward the patient's chin. The needle is inserted into the mid-line of the natal groove and then angled 45 degrees from the vertical, to enter the muscles on each side of the coccyx in turn. Throughout the injection the surgeon keeps the index finger of his left hand in the rectum, to palpate the needle through the bowel wall and so prevent perforating the rectum. Without this precaution there is a danger of carrying organisms back from the rectum and causing an abscess.

Dilatation should be gentle and of moderate degree, until four fingers can be inserted per anum. Further stretching may cause unnecessary trauma and bruising of the anal sphincter. The surgeon's finger should be well lubricated to prevent splitting the anal skin.

The symptoms generally subside gradually during the next 3 weeks, after an initial flare-up in some cases. At times there is only improvement without full recovery, and a second injection can be attempted after 6 weeks. Recovery may be aided by pelvic short-wave diathermy (provided there is no infection in the pelvic organs) and gentle pelvic and perineal exercises. In only a few patients is the condition unaffected by treatment. Even in these it should be remembered that, like other fascial inflammatory conditions, this type of coccydynia subsides spontaneously in 18 months to 2 years. If the patient's symptoms continue unabated after this length of time, the possibility of a serious psychological cause for the pain should be considered.

ENTRAPMENT SYNDROMES

Sciatic Nerve Entrapment

The entrapment usually occurs at the sciatic notch as the nerve exits from the pelvis. It is compressed against the bony edge or deep to, or as it tranverses the belly of, the pyriformis muscle. The syndrome is characterized by pain behind the greater trochanter referred down the thigh and the outer side of the leg and sole of the foot. Professor Ryosuke Katayama describes as diagnostic a positive Lasegue, hypoesthesia of the outer half of the sole, and pain behind the greater trochanter, produced when the hip and knee joints are flexed to a right angle and the thigh is forced into adduction and internal rotation.[8]

Pain on hip movement was emphasized by Kopell and Thompson as the diagnostic feature to differentiate sciatica due to a disc, where only straight-leg raising is painful, from entrapment of the nerve peripherally as it traverses the sciatic notch. When the nerve is stretched by straight-leg raising, pain is aggravated by internal rotation and relieved by external rotation.

Also, sensory changes, when present, are below the buttock and in the sole of the foot, whereas pressure on the roots by a disc may involve the peroneal distribution above the ankle and the buttock itself. The condition is not common and

may coexist with a prolapsed disc. The diagnosis is frequently missed initially and recognized only when the sciatica persists after excision of the disc.

The nerve is tender in and below the notch. The injection of local anesthetic around the nerve aids diagnosis, and the addition of corticosteroids may give more lasting comfort. Katayama finds neurography of value. After injecting contrast medium into the nerve sheath 5 cm. below the notch, the point of compression is marked by the block to the flow of fluid.

Conservative treatment, avoiding pressure on the nerve, and antiinflammatory drugs, are helpful, but the only satisfactory treatment when neurologic change is present is neurolysis. After reflecting the gluteus maximus from the femur the sciatic nerve is exposed and freed.[7] It may be necessary also to divide the tendinous belly of the pyriformis, which is, on occasion, the compressing structure.

Entrapment of the Lateral Femoral Cutaneous Nerve—Meralgia Paresthetica

The lateral femoral cutaneous nerve arises from the second and third lumbar roots and emerges from the lateral border of the psoas muscle to descend on the posterior wall of the abdomen. From its investment by the iliacus fascia, it enters the thigh medial to the anterior superior iliac spine, between the two lateral attachments of the inguinal ligament. The nerve pierces the deep fascia a short distance below, to become subcutaneous, where its branches supply the skin of the anterior and lateral portions of the thigh as far as the knee. Koppell and Thompson aptly describe the tunnel under the inguinal ligament and the point at which it pierces the fascia lata as the binding points of the nerve, for between these points it is held firmly, so that movement of the trunk above or the thigh below may produce tension and, in certain circumstances, pain.[9] Adduction of the thigh, by crossing the legs or from shortening of the opposite limb, would tense the nerve against the entrapment points and so cause dysesthesia, often severe and burning in character, over the anterior and lateral thigh. This is characteristic and suggests the diagnosis.

Koppell and Thompson instanced a psychiatrist who sat listening to patients with one leg crossed over the other.[9] He developed the typical symptoms of pain and paresthesia in the upper (crossing) thigh. The reason was explained to him; he changed his posture and had no further discomfort.

Presssure over the nerve against the medial side of the iliac spine reproduces or aggravates the pain. Injection of local anesthetic gives immediate, though usually transient relief.

The nerve may suffer compression or irritation in its course by tumor or infection but the commonest cause of the symptoms is compression or entrapment at the exit under the inguinal ligament by injury or by a tight corset or brace. It is sometimes associated with lumbar disc protrusion.

Treatment. Meralgia paresthetica, in most instances, may be relieved without surgery. Correction of lumbar spine lordosis, raising the heel on the shoe of the short leg, a suitable corset or brace if the lumbar spine is at fault, plus antiinflammatory medication, should be tried. If these measures fail, neurolysis is usually successful. The nerve should be decompressed behind the inguinal ligament and released from the iliacus fascia and the fascia lata.

Neuropathy of the Peroneal Nerve

Neuropathy of the peroneal nerve at the neck of the fibula, from direct trauma or compression by fibrous scar, or intermittent injury from recurrent dislocation of the head of the fibula, may give rise to pain at the knee and down the leg to the ankle, with paresthesia, loss of sensation, or weakness, as demonstrated by partial or complete foot-drop. It is likely to be mistaken for derangement of the lateral semilunar cartilage, but the pain may also shoot up the thigh and occasionally may be diagnosed as sciatica. This is particularly true of recurrent dislocation of the superior tibiofibular joint.[6] Freeing the nerve at the neck of the fibula usually cures, but it may be necessary to stabilize the superior tibiofibular joint.

REFERENCES

1. Apley, A. G.: A System of Orthopaedics and Fractures. London, Butterworth, 1975.
2. Butler, R. W.: Long-term follow-up of lumbar vertebral osteochondritis. J. Bone Joint Surg., *48-B*:585, 1965.
3. Fidler, M. W., Jowett, R. L., and Troup, J. D. G.: Myosin ATPase activity in multifidas muscle from cases of lumbar spinal derangement. J. Bone Joint Surg., *57B*:220, 1975.
4. Goldthwait, J. E.: Essentials of Body Med. Philadelphia, J. B. Lippincott, 1937.
5. Handlesman, J.: [Paper read at the International Orthopaedic Congress] London, Autumn, 1976.
5a. Harris, N. H.: Lesions of the symphysis pubis in women. Brit. Med. J., *4*:209, 1974.
5b. Harris, N. H., and Murray, R. O.: Lesions of the symphysis pubis in athletes. Brit. Med. J., *4*:211, 1974.
6. Helfet, A. J.: Disorders of the Knee. Philadelphia, J. B. Lippincott, 1974.
7. Henry, A. K.: Extensile Exposure. Edinburgh, E. & S. Livingstone, 1948.
8. Katayama, R.: Orthopaedic Correspondence Club Letter, 1972.
9. Koppell, H. P., and Thompson, W. A. L.: Peripheral Entrapment Neuropathies, Baltimore, Williams & Wilkins, 1963.

4 Pathological Anatomy of the Lumbar Spine

John Reilly, K. Yong-Hing, R. W. MacKay, and W. H. Kirkaldy-Willis

There is an underlying theme throughout this chapter, which will be appreciated more easily if an overall view is given at the start. Pathological change, initiated by repeated episodes of minor trauma, advances from rotatory strains of the posterior joints and discs to early degenerative changes. At first they affect either the L4–5 or L5–S1 level only. Later, still at one level, there is marked degeneration of posterior joints, disintegration of the disc, and, consequently, instability of the three parts of the intervertebral joint complex. Compression injuries may damage or fracture the cartilage end-plates. This leads slowly but certainly to disruption of the disc and concomitant changes in the posterior joints. After many years the new bone formation, which is especially marked on the surface of the posterior articular processes, produces degenerative spinal stenosis—at one level only. Eventually, strain is thrown on the joints at the levels above and below the first lesion. The result is, firstly degenerative arthritis and then multi-level segmental spinal stenosis.

At each level there are three joints: two posterior synovial joints and one anterior, formed by the intervertebral disc. Trauma or degenerative disease may primarily affect any one or all three. Lesions of the posterior joints always have an effect on the disc; lesions which primarily affect the disc always have an effect on the posterior joints. When considering a lesion at any level, attention must be directed to the changes in all three joints, even when only one of these appears to be affected.

INTRODUCTION

The Spinal Canal

The posterior wall of the spinal canal is formed by the laminae and ligamenta flava; and lateral walls, by the medial aspect of the pedicles, the medial aspect of the posterior joints (lined by ligamenta flava) and the intervertebral foramina; the anterior walls, by the posterior aspects of the vertebral bodies, the annulus fibrosus of the discs and the posterior longitudinal ligament.

Figure 4-1 demonstrates the differences in cross-section in the upper and lower parts of the lumbar spinal canal. At the L4–5 and L5–S1 levels there is a well-formed lateral recess or gutter. Encroachment by soft tissue or bone in this recess can, and often does, produce spinal nerve entrapment; one reason why the fourth and fifth spinal nerves are more liable to compression than those at higher levels.

26

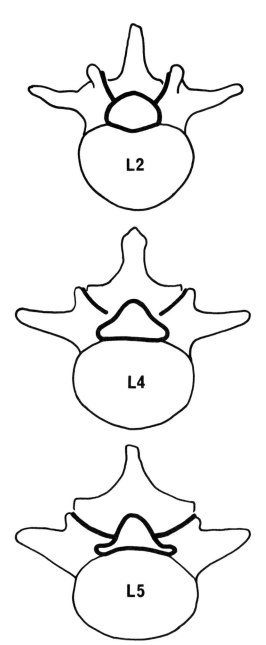

FIG. 4-1. Cross-sectional views of the normal spinal canal. At the L2 level the canal is almost circular. At L5 there are well-formed lateral recesses.

The Nerve Canal

The nerve canal is important anatomically, since it is recognized as a site where the spinal nerves can be trapped. At each level this canal begins at the point where the nerve leaves the dural sac. Because it runs obliquely downward and outward to the foramen, it has posterior, anterior, medial, and lateral walls.

The posterior wall of each canal is formed by the ligamentum flavum, the superior part of the lamina corresponding in number to the nerve and the superior articular process of the vertebra below.

The anterior wall is formed by the posterior surface of the vertebral body and its soft-tissue coverings and by the annulus fibrosus above or below.

The medial wall is the dural sac and extradural fat with blood vessels and nerves within it.

The lateral wall is formed by the medial side and the inferior aspect of the pedicle (Figs. 4-2; and 4-3).

The Intervertebral Foramen

This is shaped like an inverted teardrop. Its superior margin is the pedicle of the vertebra above. The anterior margin is the posterior aspect of the vertebral body above, then the disc and the body below. The inferior margin is the pedicle below the nerve. The posterior margin is formed of the pars, the ligamentum flavum, and the apex of the superior articular process of the lower vertebra (Fig. 4-3).

THE INTERVERTEBRAL JOINTS

For simplicity the posterior joints will be considered first, then the discs, followed by the combined lesions of all three joints. (In doing so we realize that a lesion primarily affecting one joint also affects the other joints to some degree.)

Some authors have stated that the posterior joints are affected first and the disc later.[14,15,23,39] Others have taken the opposite view.[4,8,21,35,40] It appears likely that either may occur but that posterior joint and disc injury take place simultaneously.

The posterior joints—discs as well as the vertebral bodies of the lumbar

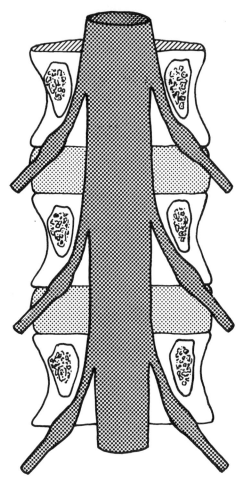

FIG. 4-2. Posterior view of nerve canals showing the relation of nerves to pedicles.

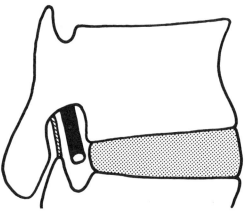

FIG. 4-3. Lateral view of the relations of spinal nerves in the canal.

spine—are most susceptible to rotational strains and resistant to compression, flexion, and extension.[13] Major compressive trauma is required to fracture the vertebral bodies and the end-plates.

The Posterior Joints

At the upper three levels these joints lie mainly in the sagittal plane. Their structure permits some flexion-extension movement but little lateral flexion or rotation, which protects both the posterior and intervertebral disc joints from rotatory strains. At the two lowest levels these joints lie mainly in the coronal plane. Flexion-extension, lateral flexion, and rotation all occur. Rotation occurs mainly at the lower two joints (see Fig. 4-1). All types of movement, particularly rotation when forced or excessive, can strain these joints, which is why posterior joint pathology affects chiefly these two levels.

The most minor strains produce synovitis of one or both posterior joints. When the synovium is torn, hemarthrosis results. On the side where tension is exerted there may be a tear of the capsule and a posterior joint with a lax capsule subject to further strain. Small fragments of articular cartilage and underlying bone may be broken off the joint surface and form loose bodies, which are responsible for recurrent or chronic pain.[20] Uneven compression of joint surfaces may damage the articular cartilage and lead to small subchondral fractures that distort the joint surfaces permanently. More severe injuries may fracture the inferior articular process, causing permanent instability of the joint (Fig. 4-4).

As in all diarthrodial joints, fibrillation and degeneration of cartilage occurs, with erosion. Reactionary new bone or osteophytosis is formed at the periphery of the joints. One or more of these may fracture. The articular processes increase in size. Repeated minor trauma, interspersed with one or more episodes of

FIG. 4.4. In this longitudinal mid-line section at the L4–5 level, note the large synovial tag (*arrow*), the irregular articular surfaces, the loss of articular cartilage, isolated disc resorption, and narrowing of the lateral recess.

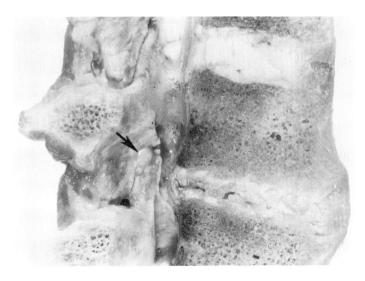

more severe injury, predispose to this typical degenerative arthritis of the posterior joints.

These changes can be seen clearly at laminectomy. After retraction of the erector spinae muscles the posterior articular processes are seen to be much enlarged and projecting posteriorly. They are apparently displaced toward the mid-line, with craggy irregular surfaces. After removal of the laminae, the inferior articular processes are seen to bulge into the spinal canal, producing a fleur-de-lis appearance on cross-section. The superior articular processes of the lower vertebrae are often enlarged and irregular, with marked narrowing of the anteroposterior dimension of the lateral recess. The branches of the posterior primary rami of the spinal nerves may undergo compression or traction as they lie in close proximity to the posterior processes. There is entrapment of the spinal nerves in the cauda equina by enlarged inferior articular processes and of spinal nerves in the lateral recesses by enlarged superior articular processes. In all these sites the circulation in arteries, veins, and capillaries may be impeded in a similar way by pressure from new bone (Fig. 4-5; 4-6).

It is possible that chiropractic manipu-

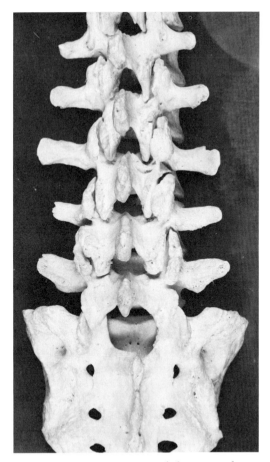

FIG. 4-5. A posterior view of the spine shows an enlarged and irregular posterior joint at the L4–5 level.

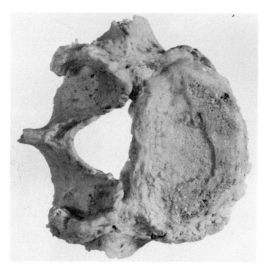

FIG. 4-6. A cross-section of L5 showing "fleur-de-lis" appearance and marked lateral recess narrowing. (Courtesy Dr. H. F. Farfan)

lations work by reducing minor subluxations of a lax posterior joint. This laxity would also explain the tendency to recurrent episodes of low back pain. When the pain is disabling at one level, posterior joint fusion results in relief in 85 per cent of patients.[17]

The Intervertebral Discs

The boundary walls are formed by the cartilage plates and the annulus fibrosus. The cartilage plates are supported by the cancellous bone of the vertebral bodies, strengthened at the periphery by the ring epiphyses. The plates and nucleus obtain their nutrition from the vasculature of the underlying bone. There is a constant exchange of fluid across the cartilage plates. Normally, no vessels cross the cartilage plate after the first 2 years of life. The annulus fibrosus is laminated. The fibers of each lamina cross one another obliquely to be inserted into the bone of the vertebral body.[21]

In the center of the disc lies the nucleus pulposus. In the lower lumbar spine it is placed eccentrically, nearer the posterior

margin. It is composed of stellate cells, sparsely scattered throughout a matrix of fine interlacing collagen fibers and mucopolysaccharides.

In the embryologic development of the nucleus a fibrous septum is formed that passes more than half-way across in the coronal plane. Frequently this persists, to give a horse-shoe appearance on discography. The biochemical and histological changes of aging and degeneration of the nucleus have been described by several authors.[5,6,9,18,22,36] There is no consensus; all that can be said is that the nature of the protein-polysaccharide chains alters and their water-binding properties decrease with progressive dessication of the disc. In the normal adult disc, no blood vessels cross the cartilage plates, into the nucleus, or the annulus fibrosus.

Tears occur in a number of different ways. The earliest are small circumferential lesions or clefts separating the lamellae of the annulus. As the lesion advances these tears enlarge and coalesce until they are radial.[4] Finally, either the inner annular fibers or the whole thickness of these fibers ruptures at one site, with herniation of the disc. When a radial tear penetrates the outer layer of the annulus, there is an attempt at healing by ingrowth of granulation tissue. Naked endings of the sinuvertebral nerve have been identified in this granulation tissue.[34] These may be pain receptors, which would explain discogenic pain in the absence of herniation (Figs. 4-7; 4-8).

Herniations are of two types: (1) localized protrusion of the nucleus pulposus beneath the thin, weakened annulus; of which in this case the superficial annular fibers are intact, and (2) complete tears of all the annular fibers with extrusion of the nucleus into the spinal canal. Posterolateral herniation is most common, but it can be central or lateral. Central herniation results in compression of the cauda equina; posterolateral herniation, in pressure on the nerve root leav-

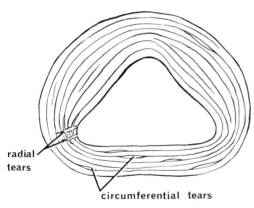

radial
tears

circumferential tears

FIG. 4-7. A cross-section of the disc shows crowding of the fibers of the annulus posteriorly, circumferential clefts, and radial tears.

ing the canal one level lower (i.e., on L4–5 herniation traps the fifth lumbar nerve); lateral herniations usually press on the nerve of the same level (i.e., an L4–5 herniation entraps the fourth lumbar nerve).

Tears and herniations of the annulus fibrosus almost always occur at the poste-

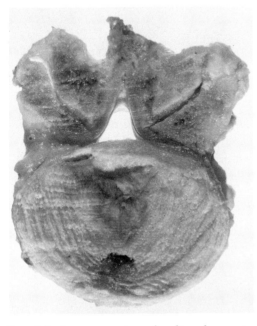

FIG. 4-8. A cross-section of a disc shows circumferential clefts and radial tears.

rior and posterolateral aspects of the discs, and tears are more common at the lower lumbar levels. Several factors dictate this pattern.

In the normal disc the layers of the annulus are more compact posteriorly, and the nucleus is displaced posteriorly. As a result the annulus is thinnest posteriorly and posterolaterally. This feature becomes more marked at the lower lumbar levels and with aging.

As seen in the lateral view, the lower lumbar discs are wedge-shaped. This is most marked at the lumbosacral junction (Fig. 4-9).

The cross-sectional shape of the discs varies with the lumbar level (see Fig. 4-1), and on this depends the site of the radial tear. Stress studies show a correlation between the site of maximum stress and the position of radial tears. In discs with a slightly concave posterior surface (midlumbar level) the maximal stress is on the posterolateral aspect, where radial tears and disc herniations are more frequent.[14] Discs with a convex posterior surface (the lumbosacral junction) are susceptible to mid-line posterior tears and disc herniations.

Reduced turgidity of the nucleus pulposus predisposes to annular tears. A reduction in volume can occur with herniation of the nucleus pulposus through a fractured end-plate[33] or with the disc dessication of aging and degeneration.

Posture is important in two ways: endplate fractures occur more frequently when the lumbar spine is less lordotic. When there is marked lordosis, wedging of discs is accentuated, and annular tears are more likely. This latter is considered of more significance.

Disruption of the Disc. Plain roentgenographs show either a normal appearance or slight loss of disc height. Discograms (Fig. 4-10) reveal a large cleft that extends from front to back and from side to side of the disc. At operation, after incision of the annulus, a large cleft may

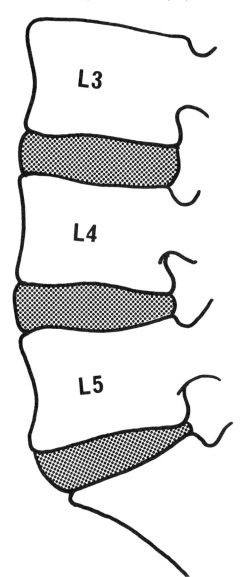

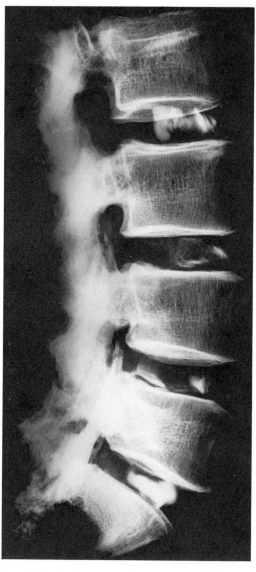

FIG. 4-9. A lateral view of the lumbar spine shows wedging of the lower discs, most marked at L5–S1.

FIG. 4-10. A discogram shows internal disruption of the disc at the L4–5 level. Note the normal disc height.

be seen crossing the interior of the disc. Large, sequestered fragments, composed mainly of collagen, may be found within the cleft. At autopsy a similar large and extensive cleft, or several clefts, may be found.

The cause is the subject of controversy. There may be coalescence of many clefts to form one large crevice, with or without herniation of the nucleus. Alternatively, it may represent the condition, described by Crock, of "internal disc disruption."[7] He considered this to be a completely separate entity, presenting with systemic symptoms and having as its basis either biochemical or immunologic changes.

Isolated disc resorption, also described by Crock, is characterized by marked loss of disc height in straight roentgenographs. Further reference to this will be made in discussing combined lesions (see Fig. 4-4).

Fractures of cartilage end-plates are the result of compression injuries after minor trauma and are more common after loss of lumbar lordosis. Plain roentgenographs may not show any abnormality. It is thought that these fractures occur at points of penetration by the embryonic blood vessels. They provide a pathway for the ingrowth of new vessels from the vertebral body to the disc. At autopsy distortion of one or more cartilage plates may be present. Sometimes definite fractures are found, associated with herniations of the nucleus into the vertebral body (Schmorl's nodes; Fig. 4-11)

Combined Lesions

The primary lesion may be in the posterior joints or disc, or both. Because of the interdependence of these three components, altered mechanics in one nearly always leads to changes in the other two.

This has been supported by experimental work. Sullivan, Farfan, and Kahn have shown that creating instability of posterior joints in rabbits by facetectomy produced degenerative changes in the disc at the same level.[39] Thomas and co-workers have demonstrated that after operations on the discs of guinea pigs and dogs, early instability is followed by an increasing immobility leading to marked degenerative changes and even to fusion of posterior joints at that level.[40] They have also shown that operations on the posterior elements result in marked changes in the disc at the same level (Fig. 4-12).

In the past the treatment of intervertebral disc herniations has been oversimplified. Other lesions may coexist with herniation and contribute to nerve entrapment. Current diagnostic techniques may lead the surgeon to suspect the presence of such lesions, but only

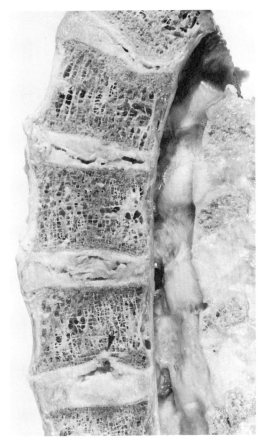

FIG. 4-11. A fracture of a cartilage end-plate (*arrow*). All the discs show disruption. The L5–S1 disc also shows resorption.

careful exploration of the lateral recesses will identify them. Failure to observe and treat all the lesions at the first operation leads to poor results after removal of the disc alone.

Rotational Lesions

Rotational lesions are common, causing changes in both posterior joints and the disc. It is rarely possible to determine which is primary and which is secondary. Of major importance is the identification and treatment of the causal lesion. The development of instability is due to the comparative thinness of the posterior part of the posterior joint capsule, while the

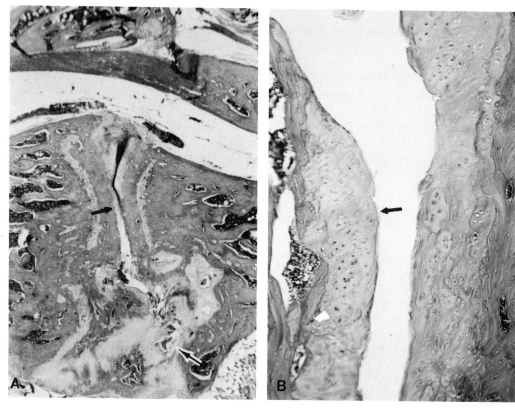

FIG. 4-12. *(A)* Anterior fusion in the guinea pig. Fusion between the vertebral bodies is by cartilage *(black and white arrow)* but has not occurred across the whole disc *(black arrow). (B)* The cartilage of the posterior joint of the same guinea pig specimen shows marked degenerative changes.

anteromedial part is stronger, being formed by the elastic lateral extension of the ligamentum flavum (see page 27).

Rotational strain to one side or the other affects mainly the posterior joints but leads also to early disc changes. On one side the capsule is stretched and may be torn (tension), while on the other there is abnormal approximation of the two posterior joint surfaces (compression). Manipulation may relieve this type of strain, but it is liable to recur. The pain is mediated by the posterior primary ramus.

This reducible lesion of the posterior joints may be accompanied by changes in the turgidity of the disc. The joint complex becomes unstable; a greater range of rotatory movement is possible than the normal 9 degrees. Rotation of the L5 to the right, for example, results in anterior displacement of the superior articular process of L5 on the left, with narrowing of the lateral recess on the left. As this movement takes place, recurrent entrapment of the fifth lumbar nerve on the left occurs and sciatic pain results. The entrapment may be accentuated if there is bulging of the disc, internal disruption, or isolated disc resorption. This may explain the effect of manipulation in the relief of sciatic pain: the rotatory strain is reduced.

Fixed rotational deformity may be due to congenital asymmetry of the posterior arch or to trauma or to progressive altera-

FIG. 4-13. Asymmetry of posterior joints. Note that the lamina on the left is short compared with that on the right.

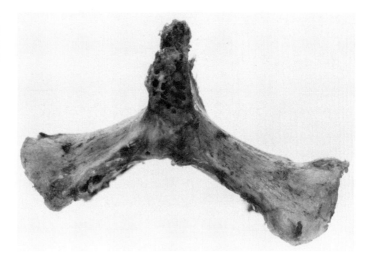

tion under repeated deforming forces. On one side the posterior joint capsule is torn; on the other, the articular cartilage is injured or the lamina fractured near the joint. The fracture heals, with permanent asymmetry of the posterior joints. These rotational strains may, by progressive degenerative change, lead to permanent fixed deformity. If symptoms are severe, posterior joint fusion, as described by Farfan, may be required (Fig. 4-13).

This type of fixed deformity may involve not only subluxation of the posterior joints with anterior displacement of the superior articular process of the lower vertebra but also advanced changes in the disc, resulting in marked narrowing of the recess and lateral entrapment of the lumbar nerve. Frequently laminectomy is required. At the same time the lateral recess is explored and the anterior margin of the superior articular process removed, thus relieving the nerve entrapment. On occasion it is wise to follow this procedure with posterior facet fusion.

Roentgen examination reveals three changes: In the anteroposterior view the spinous process of the L4 may be displaced a few millimeters laterally on that of L5, or L5 displaced on S1 (Fig. 4-14). A true lateral view of the lumbosacral joint may show the presence of a double shadow of the vertebrae above the level of the lesion. This is the result of rotation, which permits part of the posterior aspect of the upper vertebral bodies to be seen (Fig. 4-14-C). Standing lateral views may reveal that, whereas in flexion the bodies are in normal alignment, in extension the upper body is displaced posteriorly on the lower (retrospondylolisthesis). These changes are rotational, but the instability is shown as retrospondylolisthesis.

Isolated Disc Resorption

In this condition[7] the height of the L4–5 or L5–S1 disc, or both, is reduced. The cause of the resorption of the nucleus pulposus is not known. Loss of resistance of the disc, however, permits rotational, lateral, flexion-extension, and compression forces to be transmitted to the posterior joints (Fig. 4-15). Approximation of the two vertebral bodies results in overriding of the posterior joint facets. The superior articular process of the lower vertebra slides upward and anteriorly on the inferior articular process of the upper vertebra. That portion of the ligamentum

(Text continues on p. 38)

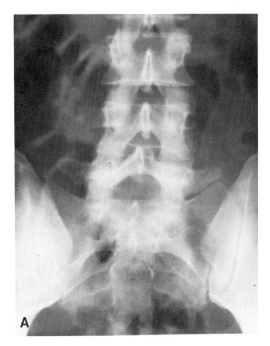

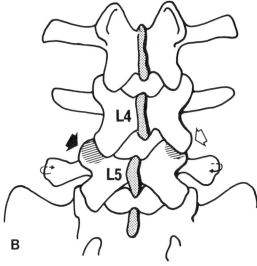

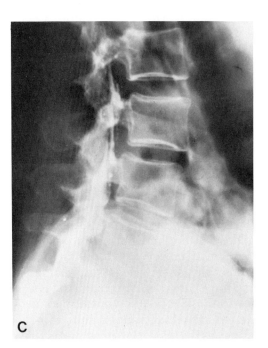

FIG. 4-14. *(A)* This anteroposterior roentgeno-graph shows rotatory subluxation. The spinous process of L4 is displaced to the patient's left and that of L5 to the patient's right. *(B)* The diagram illustrates the displacement. *(C)* A double shadow is seen at the back of the bodies of L2 and L3. No double shadow is seen at the back of the bodies of L4 and L5. L3 is displaced slightly forward on L4. These signs indicate a rotational strain at the L3–4 level.

FIG. 4-15. Longitudinal mid-line section to show isolated disc resorption with concomitant degeneration of the posterior joints and rotatory subluxation leading to narrowing of the lateral recess. Note that the lateral extensions of the ligamentum flavum form the anteromedial capsule of the posterior joints. *(A)* The posterior joint is in normal alignment, with some narrowing of the lateral recess due to posterior bulging of the annulus. *(B)* Posterior joint subluxation by a rotational force shows further narrowing of the lateral recess due to anterior displacement of the superior articular process. *(C,D)* Comparable views to those of *A* and *B*, with the ligamentum flavum excised.

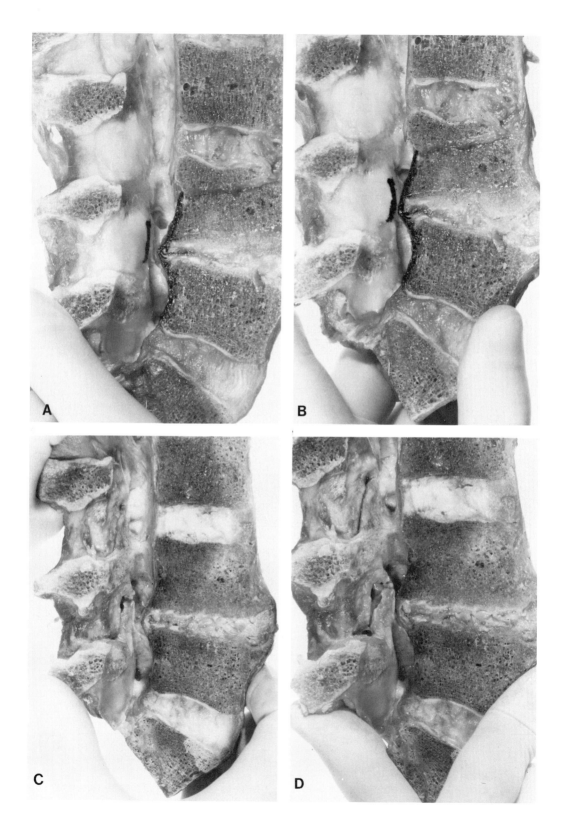

flavum attached to the upper pole of the superior articular process is shortened and thickened. In this way the lateral recess is narrowed, and there may be entrapment of the spinal nerve at this level.

PROGRESSION TO MULTILEVEL PATHOLOGY

Up to this point we have considered changes that take place at one level only as they affect the three-joint complex. We now proceed to consider more generalized lesions. Such generalized spondylosis may arise in two ways: simultaneous pathological changes at several levels, commonly considered to be the end-result of aging, and progression of changes from one level to those immediately above and below. Altered mechanics at one level due to instability or decreased mobility may throw abnormal forces on adjacent joints (Fig. 4-16).

Clinical observation supports this concept. When carrying out posterior spinal fusion 6 months after anterior fusion in patients with tuberculosis of the spine, Baker and co-workers observed that in many cases spontaneous fusion of the two laminae at the level of the anterior fusion had occurred.[4] At the levels just above and just below there were marked degenerative changes in the posterior joints. Furthermore, in Farfan's experimental work; (quoted above), when they created instability of posterior joints in rabbits, marked changes were seen to develop in a disc distant from the lesions.[15]

Degenerative spinal stenosis (see Chap. 5) occurs in some cases of spondylosis, with the difference that those parts of the stenotic spine contiguous to the cauda equina or spinal nerves undergo the greatest osteophytic new bone formation.

Degenerative Spondylosis

In spondylosis, as in other degenerative joint lesions, the main changes are degeneration and disintegration of the articular cartilage of the posterior joints and of the constituents of the discs, and osteophyte formation.

The Posterior Joints. The articular cartilage undergoes progressive degeneration as in other joints. Small fragments of separated articular cartilage may form loose bodies in the joints. Osteophytes and new bone on the surfaces of the facet joints result in large irregular processes which extend toward the midline. The enlarged articular processes bulge posterolaterally into the spinal canal (see Fig. 4-5).

The Intervertebral Disc. The discs undergo degeneration, with reduction in height and loss of disc space. Not infrequently there is fragmentation of the cartilage plates. Both radial and crescentic fissures are seen in the annulus fibrosus, and the nucleus pulposus shrivels.

Scoliosis. Degeneration of the discs and deformity of the vertebral bodies not infrequently results in scoliosis with rotational deformity of the spine (Fig. 4-16).

Subperiosteal new bone formation results in a number of changes; among them the formation of osteophytes at the edges of the vertebral bodies, which may, in the end, produce fusion of one or more vertebrae by bone. Traction spurs may form at the site of the insertion of the annulus into bone, probably owing to segmental instability.[25] The vertebral bodies enlarge and may have an irregular, craggy surface. There is thickening of the lamina with reduction of the intralaminar space. The ligamentum flavum is displaced anteriorly by the thickened lamina behind. The surfaces of the articular processes become large and irregular. At the L4–5 and L5–S1 levels, the lateral recesses become markedly narrowed, with sharp-edged osteophytes producing an irregular contour. The spinous processes are enlarged and the interspinous spaces are reduced in size.

Severe low back pain may occur in several ways. The posterior primary rami

F<small>IG</small>. 4-16. This roentgeno-graph shows severe degener-ative spondylosis with scoliosis.

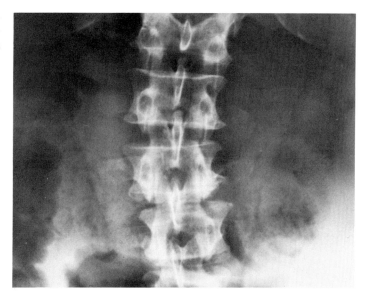

may be compressed, irritated, or stretched by irregularities of the transverse processes and posterior articular processes. There may be compression or irritation of the branches of the sinuvertebral nerves in the foramina or lateral recesses; they may be affected by osteophytes at the posterior margins of the vertebral bodies adjacent to the discs.

Leg pain may be referred from the posterior primary ramus or sinuvertebral nerve, or due to irritation or compression of the spinal nerves at any site in the nerve canal.

It is an interesting observation that when spontaneous fusion has occurred, low back pain tends to diminish.

SPONDYLOLISTHESIS

In the normal spine the orientation of the posterior joints prevents forward slipping of one vertebra on another. Spondylolisthesis can occur only because of an abnormality of the posterior joints due to separation of a defect in the pars interarticularis. Recently Newman and Wiltse produced a comprehensive classification of this condition:

Classification of Spondylolisthesis

Isthmic
  Lytic
  Elongated
  Acquisita (following fusion)
  Acute fracture
Dysplastic (congenital)
Degenerative
Traumatic
Pathological
  General
  Local

Most commonly this occurs at the L4–5 or L5–S1 level. Slips may be classified most usefully as those measuring less than 25 per cent of the anteroposterior diameter of the vertebral body, those between 25 and 50 per cent, those between 50 and 75 per cent, and total displacement (spondylolisthesis).

It is convenient to limit discussion to three types—dysplastic, isthmic and degenerative—which are most common.

Dysplastic Spondylolisthesis[28,42,43]

The primary congenital abnormality is aplasia of the proximal sacral neural arches and superior facets, resulting in abnormal orientation and shape of the

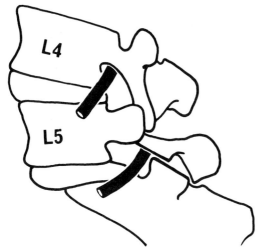

FIG. 4-17. Dysplastic spondylolisthesis. Note the abnormal alignment of the superior facet of the sacrum and the elongated pars interarticularis.

posterior facets at the L5–S1 level. This allows forward slipping of the inferior facet of L5 on the superior facet of the sacrum. Thus the whole lumbar spine above the abnormality slips forward on the sacrum. The spinous process of L5 comes to rest on the dorsal aspect of the sacrum. In some cases elongation of the pars interarticularis takes place, permitting further forward slipping of the vertebral body of L5 (Fig. 4-17).

Isthmic Spondylolisthesis

Isthmic spondylolisthesis is a defect in the pars. The posterior joints are normal.

The pathological abnormality is a bilateral defect in the pars interarticularis.

Usually it occurs without a definite history of severe injury, although it is probably due to a stress fracture. Sometimes the stress fracture heals with elongation of the pars.[44] Occasionally the cause is a single episode of severe trauma. Rarely, it is due to a local pathological condition in the bone or to generalized bone disease.

When the slip is at the L5–S1 level the defect is in the pars of L5. The body of the L5, together with the superior articular processes, the pedicles and the transverse process, slip anteriorly on the sacrum. The loose fragment (the rattler) which is formed of the lower parts of the laminae of L5, the spinous process, and the inferior articular processes, remains in normal position. The degree of displacement depends on the size of the gap between the two portions of the pars. An "attempt" is made at union: fibrocartilaginous tissue forms around both fracture surfaces. The upper fragment with this fibrocartilaginous nubbin comes to lie near the fifth spinal nerve in its canal and may compress the nerve (Fig. 4-18A).

Cause of Pain. A thorough understanding of the pathology is important for an accurate assessment of the cause of pain and muscle weakness.

Low back pain without leg pain is due to entrapment of or traction on the posterior primary ramus or on the branches of the sinuvertebral nerve (see Innervation,

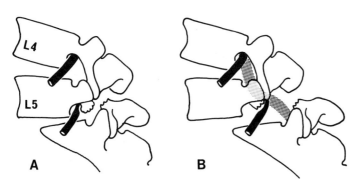

FIG. 4-18. Isthmic spondylolisthesis. *(A)* The common form of entrapment is of the fifth lumbar nerve by the superior fragment and fibrocartilaginous tissue. *(B)* An unusual form of entrapment of the nerve is due to posterior displacement of the dura. The nerve is posterior to the upper fragment.

below). If sufficiently severe, this can usually be relieved by spinal fusion.

Leg Pain. The presence of leg pain presents a much more difficult problem. It may be due to one or more of the following: Pressure on the posteriorly displaced nerve by the anteriorly displaced upper fragment causes pain as the nerve is pulled backward against this fragment (mirror image of the rattler), because the dura is kinked backward. This is more severe when the origin of the nerve from the dura is lower then normal (Fig. 4-18B). It is thus vitally important, in performing the Gill procedure, not only to remove the loose fragment in its entirety but also to remove all bone and fibrocartilage from the upper fragment and to be sure that no tissue is left pressing on the nerve (the fifth nerve with an L5–S1 slip and the fourth nerve with an L4–5 slip).

The fifth lumbar nerve may be trapped between the pedicle of L5 and the sacrum, particularly when the disc has almost disappeared and the pedicle, including half the foramen of L5, is abutting on the body of the sacrum (Fig. 4-15A). In cases of doubt, it is essential, therefore, to trace the nerve laterally and to make certain that there is no entrapment in its course through the bony canal.

Degenerative changes in the disc, posterior joints, and laminae above the level of the slip may result in localized spinal stenosis with pressure on the cauda equina. This is relieved only by laminectomy one level above the slip.

Inadequate or ill-planned previous surgery may make assessment of the site of nerve compression difficult. The authors recall one patient who previously had an operation in which removal of the loose fragment was followed by posterior spinal fusion. After some months the leg pain returned, more severe than before the operation. At a subsequent operation it was found that a remnant of the loose fragment on the left side had not been removed and was compressing the fifth spi-

nal nerve. On the right side the fifth nerve, which emerged from the dura 1.5 cm. lower than normal, had slipped posterior to the superior articular process of L5; the articular process was compressing the nerve (Fig. 4-18).

Degenerative Spondylolisthesis

This condition (Fig. 4-19, 4-20), which occurs in some cases of degenerative disease of the lumbar spine, causes one type of spinal stenosis. In some parts of the world it is relatively common, and in others, rare. It has not been noted in patients under 40 years of age. It is three times more common in women. It is not possible to account for the geographical or sexual distribution. Despite the absence of a defect in the pars interarticularis, the upper vertebra slips forward on the lower. The condition is more frequently encountered at the L4–5 level and occasionally at the L3–4 or L5–S1 level. In rare instances it is present at all three levels.

The striking feature is marked erosion of the superior articular process of the lower vertebra, with some degree of erosion of the inferior articular process of the upper vertebra. It is the erosion of the articular processes that, as the disc yields, permits the upper vertebra to slip forward. The articular processes are greatly widened and enlarged and present a scalloped appearance. Their margins are very irregular due to osteophytic new bone.

Marked degeneration of the intervertebral disc results in approximation of the two vertebral bodies. The lateral recesses of both vertebrae are narrowed from the formation of craggy, irregular, new bone, particularly affecting the anterior surface of the superior articular processes. The enlarged articular processes bulge posterolaterally into the spinal canal. The whole surface of each vertebra is irregular from new bone formation. When there has been more erosion of the bone of the superior articular process on one side than on the other, marked rotation of the upper

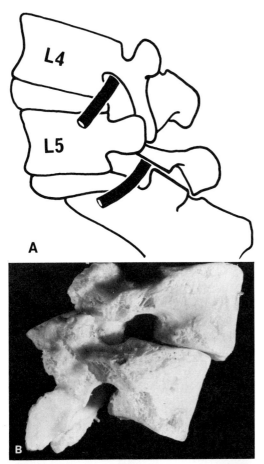

A

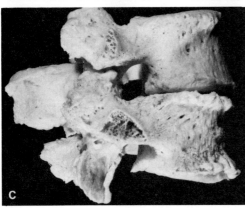

B

vertebra on the lower results, with increased narrowing of the spinal canal, the lateral recess and foramen.

It is difficult to account for the changes in bony surfaces of the articular processes at one level in a lesion that characteristically produces erosion of articular cartilage with sclerosis of subchondral bone and the formation of new bone in the form of osteophytes. Possibly there is osteoporosis coexisting with the degenerative process (Fig. 4-19).

The most important feature of degenerative spondylolisthesis is nerve entrapment. This can occur in any of four ways: (1) from pressure on the L4 nerve at the foramen by osteophytes arising from the posteroinferior surface of the vertebral body of L4 (Fig. 4-20A1); (2) pressure on the L5 nerve from posterior displacement of L5 on L4 forming a bony ridge in the region of the lateral recess (Fig. 4-20A2); (3) pressure on the L5 nerve in a narrow lateral recess at the lower border of the L5 vertebra (Fig. 4-20A3); (4) pressure on the L5 nerve by the anteriorly displaced inferior articular process of L4 (Fig. 4-20A4).

THE LIGAMENTUM FLAVUM

Special mention is made of this structure because of misconceptions as to its role in producing pressure on the cauda equina and entrapment of spinal nerves.

At each level the upper attachment of the ligamentum flavum is to the anterior surface of the lamina halfway between its upper and lower border. The lower attachment is to the upper border of the lamina below. In the mid-line, between one lamina and the next, it blends with the anterior margin of the interspinous ligament. Posteriorly it is covered by fat, which separates it from the paraspinal muscles (Fig. 4-21). It has lateral extensions between one pedicle and the next. These lie medial first, and then anterior to the posterior joints, and extend laterally

Fig. 4-19: Two specimens demonstrating degenerative spondylolisthesis. *(B)* There is a marked slip of L4 anteriorly on L5. Note that the inferior articular process of L4 has markedly narrowed the L5 lateral recess. *(C)* Minor slip of L4 on L5. There are marked degenerative changes. *(B,C,* Courtesy Dr. H. F. Farfan)

FIG. 4-20. Degenerative spondylolisthesis. *(A)* The ways in which the nerves can be entrapped: *(1)* the fourth nerve by osteophytes from the posterior body of L4; *(2)* the fifth nerve by the bony ridge of L5; *(3)* the fifth nerve in a narrow lateral recess; *(4)* the fifth nerve by the displaced inferior articular process of L4. *(B)* Marked erosion of the superior articular process of L5. *(C)* Marked rotation of L4 on L5.

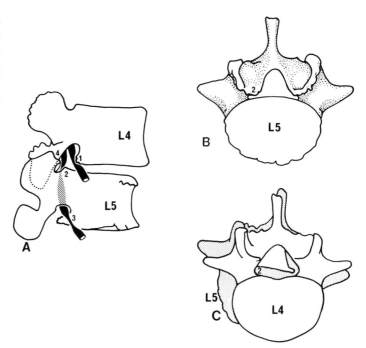

as far as the intervertebral foramen, thus forming the anteromedial part of the posterior joint capsule (Fig. 4-22).

Over the past 40 years much has been written on the subjects of thickening, hypertrophy, and buckling of the ligamentum flavum.[27,29,31,37,38,46] In 107 laminectomies we have measured the thickness of the ligamentum flavum through a longitudinal incision in the midline (with the spine held midway between full flexion and full extension). The average thickness is 2 mm. Rarely is it more than 3 mm. After division of upper or lower attachments, the ligament shortens, buckles, and thickens. Confusion may have arisen because the ligament was not measured before removal. In degenerative arthritis there is frequently a layer of fibrous tissue superficial to the ligament, and this may have led to further error. Laterally, because its upper and lower attachments have not been disturbed, the ligament does not shorten. Again, the average thickness is 2

to 3 mm. and in no instance have we seen thickening or hypertrophy of the ligament. In over 52 cases we have examined the ligamentum flavum histologically, using the Gomori aldehyde fuchsin stain. The percentage of elastin varies from 60 to 80, the remainder being collagen. There was no correlation between age and the amount of elastin present and the existence of degenerative disease or the duration of symptoms. This is not in agreement with the findings of other workers.[30,45]

When the laminae are thickened, as in spinal stenosis, the ligamentum flavum may exert pressure on the cauda equina, without real thickening, hypertrophy, or buckling. The thickened lamina pushes the normal ligament forward against the dura. The ligament may contribute to spinal nerve entrapment laterally when there is subluxation and overriding of the posterior articular processes; the upper pole of the superior articular process lies nearer to the pedicle above and glides an-

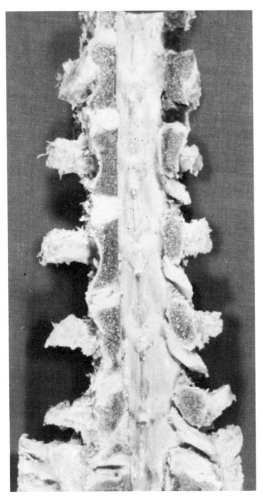

FIG. 4-21. The ligamentum flavum, showing attachments to the anterior surfaces of the laminae. (Courtesy Dr. I. Munkacsi)

teriorly. That portion of ligament forming the anterior capsule of the displaced joint (Fig. 4-22) is displaced antero-medially. When the posterior articular processes are enlarged they bulge into the spinal canal, and the portion of the ligamentum flavum forming the medial capsule is displaced medially.

THE BLOOD SUPPLY OF THE LUMBAR SPINE

The vascular supply of the vertebrae and intervertebral discs has been fully described by Crock[8]; that of the cauda equina and spinal nerves as clearly by Dommisse.[10] Here we will do no more than discuss some of the practical applications that result from the detailed and magnificently illustrated work of these two authors.

Changes in the Vascular Supply

The work of Arnoldi[3] and Ficat[16] demonstrates that venous hypertension in bone frequently accompanies degenerative arthritis. Further work of Arnoldi[3] shows the same association in the spine. Vizkelety and Wouters have shown striking changes in bone, disc, and growth plate following acute venous hypertension in the rat tail.[41] In our laboratory, R. Foley has attempted to produce chronic venous hypertension in the rat tail. In his

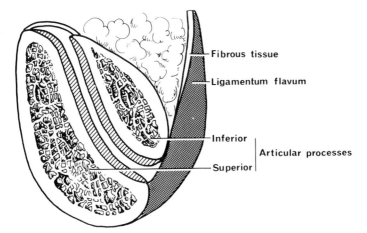

FIG. 4-22. A cross-section of a posterior joint shows that the lateral extension of the ligamentum flavum forms the anteromedial capsule of the joint.

studies, similar changes occur, but they are uncommon. It is at least possible that arteriolar thrombosis and/or venous obstruction in the vessels supplying cencellous bone deep to the end-plates interferes with the nutrition of the annulus fibrosus and nucleus pulposus.

Such changes may well be the underlying cause both of isolated disc resorption and of internal disc disruption. Certainly degenerative lesions at one level follow both these conditions. Degenerative changes at one level may represent the start of a generalized degenerative process due to venous hypertension. In other cases similar vascular changes may affect several levels simultaneously and so produce generalized degenerative lesions of the lumbar spine. None of this experimental work has proved conclusively whether venous pressure changes are cause or effect.

The Effect of Degenerative Changes in Soft Tissues and Bone on the Vascular Supply of the Lumbar Spine

In degenerative spondylosis, and particularly in spinal stenosis, several factors cause occlusion or partial occlusion by pressure on the intermediate spinal arteries, which supply the contents of the spinal canal; on the radicular arteries, supplying the nerves in the canal, and the internal venous plexus of Batson. These are: osteophyte formation, narrowing of the discs, thickening of the laminae, internal protrusion of enlarged posterior articular processes, and narrowing of the lateral recesses and foramina. It is of interest to note that the radicular veins have valves but those of Batson's plexus are without valves. As observed by Dommisse, the normal pressure in the arterioles supplying the cauda equina and spinal nerves is only slightly higher than the colloid osmotic pressure. The funiculi of the spinal nerves carry an abundant blood supply from radicular arterioles and capillaries. The blood vessels supplying the nerves (vasa nervorum) are extremely sensitive to compressive changes. The ischemic changes in nerves in spinal stenosis may be such that no recovery of neural function is possible, even after removal of the cause of compression.

Attention to Blood Vessels During Operations to Decompress the Cauda Equina and Spinal Nerves

Hemorrhage during laminectomy can be reduced considerably by placing the patient on a Hasting's frame, thus reducing pressure on the abdomen and in Batson's plexus. Both Crock[8] and Dommisse[10] have stressed the importance of avoiding damage to the intermediate neural branches of each segmental spinal artery by very careful operative technique, often using either a loupe or an operating microscope, and by controlling arterial and venous bleeding both through a thorough knowledge of the vascular supply and by using low-voltage diathermy. Care must be observed to avoid damage to the branches of the intermediate spinal artery by diathermy, to the posterior spinal branch of each lumbar artery on a level with and anterior to the pars, and to the radicular veins just inside the spinal canal. The blood vessels at the level of the foramen are particularly vulnerable. A careless operative technique with trauma to the delicately balanced vascular supply to the cauda equina and spinal nerves results in the formation of adhesions around the nerves and between the posterior dura and overlying erector spinae muscles. Ischemia of segments of the nerves may result, with the production of new pain syndromes, sensory changes, and loss of muscle power.

INNERVATION OF THE LUMBAR SPINE

A full description of innervation of the lumbar spine, together with discussion of the clinical applications and bibliography, have been given by Edgar and Ghadially.[11]

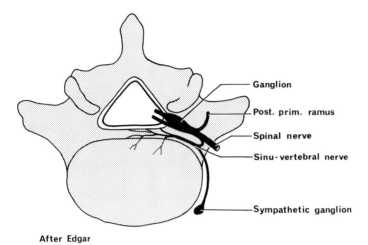

FIG. 4-23. A cross-section of the lumbar spine shows the origin, course, and structures supplied by the sinuvertebral nerve.

Ganglion

Post. prim. ramus

Spinal nerve

Sinu-vertebral nerve

Sympathetic ganglion

After Edgar

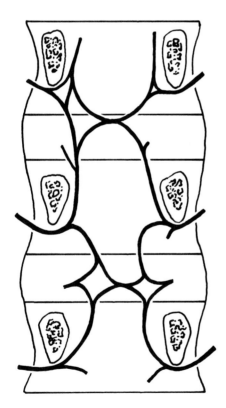

After Finneson et al

FIG. 4-24. A longitudinal section demonstrates that the branches of the sinuvertebral nerve form anastomoses with those above and below and with those of the contralateral side. (After Finneson. B.: Low Back Pain. Philadelphia, J. B. Lippincott, 1973)

Innervation of the lumbar spine is by the sinuvertebral nerve and the posterior primary ramus.

The sinuvertebral nerve (Figs. 4-23, 4-24) was first described by von Luschka.[24] It arises from the anterior aspect of the spinal nerve, a few millimeters distal to the dorsal root ganglion. It is joined almost immediately by a branch from the sympathetic ramus communicans. The composite nerve, 0.5 to 1 mm. thick, then passes back through the intervertebral foramen into the spinal canal. In the region of the posterior longitudinal ligament each sinuvertebral nerve divides into ascending, descending, and transverse branches which anastomose with the nerves of the contralateral side and with those from adjacent levels.

Branches of this nerve supply the outer layers of the annulus fibrosus. Most of the terminations are naked nerve endings and probably mediate pain sensation. Fine nerve fibers can be seen in the granulation tissue in the deeper layers of the annulus of a degenerative disc.[36] The pain-provocation test during discography is probably mediated by these branches.

The posterior longitudinal ligament has an abundant nerve supply from the

FIG. 4-25. A diagrammatic view of the lumbar spine shows the origin, course, and branches of the posterior primary rami. (Adapted from Lewin, T.: Acta Orthop. Scand., Suppl. 73: 1964)

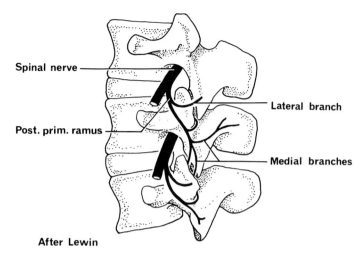

Spinal nerve

Post. prim. ramus

Lateral branch

Medial branches

After Lewin

sinuvertebral nerve with both naked and encapsulated nerve endings. This ligament is probably responsible for much of what is called discogenic pain, as it is the first structure impinged on by disc herniation outside the annulus fibrosus.

The anterior longitudinal ligament is supplied by a few anterior branches of the sinuvertebral nerve, though its main innervation is by direct branches from the sympathetic chain.

The anterior dura mater is innervated by branches of the sinuvertebral nerve that ascend one level and descend two. The terminations are naked nerve endings. The posterior dura has a scanty nerve supply from the autonomic plexus. Pressure on the dura, for example by a disc herniation, produces a pattern of pain similar to that from the posterior longitudinal ligament.

Branches of the sinuvertebral nerve supply the posterior periosteum, and probably also the bone, of the vertebral bodies.

The Posterior Primary Ramus

The posterior primary ramus arises from each spinal nerve outside the foramen and divides into medial and lateral branches (Fig. 4-25). The medial branch descends at the back of the transverse process and superior articular process, lying in a groove formed by these structures. It sends a small branch to the inferior capsule of the posterior joint. It then passes caudad to supply the dorsal spinal muscles and anastomoses with nerves from adjacent levels. It also supplies the superior part of the capsule of the posterior joint below.

The lateral branches of the posterior primary rami of the upper three lumbar levels supply the skin as far distally as the greater trochanter, but there is no cutaneous supply from the lower two posterior rami.

The spinous processes and laminae are probably supplied by branches from the posterior primary rami. Free endings have been seen on the surface and in the outermost dorsal layer of the ligamentum flavum, but none in its substance. The lumbodorsal fascia has a nerve supply from the same source, without overlap, but the origin of the nerves appears to be one level cephalad. The interspinous and supraspinous ligaments are also supplied by branches derived from nerves to the surrounding muscles.

The posterior joints are supplied by the medial branches of the posterior primary rami. There is an overlap of innervation. At each level the ramus supplies branches to that level and also to the joint at the level below. Free and complex unencapsulated nerve endings are found in the capsule, probably mediating pain and proprioception.

Clinical Application

The poor localization and radiation of low back pain may well be related to the fact that each sinuvertebral nerve and each posterior primary ramus supplies at least two levels.

Entrapment of spinal nerves is an obvious cause of pain, sensory disturbances, and muscle weakness, but the distribution of the branches of the sinuvertebral nerve and of the posterior primary rami give rise to a more complex problem. Irritation of the branches of the sinuvertebral nerve may be relevant in the pain of disc degeneration and herniation, and in spinal stenosis. On the other hand, irritation of the posterior primary rami is a feature of segmental instability. Impulses reaching the spinal nerve via the branches of the sinuvertebral nerve and the posterior primary ramus may potentiate the irritability of the spinal nerve.

In performing an intertransverse spinal fusion, the posterior primary rami are nearly always sectioned. This may be one of the beneficial effects of this operation.

Irritation of the sinuvertebral nerve may cause back pain and sciatica. This has special relevance to the variety of conditions that produce lateral recess narrowing at the L4–5 and L5–S1 levels.

As postulated by Arnoldi and co-workers[23] and by Ficat and colleagues,[16] increased intraosseous venous pressure may produce pain by pressure on nerve endings in bone. Thus laminectomy may relieve pain not only by removing pressure and irritation by soft tissue and bone on the spinal nerves and on the branches of the sinuvertebral nerve, but also by lowering the venous pressure.

Differentiation of pain referred from the posterior joints to one or both legs from that of disc herniations with no leg pain or atypical leg pain presents a great diagnostic challenge. Adequate decompression in cases of spinal stenosis is still most difficult to achieve. An increased understanding of the role of the sinuvertebral nerve and posterior primary ramus seems most likely to produce solutions to these problems.

THE MUSCULATURE

Bruising

Bruising of the extensors of the lumbar spine is not uncommon. It is usually caused by a direct blow. The pathological changes are probably those of rupture of small blood vessels and of individual muscle fibers. On rest, analgesics, and antispasmodic drugs the patient usually makes a full and rapid recovery.

Atrophy and Weakness

Atrophy and weakness of the spinal muscles is commonly encountered. Weak abdominal muscles (the spinal flexors) result in a faulty posture with marked lumbar lordosis. This places the three-joint complex at the lower two levels at risk and predisposes to joint strains, degeneration, and low back pain. In the same way weak quadriceps put the knee joint at risk. Weakness of the quadratus lumborum muscles causes abnormality in lateral bending and may itself be a cause of pain. Weakness of the erector spinae muscles is less common, as these muscles act together with the ligamentum flavum to extend the spine.

Muscle Spasm

Spasm of the posterior muscles, sometimes accompanied by functional scoliosis and often by pain, usually indicates an underlying strain of posterior joints or disc or both of these. Unilateral spasm is suggestive of a unilateral posterior joint strain. Lesions involving both disc and posterior joints are often accompanied by spasm of the spinal flexors, producing a straight or slightly kyphotic lumbar spine. Psoas spasm produces flexion deformity of the hip, and this may be missed in the initial examination. Spasm of the piriform, a common cause of buttock pain, can be diagnosed by palpation medial to the lower part of the neck of the femur.

Shortening

Shortening (or tightness) of the hamstrings and triceps surae results from faulty posture and is a not uncommon cause of thigh and leg aching, which must be distinguished from sciatica. Chronic low back and leg pain due to marked degenerative changes and herniations of the nucleus pulposus, and spinal stenosis often leads to shortening of these muscles. Treatment of the underlying condition must be followed by stretching exercises to restore these muscles to their normal length.

Muscle Strain

Acute and chronic muscle strain is, in our opinion, an uncommon entity. Admittedly this diagnosis is made by many clinicians. When there is pain, tenderness, and spasm of muscles over a posterior joint it is often difficult to assess whether the symptoms come from muscle or from joint.

We wish to record our thanks to Miss Jean MacGregor, Mrs. Cecile Mason, Mr. John Junor and Mr. Bob van den Beuken for a great deal of assistance with the illustrations.

REFERENCES

1. Arnoldi, C. C.: Intravertebral pressures in patients with lumbar pain. Acta Orthop. Scand., *43*:109, 1972.
2. ———: Intraosseous hypertension a possible cause of low back pain. Clin. Orthop., *115*:30, 1976.
3. Arnoldi, C. C., Lindesholm, H., and Miissbichler, H.: Venous engorgement and intraosseous hypertension in osteoarthritis of the hip. J. Bone Joint Surg., *54B*:409, 1972.
4. Baker, W. de C., Thomas, T. G., and Kirkaldy-Willis, W. H.: Changes in the cartilage of posterior intervertebral joints after anterior fusion. J. Bone Joint Surg., *51B*:736, 1969.
5. Colve, J. C., and Golland, M.: The intervertebral nucleus pulposus, its anatomy, its physiology, its pathology. J. Bone Joint Surg., *12*:555, 1930.
6. Compere, E. L.: Origin, anatomy, physiology and pathology of the intervertebral disc. A.A.O.S. Instructional Course Lectures, vol. 18. St. Louis, C. V. Mosby, 1961.
7. Crock, H. V.: A reappraisal of intervertebral disc lesions. Med. J. Austral. *1*:983, 1970.
8. ———: Blood supply of the spine. Clin. Orthop., [In press].
9. DePalma, A. F., and Rothman, R. H.: The Lumbar Disc. Philadelphia, W. B. Saunders, 1970.
10. Dommisse, G. F.: The Arteries and Veins of the Human Spinal Cord from Birth. London, Churchill Livingstone, 1975.
11. Edgar, M. A., and Ghadially, J. A.: Innervation of the lumbar spine. Clin. Orthop., [In press].
12. Ehni, G.: Significance of the small lumbar spinal canal: cauda equina compression syndromes due to spondylosis. J. Neurosurg., *31*:490, 1969.
13. Farfan, H. F.: Effects of torsion on the intervertebral joints. Can. J. Surg., *12*:336, 1969.
14. Farfan, H. F., and Sullivan, J. B.: The relation of facet orientation to intervertebral disc failure. Can. J. Surg., *10*:179, 1967.
15. Farfan, H. F., Huberdeau, R. M., and Dubow, H. I.: Lumbar intervertebral disc degeneration. J. Bone Joint Surg., *54A*:492, 1972.
16. Ficat, P., and Arlet, J.: Coxopathies Ischemique. Rev. Chir. Orthop., *58*:543, 1972.
17. Forbes, D. B.: The Farfan back operation, technique and results. Can. J. Surg., *18*:546, 1975.
18. Gill, G. G., Manning, J. G., and White, H. L.: Surgical treatment of spondylolisthesis without spine fusion. J. Bone Joint Surg., *37A*:493, 1955.
19. Golante, J. O.: Tensile properties of the lumbar annulus fibrosus. Acta Orthop. Scand., Suppl. *100*: 1976.
20. Harris, R. I., and Macnab, I.: Structural changes in the lumbar intervertebral discs. J. Bone Joint Surg., *36B*:304, 1954.
21. Hirsch, C.: Studies on the pathology of low back pain. J. Bone Joint Surg., *41B*:237, 1959.
22. Hirsch, C., and Schajowicz, F.: Studies on structrual changes in the lumbar annulus fibrosus. Acta Orthop. Scand., *23*:184, 1953.

23. Lewin, O. A.: Osteoarthritis in lumbar synovial joints. Acta Orthop. Scand., Supp. 73: 1964.

24. von Luschka, H.: Die Nerven des Menschlichen Wirbenkanales. Tübingen, Hlaupp., 1850.

25. Mcnab, I.: The traction spur. J. Bone Joint Surg., *53A*:663, 1971.

26. ———: Negative disc exploration. J. Bone Joint Surg., *53A*:891, 1971.

27. Naffziger, H. C., Inman, V., and Saunders, J. B. de C. M.: Lesions of the intervertebral disc and ligamenta flava. J. Surg. Gynaecol. Obstet., *66*:288, 1932.

28. Newman, P. S.: Etiology of spondylolisthesis. J. Bone Joint Surg., *45B*:39, 1963.

29. Pheasant, H. C.: Ligamentum flavum intrusion: a source of back and radicular disability. J. Bone Joint Surg., *37A*:408, 1955.

30. Pickett, J. C.: Some studies on the ligamentum flavum. J. Bone Joint Surg., *44A*:794, 1962.

31. Ramsay, R. H.: Anatomy of the ligamenta flava. J. Bone Joint Surg., *46A*:921, 1964.

32. Ritchie, J. H., and Fahrni, W. H.: Age changes in lumbar intervertebral discs. Can. J. Surg., *13*:65, 1970.

33. Roaf, R. O.: A study of the mechanics of spinal injuries. J. Bone Joint Surg., *42B*:810, 1960.

34. Shinohara, H.: A study of lumbar disc lesions. J. Jap. Orthop. Assn., *44*:553, 1970.

35. Singh, S. H., and Kirkaldy-Willis, W. H.: Experimental "anterior" spinal fusion in guinea pigs: a histologic study of the changes in the anterior and posterior elements. Can. J. Surg., *15*:239, 1972.

36. Souter, W. A., and Taylor, T. K. F.: Sulphated mucopolysaccharide metabolism in the rabbit intervertebral disc. J. Bone Joint Surg., *52B*:371, 1970.

37. Spurling, R. G., Mayfield, F. H., and Rogers, J. B.: Hypertrophy of the ligamenta flava as a cause of low back pain. J.A.M.A., *109*:928, 1937.

38. Stoltman, H. F., and Blackwood, W.: The role of the ligamenta flava in the pathogenesis of myelopathy in cervical spondylosis. Brain, *87*:45, 1964.

39. Sullivan, J. D., Farfan, H. F., and Kahn, D. S.: Pathological changes with intervertebral joint rotational instability in the rabbit. Can. J. Surg., *14*:71, 1971.

40. Thomas, I., Kirkaldy-Willis, W. H., Singh, S., and Paine, K. W. E.: Experimental spinal fusion in guinea pigs and dogs. Clin. Orthop., *112*:363, 1975.

41. Vizkelety, T., and Wouters, H. W.: Recherches experimentales sur le development de la necrose aseptique schemique de l'os. Rev. Chir. Orthop., *55*:40, 1969.

42. Wiltse, L. L.: The etiology of spondylolisthesis. J. Bone Joint Surg., *44A*:539, 1962.

43. ———: Spondylolisthesis: classification and etiology. Symposium on the spine: A.A.O.S. Instructional Course Lecture. vol. 143. St. Louis, C. V. Mosby, 1969.

44. Wiltse, L. L., Widell, E. H., and Jackson, D. W.: Fatigue fracture the basic lesion in isthmic spondylolisthesis. Presented at A.A.O.S., Las Vegas, Nevada, February 6, 1973.

45. Yamashita, H., and Kato (Nagoya) A.: Pathohistological study of abnormal ligamenta flava. J. Bone Joint Surg., *40A*:224, 1958.

46. Yamoda, H., Ohya, M., Okada, T., and Shiozawa, Z.: Intermittent cauda equina compression due to narrow spinal canal. J. Neurosurg., *37*:83, 1972.

5 Lumbar Spinal Stenosis

John H. Wedge, W. H. Kirkaldy-Willis, and P. Kinnard

THE CONCEPT

Pathological changes involving the spinal canal other than simple herniation of the nucleus pulposus have been recorded by numerous authors during the past 75 years.[18,25] In 1900 Sachs and Fraenkel described a case in which at laminectomy a thick lamina was encountered. Elsberg reported 60 laminectomies in which he thought good results were due to improved circulation of blood to the cauda equina.[10] Twenty-six cases of hypertrophic arthritis were described in 1934 by Cramer with edema and hyperemia of the spinal nerves.[5] Sarpenyer described congenital narrowing of the spinal canal.[30] Munro believed that other causes of narrowing of the canal than disc herniations were equally important.[24] Pennal and Schatzker reported 21 cases of narrowing of the canal due, in their opinion, to an abnormality of development.[27] Cauchoix described narrowing of the spinal canal following spinal fusion.[4]

Recently Paine and Huang recorded 227 cases of herniation of the nucleus pulposus and of developmental and degenerative stenosis.[25] Herniation alone formed less than one third of their series. Kirkaldy-Willis, Paine, Cauchoix and McIvor together with Brodsky and Dombrowski, recorded 973 cases.[3,18] In these series only 126 cases were of uncomplicated herniation of the nucleus pulposus. Thus, stenosis of the central spinal canal has gradually been emphasized as an important cause of cauda equina and spinal nerve compression.

During the past few years attention has focused on spinal nerve entrapment in the nerve canals and lateral recesses (See Chap. 4). Dandy[8] discussed the "concealed" disc and Macnab[22] described the causes of nerve entrapment in what he called "negative disc exploration." Recently Crock has described isolated disc resorption with lateral entrapment of spinal nerves by the superior articular processes.[6]

Thus, whatever the cause, there are two kinds of nerve entrapment. The first is in the main spinal canal, affecting mainly the cauda equina but also the nerves in the medial part of the nerve canal. The second affects mainly the spinal nerves in the lateral part of the nerve canal. A single underlying pathological process can cause both central and lateral compression.

DEFINITION

Of necessity, any definition of spinal stenosis is arbitrary. As a working hypothesis the following has been suggested by Arnoldi and co-workers.

Spinal stenosis is narrowing of any region or regions of the spinal canal or nerve foramina, usually with pressure on nerves or those vessels supplying the nerves.[2]

Uncomplicated herniations of the nucleus pulposus are excluded, as are inflammatory lesions due to infection, as well as primary and secondary neoplastic lesions.

CLASSIFICATION

Recently Arnoldi and co-workers put forward a comprehensive classification of spinal stenosis, both of the spinal and nerve canals.[2] They divide the syndrome into the following types:

Classification of Spinal Stenoses

Congenital and Developmental
  Achondroplasia
  Idiopathic
Degenerative
  Central
  Peripheral
  Degenerative spondylolisthesis
Combined
  Any combination of developmental and degenerative spinal stenosis and herniations of the nucleus pulposus
Spondylolisthesis and spondylolysis
Iatrogenic
  Post-laminectomy
  Post-spinal fusion (anterior or posterior)
Traumatic (late changes)
Metabolic (fluorosis)
Other (Paget's disease)

Combined lesions (Type 3) are the most common.[33] The figures for 130 consecutive patients at the University of Saskatchewan from December 1966 to November 1975 are shown in Table 5-1.

PATHOLOGICAL ANATOMY OF SPINAL STENOSES

Developmental Stenosis

The most common type is idiopathic. Frequently the whole of the lumbar spinal canal is narrowed, especially in the an-

Table 5-1. Breakdown by Type of 130 Cases of Spinal Stenosis

Classification	Number of Patients	Per Cent
Developmental	0	0
Degenerative		
Central	10	
Peripheral	5	21
Central and peripheral	13	
Degenerative spondylolisthesis	0	
Combined		
Degenerative and disc	49	
Developmental and disc	6	49
Developmental and degenerative	7	
Developmental, degenerative and disc	1	
Spondylolisthesis	18	14
Traumatic	1	1
Iatrogenic		
Post-discoidectomy/ laminectomy	13	15
Post-fusion	7	

teroposterior diameter as seen on the lateral roentgenograph, measuring less than 12 mm. The lateral diameter is less than 2.0 centimeters (Fig. 5-1), measured on the anteroposterior view. Occasionally the narrowing affects only the lower half of the lumbar spinal canal. More rarely there is stenosis at only one level, due to shingling (obliquity) of the laminae. The cause is unknown: there may be an inborn error of growth resulting in narrowing of the canal during the years of growth. For this reason we have called this type "congenital/developmental" stenosis. Rare cases of narrowing of the whole canal with segmental narrowing at the level of the posterior articular processes are encountered in young patients. This may represent degenerative change superimposed on developmental narrowing, or it may be a special type of stenosis with developmental enlargement of the posterior articular processes, which bulge into the spinal canal. In this condition the lateral recesses may also be narrow.

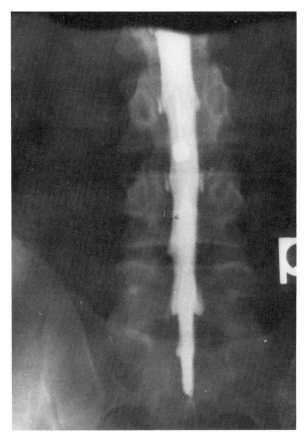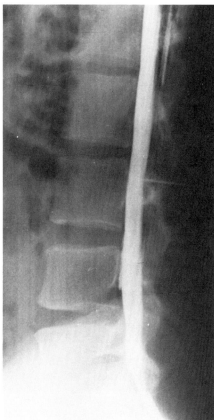

FIG. 5-1. Myelogram of a 28-year-old man with developmental stenosis. Note that the whole canal is uniformly narrowed.

Degenerative Stenosis

There are two causes: disintegration of the intervertebral discs and the articular cartilage of the facets, and new bone formation. The latter is equivalent to the osteophytic outgrowths that form in degenerative arthritis in other joints, but it is more generalized in nature (Fig. 5-2).

The laminae are thickened, usually more than 7 mm., while new bone forming their upper and lower surfaces reduces the interlaminar space to 4 mm. or less. The ligamentum flavum is not shortened or thickened but is pushed forward by thickening of the overlying lower half of the upper lamina. The posterior articular processes are enlarged and irregular in outline, projecting posteriorly under the erector spinae muscles and nearer the midline than normal. They bulge posterolaterally into the spinal canal, indenting the dura and giving a cloverleaf or fleur-de-lis cross-sectional appearance to the canal. The enlarged superior articular process, with sharp edges and forward displacement, frequently narrows the lateral recess and entraps the nerve.

The dura may be "tight" along the whole length of the lesion, and it is particularly narrowed (waisted) opposite the articular processes. At this level the extradural fat may be absent (Fig. 5-3), while in severe cases the normal dural pulse is absent.

The vertebral bodies are enlarged, and their surfaces are craggy and irregular with osteophytic outgrowths adjacent to the attachments of the annulus fibrosus

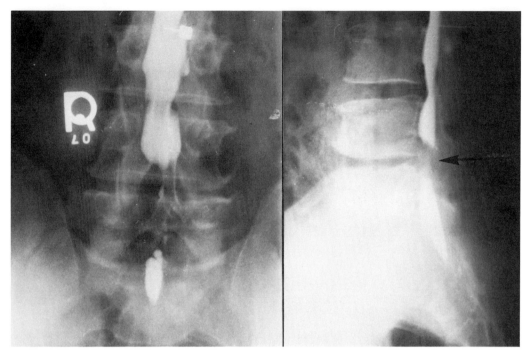

FIG. 5-2. Myelogram of a 49-year-old man with degenerative stenosis. Note the almost complete block at the L4–L5 level (*arrow*).

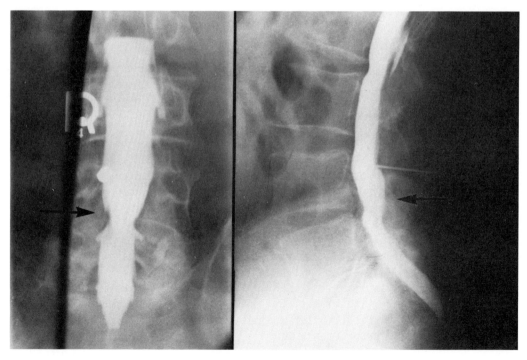

FIG. 5-3. Myelogram of a 69-year-old man with segmental degenerative stenosis. Note the narrowing of the dye column at the L4–L5 level (*arrow*).

across their margins posteriorly from side to side.

The disc space is reduced in height with marked degeneration of the nucleus pulposus, sometimes with crescentic and radial fissures. The changes in the disc and contiguous vertebral bodies produce a "hard" disc protrusion quite different from herniation of the nucleus pulposus. This is due to osteophytes from the vertebral body margins and to thickening of the annulus fibrosus. The disc height may be more reduced on one side than on the other, leading to scoliosis, which may be enhanced by wedge-shaped vertebral bodies.

Frequently the lateral recesses at the L4−5 and L5−S1 level are narrowed, mainly by subluxation and enlargement of the superior processes. Occasionally the foramen is narrowed by projecting sharp osteophytes, chiefly from the posterorlateral surface of the body, causing lateral stenosis. Rarely degenerative stenosis can produce complete block. The changes seen in degenerative spondylolisthesis and the rotational changes of one vertebra on the next have been described in Chapter 4.

Combined Stenosis

The term denotes either developmental stenosis with herniation of the nucleus pulposus, developmental with superadded degenerative stenosis (Fig. 5-4), degenerative stenosis with herniation of the nucleus pulposus (Fig. 5-5), or developmental and degenerative stenosis with

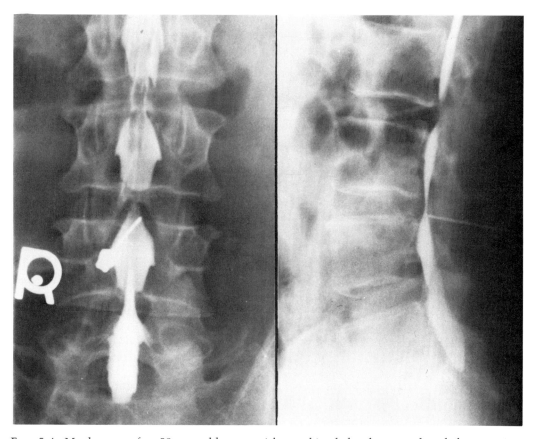

FIG. 5-4. Myelogram of a 59-year-old man with combined developmental and degenerative stenosis. Note the segmental narrowing in the anteroposterior view and the marked uniform narrowing in the lateral view. (Kirkaldy-Willis, W. H.: Clin. Orthop., *115*:75, 1976)

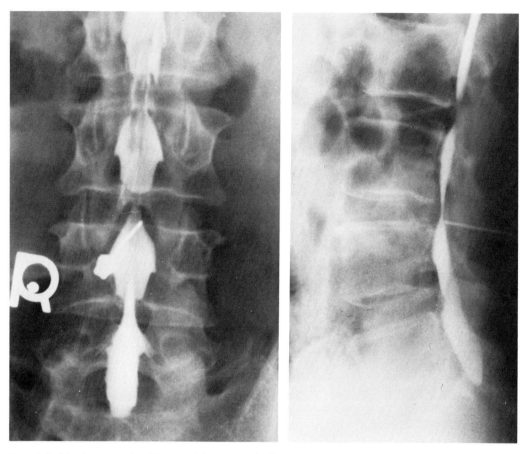

FIG. 5-5. Myelogram of a 51-year-old man with degenerative stenosis associated with a L4–L5 disc protrusion (*arrow*).

herniation of the nucleus pulposus (Fig. 5-6). In our opinion developmental stenosis rarely if ever produces symptoms unless there is added disc herniation or a mild degree of degenerative stenosis.

Spondylolisthetic Stenosis

Cauda equina compression from stenosis of the spinal canal is due to degenerative change at the level above the slip (Fig. 5-7).[18] There may be marked constriction of the dura. Lateral stenosis with entrapment of the spinal nerve may be due to pressure on the nerve of the superior part of the pars (above the defect), which is pulled backward against it, and entrapment of the nerve between the upper bony surface at the level of the defect and the intervertebral disc surface of the body below. It also occurs following operative procedures in which the "mirror image" (the bone superior to the defect) is not removed along with the loose fragment, the nerve becoming hooked over the back of the upper part of the pars. In congenital spondylolisthesis a variety of anomalies may be encountered with lateral entrapment of the nerve (Chap. 4).

Stenosis Following Laminectomy and Spinal Fusion

Recurrence of symptoms after laminectomy may be due to fibrosis between the erector spinae muscles and the back of the

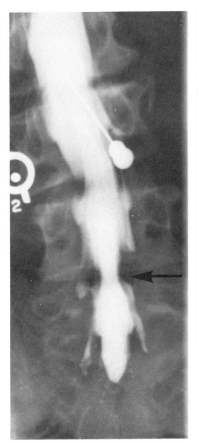 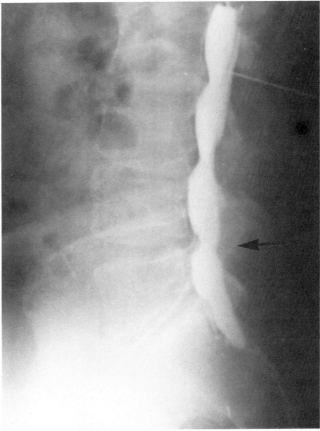

FIG. 5-6. Myelogram of a 50-year-old man with combined developmental/degenerative stenosis and L3–L4 protrusion. The anteroposterior view shows an almost complete block at L3–L4. The lateral view shows uniform narrowing of the canal with a block due to the herniation of L3–L4 (Kirkaldy-Willis, W. H.: Clin Orthop., *99*:30, 1974)

dura, especially if too wide a laminectomy has been done.[21] It may also be due to adhesions between the spinal nerves and the back of the disc, or to adhesions in the lateral recess. Rough handling at a first operation may impair the blood supply to the vessels of the spinal nerves, resulting in ischemia and intraneural fibrosis. Stenosis may also occur following posterior spinal fusion (Fig. 5-8). Thickening of the graft and new bone formation stimulated by the graft may result in stenosis over the whole length of the grafted area or mainly at the upper end of the graft. The new bone lies posterior to

the dura and anterior to the laminae and ligamenta flava. Stenosis may also follow degenerative changes at the upper end of the graft, involving both sides, the top of the grafted area, and the vertebra just above this. Of 350 cases of spinal stenosis, Brodsky recorded 67 following fusion and another 69 following laminectomy.[3]

Stenosis Following Trauma

Following a burst fracture of a vertebral body it is obvious that there must be encroachment on the spinal canal. Further narrowing of the canal may result from

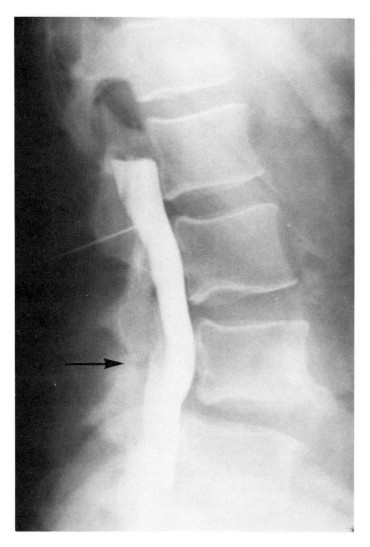

Fig. 5-7. L4–L5 spondylolisthesis with degenerative changes in a 46-year-old man. Note the defect in the pars at L4 (*arrow*).

degenerative changes, with new bone formation, over a period of years.

Metabolic Stenosis

The changes seen in fluorosis, which occurs in certain parts of India, resemble those seen in degenerative stenosis.[32] They are often severe. There is florid new bone formation, which is irregular in contour. It may affect any part of the lumbar spinal canal and may involve laminae, posterior articular processes, vertebral bodies, and foramina in an irregular way.

Paget's Disease

In this condition the whole vertebral body becomes enlarged.[29] The posterior aspect comes to protrude posteriorly and narrows the spinal canal. As a result, the cauda equina and spinal nerves may be compressed.

In summary, once the setting for stenosis is present, for whatever cause, degenerative changes progress from local disease in the intervertebral disc to posterior joint arthritis, segmental instability, then to an attempt at repair, and finally

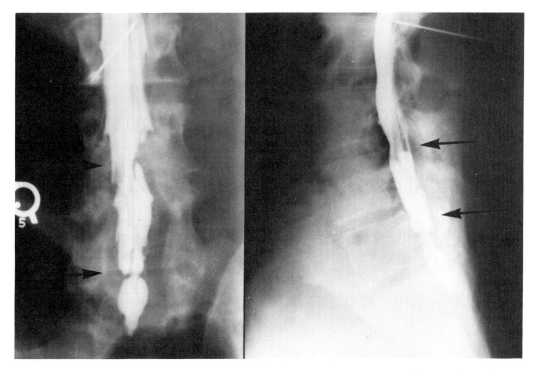

F<small>IG</small>. 5-8. Myelogram of a 30-year-old man with post-fusion stenosis. Note the irregular indentation at the L3–L4 levels in the anteroposterior views (*arrows*) and indentation from the graft in the lateral view (*arrows*).

culminate in spinal stenosis. This may be central, lateral, or a combination of both (Fig. 5-9).

PATHOPHYSIOLOGY

Our hypothesis of the sequence of events that leads to nerve entrapment and pain in the low back and legs is described in Figure 5-10. This is a combination of compression and irritation of the spinal nerves in the cauda equina and nerve canals; irritation of the network formed by the branches of the sinuvertebral nerve (see Chap 4); varying degrees of occlusion of the arteries, veins, and capillaries supplying the nerves; and possible venous hypertension in vertebral bone, irritating small intraosseous nerve endings.[2]

Sensory changes in the leg are due to pressure on and irritation of the spinal and sinuvertebral nerves and pressure on blood vessels.

Motor deficit is caused by a combination of compression on the spinal nerves centrally in the cauda equina and laterally in the nerve canals, and impairment of the vascular supply of these nerves.[9]

Thus the bizarre signs and symptoms are due to a combination of factors at several levels in the spine and very seldom fit into the pattern of single nerve root entrapment. An understanding of this complex pathophysiology is essential in producing a rational approach to treatment.

SYMPTOMS AND SIGNS

Pain

Pain may be chiefly in the back but is usually present in one or both legs. It may be constant or intermittent. Often it is

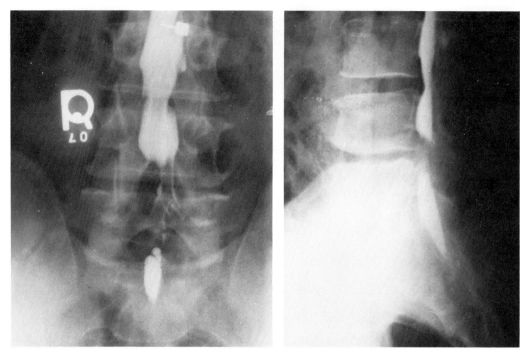

FIG. 5-9. Myelogram of a patient with combined stenosis.

made worse by exercise. The patient may have to rest after walking a short distance because of increasing leg pain, which thus resembles intermittent claudication. Exercise may also increase sensory disturbances and motor weakness. Characteristically night pain in the legs is relieved by walking for several minutes. The pain may be felt in dermatomes supplied by upper lumbar nerves in one leg and lower nerves in the other. Diffuse pain may be felt in the whole of both legs. The symptoms may be made worse by hyperextension and relieved by flexion.

Sensory Changes

Sensory changes are patchy in nature, involving different dermatomes in each leg. Altered sensation may involve the whole of both legs. The patient cannot explain the nature of these changes and may say after laminectomy that his legs now feel as though they "belong to him" again. Both legs may feel cold, although in fact they are not. The patient may complain that his legs feel as though made of rubber.

Motor Changes

Motor changes are also patchy in distribution. Most commonly they involve lower lumbar nerves, but not infrequently upper nerves are involved. A different level may be affected on each side. This weakness may be constant or intermittent. It is often increased by exercise, the patient saying that his legs feel as though they were going to let him down after he walks a short distance. Without losing consciousness he may fall because of leg weakness—a "drop attack."

Reflexes

Reflex changes occur at various levels, which may differ on the two sides. The bizarre nature of the signs and symptoms suggests the presence of spinal stenosis, but it is necessary to exclude psychoneurosis, malingering and secondary gain, as well as uncomplicated herniation of

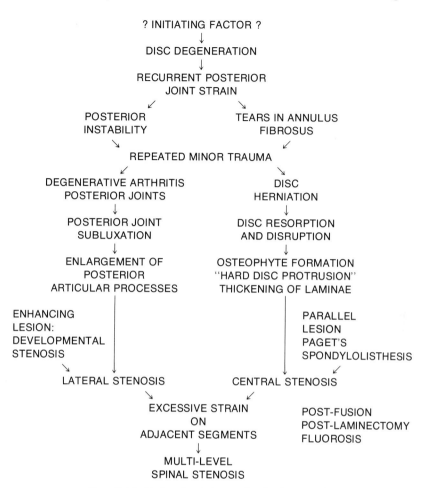

FIG. 5-10. Pathophysiology of spinal stenosis.

the nucleus pulposus and intermittent claudication.

Movement

Movement of the spine and straight-leg raising are reduced, but this is less marked in characteristic herniation of the nucleus pulposus.

DIAGNOSIS

Roentgenography

The diagnosis of spinal stenosis is supported when roentgenographs show degenerative changes in the posterior joints, articular processes larger and nearer the midline than normal, and the anteropos-

terior diameter of the canal reduced. When there is spondylolisthesis without a defect in the pars interarticularis in the presence of leg pain, the diagnosis is almost certainly degenerative spondylolisthesis with stenosis.

Tomography is helpful in the evaluation of the degenerative process and in recognition of an early slip. It may also help in assessing the size of the bony canal.

Discography is, in our opinion, of limited value in stenosis of the lumbar spine. It is advocated by some authors, to assess the number of degenerate discs present.

Myelography is essential if the symptoms and signs are severe enough for laminectomy to be considered. Enough dye should be used to fill the theca to the L1–2 level with the patient erect: it may be necessary to inject as much as 30 ml. Longitudinal streaking, previously considered to indicate arachnoiditis, may well be due to stenosis with crowding of the nerves of the cauda equina. Myelography, using oil-soluble dye, not infrequently fails to reveal the presence of stenosis, particularly when this affects mainly the nerves in the canals and lateral recesses. Water-soluble dye is now used almost exclusively in many countries. This shows the condition of the nerves as they leave the dura almost to the level of the foramina.

Transaxial tomography gives an accurate picture of the cross-section of the spinal and nerve canals at the various levels.[17] It is of special value in defining both the lateral and anteroposterior dimensions of the canal, as well as protrusion of the superior and inferior articular processes and bulging of the disc. At present this expensive and complex equipment is used only in a few centers. Its use may become more widespread, or it may be replaced by the EMI scanner.

The final diagnosis is made by correlating the clinical findings with the special methods just discussed.

TREATMENT

Nonoperative Treatment

A number of patients present with symptoms and signs suggestive of spinal stenosis that are not severe enough to warrant myelography or operative treatment. Extensive degenerative changes on plain roentgenographs suggestive of spinal stenosis may be present with remarkably minor symptoms. These patients may be helped by a number of means: exercises designed to strengthen the flexor muscles of the lumbar spine; reduction of lumbar lordosis by instruction in posture and pelvic tilting (since hyperextension increases, and flexion decreases,

the symptoms because the volume of the spinal canal is greater when the spine is flexed); instruction in the care of the low back with regard to activities of daily living, the wearing of a light elastic back support or spring brace which does not impede the existing movement of the spine and controlled manipulation by persons trained in this form of treatment.[19] It is important, however, that careful clinical supervision be maintained after initial investigations have ruled out other significant pathology. Some patients respond dramatically to these little-recognized forms of treatment.

Operative Treatment

When the patient fails to respond to conservative measures, or when from the start the symptoms are sufficiently disabling, it is necessary to consider laminectomy to decompress the nerves and vessels. Severe pain in one or both legs is a greater indication for operation than back pain alone. At this stage it is important to explain to the patient that an operation will almost certainly reduce his pain but that he will not ever have a completely normal back. He may need to seek a lighter job in the future.

LAMINECTOMY

The first operation has the best chance of success. It should be performed so carefully and so thoroughly that no further exploration will be necessary.[18] Second, third, and subsequent procedures are fraught with difficulty, and the success rate is much lower because of scarring between the dura and overlying muscles, and adhesions around and within the substance of the nerves with intraneural fibrosis and ischemia ("the battered nerve").

General Considerations

The positioning of the patient on a Hasting's frame,[16] with the table in the reversed Trendelenburg position, reduces abdominal pressure which is transmitted to the valveless veins and Batson's plexus. In this way venous congestion and intraspinal hemorrhage are greatly reduced. A dry field enables the surgeon to see exactly what he is doing, to evaluate the pathology with accuracy, and to avoid injury to the arteries and veins supplying the nerves within and outside the cauda equina, and to the branches of the sinuvertebral nerve.

Bipolar low-voltage cautery is used to coagulate vessels within the spinal and nerve canals.

Bone wax applied to raw bone surfaces reduces oozing of blood. Dissection of and cautery to the posterior branches of the segmental vessels, further reduces operative hemorrhage.[23]

A magnifying loupe or operating microscope is essential to assess the condition of and to avoid injury to the spinal nerves, arteries, and veins that lie around the dura, around the nerves in their canals, and at the foraminal levels.

A careful recording of findings at operation should always be made. Even though there may be a 10- to 25-per-cent error in quantitative measurements taken at surgery, these encourage careful definition of pathology. By so doing the surgeon learns, with experience, the significance of the thickness of lamina, the distance between laminae, the distance between articular processes, the height of the lateral recess, and the thickness of the ligamentum flavum. The presence or absence of pulsation of the dura and the amount of anteroposterior, rotatory, and flexion-extension movement of one vertebra on the next should be noted. A fine blunt probe is passed through the spinal nerve foramen to assess its diameter.

Details of Operative Technique

After retraction of the erector spinae muscles, adjacent spinous processes are grasped with towel clips and the amount of anteroposterior, rotatory, and flexion-extension movement of one vertebra upon the next is noted. The spinous processes are removed from those laminae that are to be excised. When the laminae lie close together, with only a small space between them, it is convenient to remove the lower border of the lamina with rongeurs. The ligamentum flavum is incised longitudinally in the midline, and the two halves are removed with a small scalpel. It is then easy to remove the rest of the lamina above and all the lamina below using Kerrison forceps after freeing adhesions between the back of the dura and the lamina. The absence of extradural fat and of pulsation of the dura are indicative of marked stenosis. The number of laminae to be removed is assessed by the clinical findings, by the myelographic changes, and by what is seen at operation. Normally at least two levels are decompressed, occasionally three, and rarely four. Deciding how many laminae to remove is sometimes difficult, but a good guide is pulsation of the dura. Absence of pulsation suggests occlusion of the vessels supplying the dura and cauda equina.[18] Therefore the laminectomy should be taken to the level at which there are good pulsations. It is important to note that the patient's ventilation and blood pressure are normal when assessing pulsation. The width of the laminectomy should be at least 1.5 cm. Following a very wide laminectomy there is a greater chance of postlaminectomy stenosis and instability.[14] To avoid this, the lateral portions of the ligamentum flavum are dissected free from the bone and posterior joints from a medial direction. An oblique osteotomy is then made to remove bone from the lateral recess while leaving most of the joint and the posterior articular process (Fig. 5-11).

Enough of the articular process must be removed to deal with indentation of the dura and entrapment of the nerve in the lateral recess. If more of the bone is removed anteriorly in the region of the lateral recess and less posteriorly there is little likelihood of postlaminectomy in-

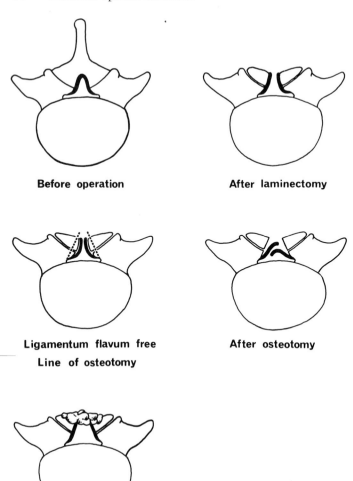

Before operation

After laminectomy

Ligamentum flavum free

Line of osteotomy

After osteotomy

Ligamentum flavum repositioned

Free fat graft posteriorly

FIG. 5-11. Technique of osteotomy. Note the oblique osteotomy to decompress the lateral recess while preserving stability of the posterior joints.

stability. When the lateral portion of the ligamentum flavum remains between the raw bone and the nerves, the chances of adhesion formation are greatly reduced. If, by gently probing of the foramina, the nerve is found to be trapped still further laterally, it is necessary to enlarge the foramen as described by Wiltse, Kirkaldy-Willis and McIvor.[34] The canal is enlarged anteriorly by removal of the osteoarthritic build-up with small osteotomes and chisels. It is preferable to complete unroofing of the nerve canal posteriorly, as this has the theoretical risk of producing instability.

Finally the intervertebral discs are inspected, and herniations of the nucleus pulposus are dealt with in the usual way. "Hard" disc protrusions which are the result of degenerative changes are best left alone, as any attempt to excise or pare them down leads to more adhesion formation.

Closure of the wound is carried out in the following way: small free subcutaneous-fat grafts, as advocated by Langenskiold and Kiviluoto, are placed between raw bone surfaces or incisions into discs and the adjacent nerves.[20] A larger free-fat graft is placed between the posterior aspect of the dura and the overlying erector spinae muscles. Experimental work suggested that the fat survives and that adhesions are less.[20] A large piece of Gelfoam is placed on top of the dural fat graft. The deep layer of the erector spinae muscles is approximated with interrupted sutures. A small polyethylene drain inserted through a small stab incision in the skin is placed superficial to this layer of sutures. The rest of the incision is closed in the usual way, another small drain being inserted in the subcutaneous tissues for oozing from the donor site of the fat grafts. The skin is closed, using one or two continuous subcuticular stainless steel sutures.

SOME SPECIAL CASES

Isolated Disc Resorption

Spinal nerve entrapment in this condition in the lateral recess at one level (see Chap. 4) needs removal of the ligamentum flavum and half of the lamina above together with half of the lamina below the level of the lesion.

Spondylolisthesis

Pressure on the spinal nerves at the L4–5 and L5–S1 level in isthmic spondylolisthesis can usually be relieved by removal of the loose fragment[15] and excision of enough of the pars interarticularis above the defect to ensure that there is no remaining entrapment of the nerve.

In degenerative spondylolisthesis, most commonly seen at the L4–5 level, adequate decompression can usually be obtained by removal of the laminae of L4 and L5. The entrapment may be above, at, or below the level of the slip. It is essential to explore the lateral recess.

Congenital spondylolisthetic stenosis presents a more difficult problem. Not infrequently nerve compression is caused by one of the anomalies that accompany the slip.

When spondylolisthesis is complicated by degenerative spondylosis above the level of the slip, there may be stenosis that necessitates the removal of the laminae above.

Stenosis Following Laminectomy or Fusion Operations

Operation is often difficult because of adhesions between the dura and the laminectomy membrane or the fusion mass.[21] It is wise first to remove the ligamentum flavum at a normal level, just above the fibrous tissue or the fusion, and from there to carry the dissection caudad.

Other Types of Stenosis

Other spinal stenoses require the same operative technique as that outlined above. In developmental stenosis the canal may be very narrow, and this presents its own problems. In fluorosis the new bone protruding into the spinal canal is probably more marked than in any other form.

POSTOPERATIVE CARE

Prophylactic antibiotics are commenced just prior to surgery and are continued for three days.[26] The patient may experience difficulty with micturition, and this may necessitate an indwelling catheter for 2 to 3 days. He is encouraged to stand for a few minutes on the day following operation, if possible, and to begin walking within 3 to 4 days. Usually he leaves hospital in about 10 days, being instructed to go very slowly for the first month at home. Straight-leg raising causes movement of the spinal nerves in their canals and appears to prevent adhesions (Fig. 5-12). A light elastic support is fitted to provide support without limiting spinal movement.[19]

At the end of a month he is encouraged to exercise at a gradually increasing tempo, to strengthen the flexor muscles. At the end of 3 months he should be ready to return to work. Farmers using tractors,

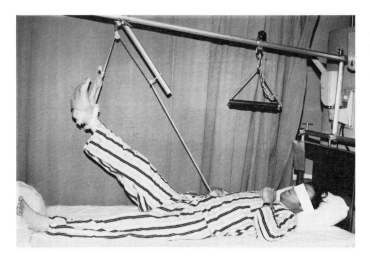

FIG. 5-12. The apparatus is used for passive straight-leg raising, which is commenced on the third postoperative day.

operators of caterpillar tractors, and those engaged in heavy manual labor may have to modify their activities or even seek work of an easier nature.

RESULTS OF SURGERY

We have reviewed our results in 101 patients operated on from 1966 to 1974. Only patients with spinal stenosis diagnosed by the criteria outlined earlier in this chapter were included. Patients undergoing surgery for "simple disc herniations" were thus excluded. The average follow-up was 34 months and the shortest, 1 year. The average age was 46.6 years, with a range from 16 years to 78 years. The duration of symptoms was longer than 5 years in 60 per cent of patients.

Eighty-three of the 101 patients felt that surgery resulted in significant alleviation of their symptoms; eleven, that their symptoms were unchanged; and five patients indicated that their symptoms were worse. Three of these were iatrogenic stenosis, one was diagnosed postoperatively as having amyotrophic lateral sclerosis, and one had two subsequent surgical procedures elsewhere, again with no benefit. Two patients were lost to follow-up.

Forty-four patients returned to their preoperative occupation. Eighteen patients were employed in lighter jobs for reasons not related to their low back. Thirty-two patients returned to less strenuous jobs because of their backs. Only five patients were unable to work.

DISCUSSION

Recent recognition of the concept of lumbar spinal stenosis has led surgeons to think of it as a compact and limited entity. Unfortunately it has been narrowly regarded by many as central spinal canal stenosis resulting mainly in compression of the cauda equina. Recent work by Crock,[6] Farfan,[11,12] Forbes,[13] Macnab,[22] and others has focused attention on nerve entrapment in the nerve canals and recesses, a lateral type of stenosis. The multiplicity of causes of the lumbar spinal stenosis syndrome should be recognized.[2] Single or multiple levels of involvement may be present. The findings vary from patient to patient, necessitating careful exploration of all potentially affected levels in the spine.

In Chapter 4 emphasis its placed on rotational strains affecting the posterior joints and intervertebral discs at one level only. It is convenient to regard these as being the initial changes in a pathological spectrum; early rotational strains, sometimes complicated by compressive injury to the disc, lead to degeneration of articular cartilage in the posterior joints and, later, to new bone formation enlarging these articular processes. Enlargement and irregularity of the superior articular processes produces lateral spinal nerve entrapment. Degenerative changes at one level cause mechanical strains leading to degenerative lesions at other levels. It seems reasonable to assume that in some cases the full-blown picture of degenerative spindylosis is produced in the lumbar spine. For reasons little understood, this not infrequently affects the bone around the spinal canal with resulting stenosis. Dissection of autopsy specimens suggests that stenosis is far from being a rare change in the elderly and aged. It is thus interesting to ask why such changes only produce symptoms sometimes.

The true incidence of symptomatic spinal stenosis is difficult to assess. Genetic and environmental factors are probably both important. In Saskatchewan there is a high incidence among farmers who spend long hours sitting on heavy machinery driving over rough terrain.

We appreciate the difficulty of accurately assessing any method of treatment for chronic low back pain. We have therefore not emphasized this strongly. In a series such as ours, with a small number of patients receiving compensation, the ability to work is probably the best criterion. As patients with simple disc herniation affecting only a single nerve root have been excluded, the results must be related to the types of patient treated, namely those with a long history of symptoms who have undergone a variety of unsuccessful treatments. This is precisely the patient excluded from most series which report the results of surgery for low back and leg pain.

The error, in the past, has been to overlook the possibility of spinal stenosis as a cause of back and leg pain. The mistake of the future, equally serious, may well be to overdiagnose this condition and undertake operative treatment when it is not indicated. The possibility of the existence of spinal stenosis should certainly be entertained in all cases of back and leg pain.

REFERENCES

1. Arnoldi, C. C.: Intraosseous hypertension: A possible cause of low back pain? Clin. Orthop., *115*:30, 1976.
2. Arnoldi, C. C., et. al.: Lumbar spinal stenosis and nerve root entrapment syndromes—definition and classification. Clin. Orthop., *115*:4, 1976.
3. Brodsky, A. E.: Iatrogenic spinal stenosis of the cauda equina. Paper read at S.I.C.O.T., Tel Aviv, 1972.
4. Cauchoix, J., Taussig, G., and Nordin, J. Y.: Sciatique et syndrome de la queue de cheval par rétrésissement du canal rachidien aprés arthrodèse lombo-sacrée postericure. Sem. Hôp. Paris, *45*:2023, 1969.
5. Cramer, F.: A note concerning the syndrome of cauda equina radiculitis. Bull. Neurol. Inst. N.Y., *3*:501, 1934.
6. Crock, H. V.: A reapprasial of intervertebral disc lesions. Med. J. Austral. *1*:983, 1970.
7. Crock, H. V., and Yoshizawa, H.: The blood supply of the lumbar vertebral column. Clin. Orthop., *115*:6, 1976.
8. Dandy, W. E.: Concealed ruptured intervertebral discs: a plea for the elimination of contrast medium in diagnosis. J.A.M.A., *117*:820, 1941.
9. Dommisse, G. F., and Grobler, L.: Arteries and veins of the lumbar nerve roots and cauda equina. Clin. Orthop., *115*:22, 1976.
10. Elsberg, C. A.: Experiences in spinal surgery. J. Surg. Gynecol. Obstet., *16*:117, 1913.
11. Farfan, H. F., and Sullivan, J. D.: The relation of facet orientation to intervertebral disc failure. Can. J. Surg., *10*:179, 1967.
12. Farfan, H. F., Huberdeau, R. M., and Dubow, H. I.: Lumbar intervertebral disc degeneration. The influence of geometric features on the pattern of the disc degeneration—A post mortem study. J. Bone Joint Surg., *54A*:492, 1972.
13. Forbes, D. B.: The Farfan back operation: technique and results. Can. J. Surg., *18*:546, 1975.
14. Funquist, B., and Schantz, B.: Influence of extensive laminectomy on the shape of the spinal canal. Acta. Orthop. Scand., Suppl. 56, 1962.
15. Gill, G. H., Manning, J. G., and White, H. L.: Surgical treatment of spondylolisthesis without spine fusion. J. Bone Joint Surg., *37A*:493, 1955.
16. Hastings, D. E.: A simple frame for operations on the lumbar spine. Can. J. Surg., *12*:251, 1969.

17. Jacobsen, R. E., Gargano, F. P. and Rosomoff, H. L.: Transverse axial tomography. J. Neurosurg., *42*:406; 412, 1975.

18. Kirkaldy-Willis, W. H., Paine, K. W. E., Cauchoix, J., and McIvor, G. W. D.: Lumbar spinal stenosis. Clin. Orthop., *99*:30, 1974.

19. Kirkaldy-Willis, W. H., and Read, S. E.: An elastic support for the lumbar and lumbosacral spine. Clin. Orthop., *59*:131, 1968.

20. Langenskiold, A., and Kiviluoto, O.: Prevention of epidural scar formation after operations on lumbar discs by means of free fat transplants. Clin. Orthop., *115*:92, 1976.

21. LaRocca, H., and Macnab, I.: The laminectomy membrane: studies in its evolution, characteristics, effects and prophylaxis in dogs. J. Bone Joint Surg., *56B*:545, 1974.

22. Macnab, I.: Negative disc exploration: an analysis of the causes of nerve root involvement in sixty-eight patients. J. Bone Joint Surg., *53A*:891, 1971.

23. Macnab, I., and Dall, D.: The blood supply of the lumbar spine and its application to the technique of intertransverse lumbar fusion. J. Bone Joint Surg., *53B*:628, 1971.

24. Munro, D.: Lumbar and sacral compression radiculitis (Herniated lumbar disc syndrome). N. Engl. J. Med., *254*:243, 1956.

25. Paine, K. W. E., and Huang, P. W. H.: Lumbar disc syndrome. J. Neurosurg., *37*:75, 1972.

26. Pavel, A., Smith, R. L., Ballard, A., and Larsen, J. J.: Prophylactic antibiotics in clean orthopaedic surgery. J. Bone Joint Surg., *56A*:777, 1974.

27. Pennal, G. F., and Schatzker, J.: Stenosis of the lumbar spinal canal. Clin. Neurosurg., *18*:86, 1971.

28. Sachs, B., and Fraenkel, J.: Progressive ankylotic rigidity of the spine. J. Nerv. Ment. Dis., *27*:1, 1900.

29. Sadar, E. S., Walton, R. J., and Grossman, H. H.: Neurological dysfunction in Paget's disease of the vertebral column. J. Neurosurg., *37*:661, 1972.

30. Sarpenyer, M. A.: Congenital stricture of the spinal canal. J. Bone Joint Surg., *27*:70, 1945.

31. Schatzker, J., and Pennal, G. F.: Spinal stenosis, a cause of cauda equina compression. J. Bone Joint Surg., *50B*:606, 1968.

32. Singh, A., and Joly, S. S.: Endemic fluorosis. Quart. J. Med., *30*:357, 1961.

33. Tile, M., McNeil, S. R., Zarins, R. K., Pennal, G. F., Garside, S. H.: Spinal stenosis; results of treatment. Clin. Orthop., *115*:104, 1976.

34. Wiltse, L. L., Kirkaldy-Willis, W. H., and McIvor, G. W. D.: The treatment of spinal stenosis. Clin. Orthop., *115*:83, 1976.

6 Segmental Intervertebral Instability and Its Treatment

LUMBAR INSTABILITY

"Instability may be defined as a loss of integrity of soft-tissue intersegmental control, causing potential weakness and liability to yield under stress," so wrote P. H. Newman in 1973. The concept of instability between vertebrae has helped greatly in the understanding of pain in the spine, as has the concept of spinal stenosis (Chap. 5).

In a careful study, Morgan and King found "primary instability" of lumbar vertebrae to be the commonest cause of low back pain.[25] (The backache of muscle strain and fatigue was not included.) This form of lumbar vertebral weakness was labelled "pseudo-spondylolisthesis" by Junghans, because there is no neural arch defect.[21] The anteroposterior slide is determined from lateral roentgenographs of the spine in full extension, with the patient sitting or standing.

Knutsson wrote "the anteroposterior sliding could be shown long before these signs of disc degeneration, such as narrowing of the disc interspaces, sclerosis of the epiphyseal rings of bone, marginal osteophytes, or rounding of the anterior margins of the bodies."[24] He considered the instability to be due to "incipient disc degeneration," a process admirably discussed by Professor Kirkaldy-Willis and

his colleagues in Chapter 4 of this volume.

"Secondary" lumbar instability is present in most derangements of the intervertebral joints, including disease and injury of the discs, osteoarthritis, spondylolisthesis, and traumatic rupture of ligaments with or without fracture. Barr believed that an unstable spine was the most frequent cause of an unsatisfactory result after operation for disc prolapse, and consequently recommended routine spinal fusion, a view in which we concur, at least in theory, as will be shown later.[2] It is the ideal, if only the practical difficulties can be overcome.

Secondary instability is seen at all ages: in the young, as in spondylolisthesis or after severe trauma, and in middle-aged and older patients, as a long-term result of trauma, or in degenerative conditions such as arthritis.

Primary instability occurs chiefly in men in their thirties and forties, when they are vulnerable to such strains as heavy lifting, repeated fatigue, or the falls and twists of games.

CASE 6-1. Figure 6-1 (a, b, c and d) shows roentgenographs of a 28-year-old man who had the symptoms of lumbar epiphyseal derangement in adolescence (see Chap. 3.) He was treated with a temporary extension brace and

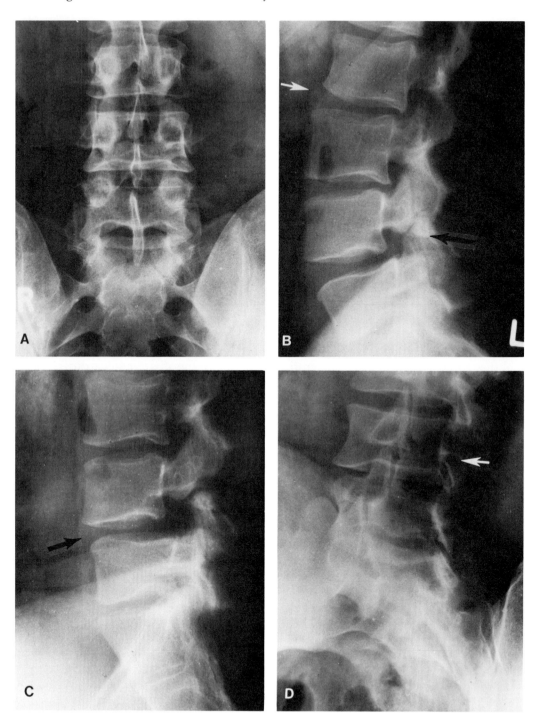

FIG. 6-1. *(A)* An anteroposterior roentgenograph of the lumbar spine, shows rotational displacement of L2 on L3 and L4 on L5. *(B)* A lateral view shows retrospondylolisthesis at the L2–3 level, and fracture of the pars interarticularis with mild displacement of L4 on L5 *(arrows)*. *(C)* A lateral view in flexion, shows reduction of retrospondylolisthesis at L2–3, but marked anterior displacement of L4 on L5 *(arrow)*. *(D)* An oblique view shows a pars interarticularis defect *(arrow)*.

exercises. Later he was able to return to games, even playing rugby.

He became a hard-working grape farmer and continued to play rugby until, at the age of 28, he was injured during a game.

The roentgenographs demonstrate retrospondylolisthesis of L2 on L3, with a stunted anterior vertebral margin, as described. The displacement was present in extension, but not in flexion. This followed the old injury. The lateral roentgenograph also shows a spondylolisthesis of L4 on L5, due to recent fracture of the pars interarticularis, with instability in flexion. The patient was able to do all his work in a spring brace.

The disc may not be an unstable element in spondylolisthesis, or after ligamentous rupture, despite the fact that it is always involved to some extent. In other cases, a deranged disc is part of the complex of instability: in some it is the only unstable element. Signs and symptoms, therefore, vary, but only in emphasis.

Clinical Features

The features of instability, both primary and secondary, that differentiate the condition from prolapsed intervertebral disc, are:

Bilateral Pain. Pain from a prolapsed disc is predominantly unilateral, whereas the pain caused by instability tends to be bilateral, even if one side may be worse than the other.

Sudden Onset. The attacks of pain begin suddenly, immediately after an incident of trauma which the patient can remember. The pain in the acute stage is severe. It subsides with rest and bracing, and the attack is usually over within 4 to 5 days. There may be a previous history of chronic ache, interspersed with such acute incidents. As the nerve roots are not necessarily involved, the ligamentous pain may be referred to an ill-defined site. Since the most common level of instability is between the L4 and L5 lumbar vertebrae, the pain usually radiates from the lower back and buttocks to the groin and down the legs, but seldom below the knees.

The onset of an attack of pain from a prolapsed disc may also be sudden, but it is more constant and persistent. Pain occurs more easily on movement than in instability. The pain of prolapse seldom subsides until the disc is reduced.

Weight-Bearing Relationship. An incident of instability may produce not only pain, but brief attacks of paresis and paresthesia in both legs, which may be severe enough to make the patient collapse to the floor. Unlike the persistence of sciatica in disc prolapse, the symptoms subside immediately if the unstable back is rested completely.

Length of Attacks. As a rule subluxation or displacement is momentary. The spinal muscles immediately splint the back, a form of "protective spasm." In addition, the patient learns to protect his back voluntarily, at the hint of pain.

Pain on Coughing and Sneezing. Pain caused by increased venous and intradural pressure is the hallmark of disc prolapse and does not occur in instability, except when an exceptionally violent sneeze causes such sudden back movement that the muscle control is inadequate.

Neurologic Signs. Persistent neurologic signs are not usually present in instability, unless related disc prolapse is present.

Straight-Leg Raising. Loss of straight-leg raising does not occur with instability, since it is caused by entrapment of the nerve root in the intervertebral canal.

The Interspinous Ligaments. The ligaments are tender after an incident of instability, whereas paraspinal tenderness, lateral to the mid-line in the interlaminar space, is indicative of disc prolapse.

Rotational Pain. In the presence of lower lumbar disc prolapse, pain is more pronounced when the lumbar spine is rotated in one direction than in the opposite. Indeed, rotation in the reverse direction may relieve the pain. This is the basis

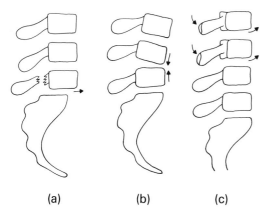

(a)   (b)   (c)

FIG. 6-2. Diagrams showing types of instability. *(A)* Spondylolisthesis with abnormal gliding of L5 on the sacrum. *(B)* Instability in flexion. *(C)* Rotational instability.

of most manipulative procedures. Intervertebral instability is not affected by rotation.

A lumbar joint may be unstable in any of three planes: horizontally forward or backward (as in spondylolisthesis when one vertebra glides on another), by tilting into flexion, or by lateral rotation (Fig. 6-2).

THE RELATION OF THE RANGE OF MOVEMENTS TO INJURY OF THE LUMBAR SPINE

We are apt to assume that flexion and extension occur evenly in the lumbar spine. In fact, in the ordinary sense, flexion is not possible at the lumbosacral joint. It is capable of a full range of extension, greater than at any other lumbar joint, but can flex, or rather straighten, only as far as the vertical (Fig. 6-3). If abnormal hinging or flexion is possible, the joint must have an injured, unstable disc.

Conversely, maximum flexion is possible at the dorsolumbar joint, but little true extension. Below this level, flexion decreases at each level until the lumbosacral joint is reached, while extension increases.

On the other hand, rotation is a feature of the movement of all intervertebral joints, each joint from the atlas downward taking part, in corkscrew fashion. This is shown in Figure 6-4, which shows the anteroposterior roentgenograph of the lumbar and lumbosacral joints of a dancer. As demonstrated previously by Steindler, it shows that the range of rotation decreases progressively in the lower lumbar joints, and, although still possible, is least at the lumbosacral level.

Figure 6-5 shows the rotation in the back of a young woman as she reaches downward with her left arm. This rotational strain or torque was described by Coplans as a potent cause of disc injury.[8] Professor Kirkaldy-Willis and co-workers concur (Chap. 4). The greatest strain, and so the greatest number of disc injuries, take place in those joints in which flexion and rotation are limited by their anchorage to the relatively immobile pelvis, viz., the lumbosacral and L4–5 joints. Some 90 per cent of injuries occur at these levels.

It is of interest to reflect on the effect of the strong iliolumbar ligaments, which stretch between the transverse processes of L5 and the ilium, in promoting this relative immobility of the lumbosacral joint. This adds to the strain taken on the mobile joint above, which explains the finding that it is the L4–5 joint that most frequently becomes unstable.

TYPES OF INSTABILITY

Rotational Instability

As described above, the main effect of rotational injuries is on the intervertebral disc itself. Simultaneous involvement of the supra- and interspinous structures is infrequent, as evidenced by the absence of mid-line swelling, while fingerpoint paraspinal tenderness is present. Rotational displacement may be detected on the anterior and lateral roentgenographs (Fig. 6-6).

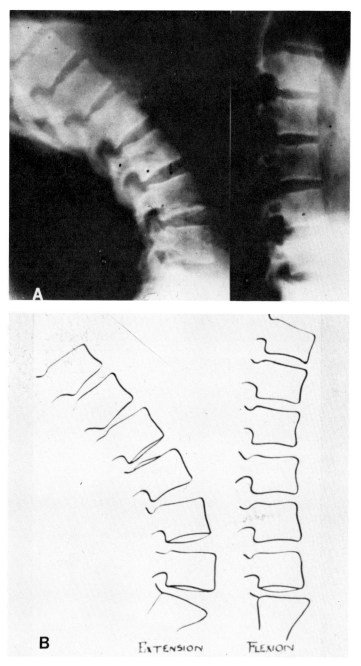

FIG. 6-3. *(A)* Lateral views of the lumbar spine in full flexion and extension. *(B)* Tracings of these roentgenographs demonstrate increasing range of flexion upward from the lumbosacral joint, and increasing extension downward.

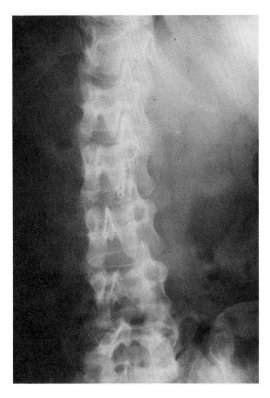

Fig. 6-4. Anteroposterior roentgenograph of the lumbar spine of a dancer, twisting to the left shows increasing rotation from the sacrum upward.

Flexion Injuries

Pure flexion injuries, without rotation, occur at the levels where the greatest flexion is possible, that is, in the mid- or upper lumbar spine, which is the apex of the curve of the flexed back (Fig. 6-7A). After trauma of this type, the supraspinous and interspinous ligaments may be torn, and if the force is excessive, the upper anterior edge of the vertebral body below is fractured (Fig. 6-7B, C).

Pure flexion injuries most often involve the first, second, and third lumbar joints. Once the acute stage is over, a careful history will show that spasms of pain occur almost solely on flexion movements. The pain may be of root distribution, usually femoral, and is usually bilateral, even if it is more pronounced on one side. Local

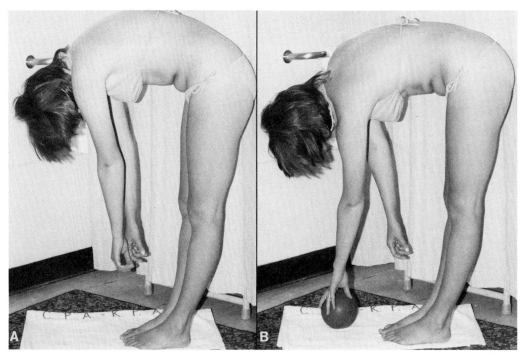

Fig. 6-5. Beyond the limit of stooping, the left hand reaches the floor only if the patient rotates the spine.

tenderness is palpable over the torn interspinous ligaments, as is paraspinal tenderness. There is localized pain on full extension, owing to impingement of the spinous processes, with compression of the tender ligament between them. With the back straight, the patient may feel pain on rotation and lateral flexion, but it is likely to be equally severe on both sides.

Diagnosis is always difficult in the acute stage, especially as, in many injuries, both flexion- and rotational strain are present. As the spasm settles, the diagnostic signs become clearer. Roentgenographs taken with the patient sitting, as well as lateral views of the lumbar spine and the lumbosacral joint in full extension and flexion are invaluable. This technique was described by Murray, Begg, and Falconer as a diagnostic aid in intervertebral disorders.

Severe flexion injuries, such as those sustained in motor vehicle accidents, in headlong somersault falls onto the shoulders, or when a heavy weight falls upon the flexed back, usually result in injury to the dorsolumbar or upper lumbar joints. The result may be a grave fracture or fracture-dislocation, with paraplegia, but more frequently it is rupture of the posterior ligament complex, with or without fracture of the anterosuperior margin of the vertebral body. Instability in flexion results. The dorsolumbar and first two lumbar intervertebral joints are the levels of maximal flexion and bear the brunt of such an injury.

CASE 6-2. A 23-year-old woman had sustained a high diving injury at the age of 14, but had had severe symptoms for 1 year only. She complained of pain on weight bearing, and even while turning in bed.

Examination revealed tenderness in the upper lumbar spine. Extension and full flexion of the spine were painful, but not rotation or lateral flexion. Straight-leg raising was full, and there were no neurologic changes in the legs.

Roentgenographs (Fig. 6-8A,B) revealed flexion instability due to rupture of the posterior ligament complex at the L2–3 level and an ununited unstable fracture of the anterosuperior border of the second lumbar vertebra.

Local spinal fusion was performed in January, 1975. She was up and walking comfortably in a brace 6 days later and returned to work 4 months later. Roentgenographs (Fig. 6-8C) taken 13 months after operation, show solid fusion and union of the fracture.

Lateral Displacement Instability

Lateral displacement instability is rare and can occur only after destruction of the disc and pedicles. The roentgenographic appearance of lateral displacement is usually of the marked rotational instability that accompanies it (Fig. 6-9). This may be corrected wholly or partially by traction.

Lateral Tilt Instability

Unless it complicates flexion instability, lateral flexion instability is unusual. Anteroposterior roentgenographs of the sitting patient, with the trunk flexed laterally, first to one side, then to the other, sometimes reveal lateral intervertebral wedging. It may be unilateral or bilateral. Figure 6-10 shows the roentgenographs in a case with such lateral tilting, in a patient with flexion instability at the L2–3 level. The films show abnormal lateral tilt at the L2–3 level on one side, and the L1-2 and L2-3 levels on the other. The movements did not hurt the patient.

Instability in Extension

Occasional patients suffer pain, localized to the small of the back, in full extension only. Flexion is free. Examination elicits tenderness between the spinous processes of the involved joint. The patient finds walking with a slight stoop to be more comfortable. Lateral stress

(Text continues on p. 78)

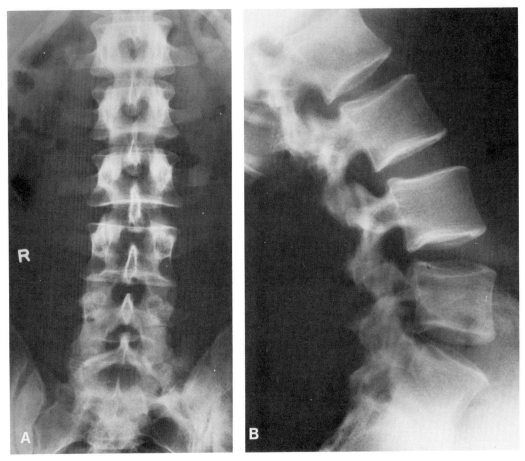

FIG. 6-6. Roentgenographs of a young man injured at sport. He felt pain on extension of the spine when rotating to the right. *(A)* The anteroposterior view shows rotation of L5 on the sacrum. *(B)* The lateral film in flexion, shows reduction of retrospondylolisthesis when L5 rotates on the

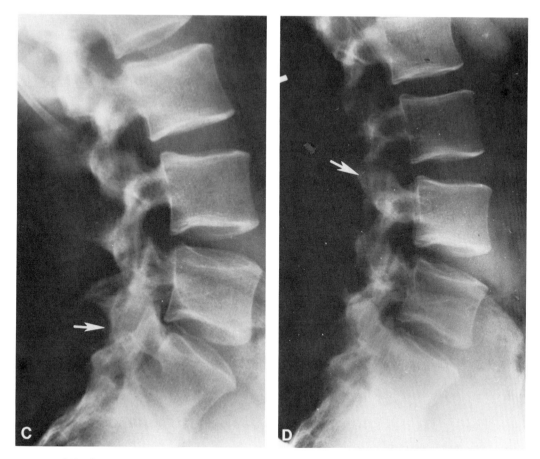

sacrum. *(C)* The same patient, shows retrospondylolisthesis on extension. When he twisted to the left, this became more severe and he felt pain *(arrow)*. *(D)* When twisting to the right, vertical rotation was easily visible by the double line presented by the back of the bodies of L3 and L4 *(arrow)*.

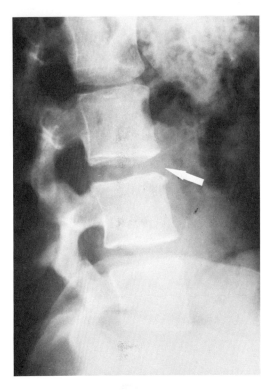

FIG. 6-7. *(A)* Roentgenographs of an old injury at the L3–4 level, demonstrating widening of the posterior intervertebral space and anterior lipping at the impact point. *(B, opposite)* Roentgenograph showing more severe injury with resulting fracture of the anterosuperior angle of the body of L4. The instability at L3-4 is seen on flexion. *(C)* Tracings of *B* show the instability and rotation.

eration completed, the lumbar spine had been fixed in a hyperextension jacket.

This is reminiscent of the 1930's, when Watson Jones introduced hyperextension plaster jackets as a treatment for fractures of the lumbar spine.[35] These were applied by suspending the patient face-down between two tables, with the head and shoulders on a higher table than the pelvis. Abdominal ileus was a troublesome complication, which could be relieved only by reducing the degree of extension.

The patient's deformity was corrected and the hyperextended joint released by excision of the fusion mass. This solved the problem of constipation, but a mild backache persisted, although not as severe as before. The patient felt better in a well-fitting corset.

roentgenographs show normal alignment in flexion, but retrospondylolisthesis occurs on extension (Fig. 6-11). A Goldthwait brace (which limits lordosis) or, in severe cases, local fusion, relieves the symptoms.

HYPEREXTENSION OR LOCALIZED HYPERLORDOSIS OF THE LUMBOSACRAL JOINT

Eighteen months after an operation for lumbosacral fusion, a patient complained of low backache and intractable constipation. Examination revealed fixed localized hyperlordosis with tenderness of the lowest lumbar joint. The abdomen was tense. Some relief was obtained by flexing the lumbar spine above the level of the lumbosacral joint, which was remarkably hyperextended. The technique of the operation was not known, but presumably, after the grafts were inserted and the op-

SPINOUS PROCESS IMPINGEMENT

Another cause of pain on extension of the lumbar spine is impingement of the lumbar spinous processes, the so-called kissing spines. The pain is relieved by flexion. In most instances the lowest lumbar or first sacral processes are longer than normal. Brailsford described vagaries in shape of the spinous process of L5, which is normally shorter than L4, but is sometimes longer when associated with spondylolisthesis. If for any reason lordosis is increased or the lumbosacral angle diminished, the spinous processes are approximated. This may also be a feature of retrospondylolisthesis.

The bone on the contacting surfaces, in

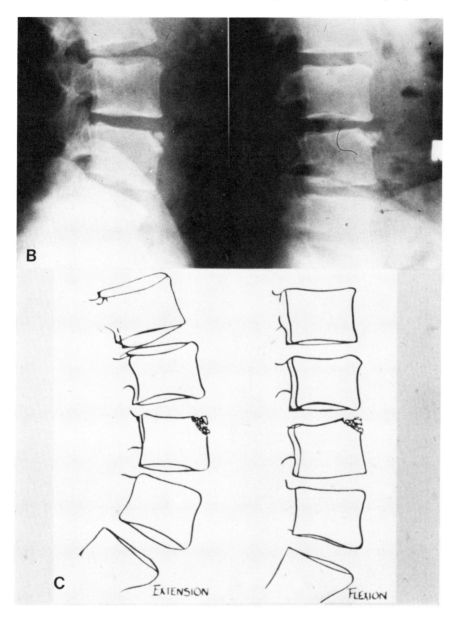

B

C   EXTENSION   FLEXION

time, becomes burnished, molded, and faceted, the roentgenographs showing sclerosis of the margins (Fig. 6-12). The condition may cause symptoms, when middle-age loss of postural tone leads to spinal sag and increasing lordosis. The patients flatten the lumbar spine and walk with a stoop, because that attitude is more comfortable. Examination reveals a thickened tender interspinous ligament.

An intervening bursitis, or pseudarthrosis with erosive "arthritic" change, may develop.

Treatment includes exercises to correct the lordosis of spinal sag, and injections of local anesthetic and corticosteroids into the supraspinous ligament. Finally, wedge excision of the contacting surfaces of the involved spinous processes may be indicated. *(Text continues on p. 83)*

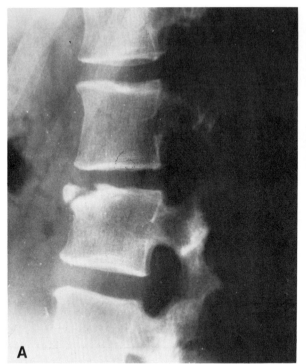

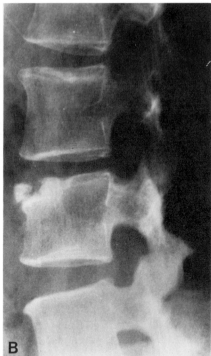

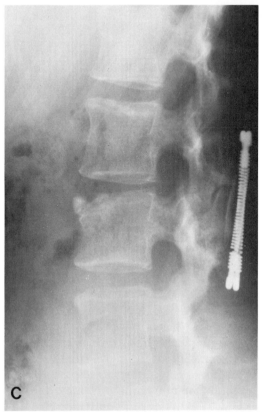

FIG. 6-8. *(A,B)* Lateral views of the lumbar spine in flexion and extension demonstrate instability in flexion of L1 on L2 with a fracture of the anterosuperior angle of the body of L2. The fragment is unstable and moves with flexion. *(C)* A lateral film made 13 months after solid posterior fusion with compression springs. The fracture appears to be uniting and the sclerosis is resolved.

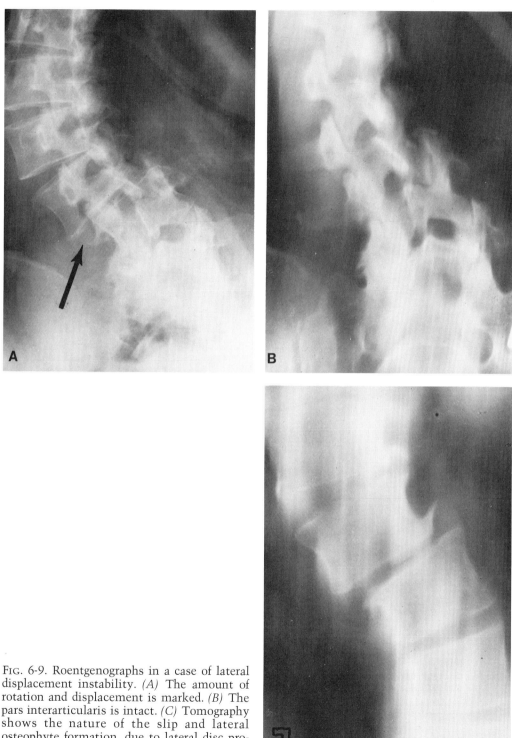

FIG. 6-9. Roentgenographs in a case of lateral displacement instability. *(A)* The amount of rotation and displacement is marked. *(B)* The pars interarticularis is intact. *(C)* Tomography shows the nature of the slip and lateral osteophyte formation, due to lateral disc prolapse.

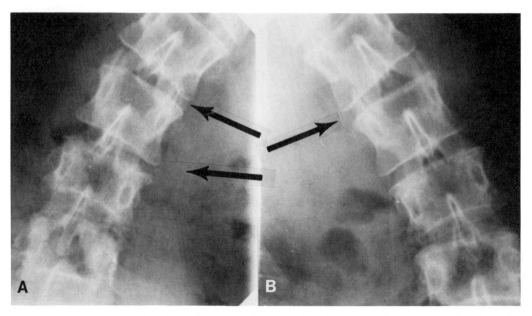

FIG. 6-10. Roentgenographs show abnormal tilt at two levels to one side and at one level on the other.

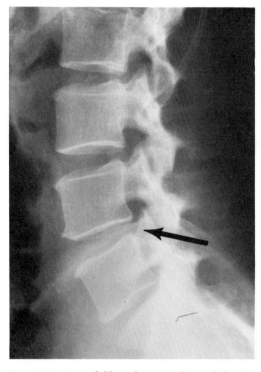

FIG. 6-11. Lateral film of a case of instability in extension. Retrospondylolisthesis is seen at the L4–5 level on extension. There are anterior osteophytes.

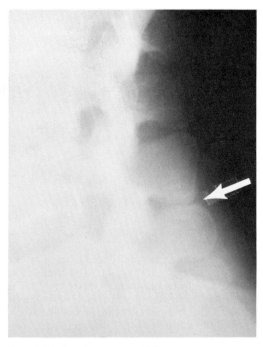

FIG. 6-12. Impingement of the spinous process of L4 and L5 *(arrow).*

SPONDYLOLYSIS AND SPONDYLOLISTHESIS

Newman's classification of spondylolisthesis is described in Chapter 5.[27] The upper lumbar vertebral body usually slips forward on the next, but occasionally a backward slip of the upper vertebra occurs, the condition being called retrospondylolisthesis.

In rare instances roentgenographs show lateral displacement. This is usually due to a gross rotational movement of one vertebra on the next and can only be reduced by a rotational force.

NEURAL ARCH SPONDYLOLISTHESIS

In this condition forward displacement occurs because of a bilateral structural defect in the pars interarticularis of the neural arch. The affected vertebra separates into two parts, the anterior comprising the body, pedicles, transverse processes, and superior articular facets. The posterior fragment includes the spinous process, laminae, and inferior articular facets. Spondylolysis is the name given to the condition of a vertebra with such a defect, but without separation. Spondylolisthesis may be stable or unstable. Pain in spondylolisthesis is sometimes a consequence of an ill-defined fibrous mass or of chondrophytes or osteophytes which form around the edges of the defects in the neural arch and which may press on the nerve roots, giving rise to sciatic pain.

The fibrous bond that bridges the defect in the pars interarticularis is subject to considerable stress during weight bearing and other movements. The back may be able to deal with this stress for many years, even for the lifetime of the patient. In this event the condition is symptomless and is discovered only by accident. When it gives way through injury or repeated stress, the clinical picture of pain and deformity develops. Frequently injury is the final disrupting force.

The vertebra most often involved is L5. Displacement may be slight or considerable. In a personal series of 160 cases of spondylolisthesis of L5, Harris recorded: a defect in the neural arch present but without displacement of the vertebral body (spondylolysis) in 37.5 per cent; slight to moderate displacement of the body of L5 (not more than a third of the width of the top of the sacrum) in 52 per cent; displacement greater than a third of the width of the top of the sacrum in 8 per cent, and the vertebral body completely off the top of the sacrum in 2.5 per cent.[16] Harris went on to say, "The factors that determine the amount of displacement of the involved vertebra, the rapidity with which it develops, and the uniformity of progression are obscure."

It was possible to follow the development of a spondylolisthesis deformity over a period of years in one patient. But in many patients the joint is strong enough to allow the patient to continue for many years, even for life, without symptoms of deformity. Symptoms and signs depend on the degree of stability.

In the same chapter Harris gave this admirable description: "The *deformity* is the result of the forward displacement of the body of the involved vertebra. It carries with it all the vertebrae above it, leaving behind its own spinous process. Consequently this projects prominently in relation to the spinous process above it, forming a step kyphosis in contrast to the angular kyphosis of Pott's disease. The pelvis is rotated about a transverse axis passing through the hip joints, so that the antero-superior spines of the ilium are raised to the same level as the posterosuperior spines or even higher, a remarkably constant sign in spondylolisthesis, even when the vertebral displacement is slight (Fig. 6-13). It occurs also in certain lumbosacral disc lesions, but in combination with the step kyphosis and other signs of spondylolisthesis, it is a valuable aid to diagnosis.

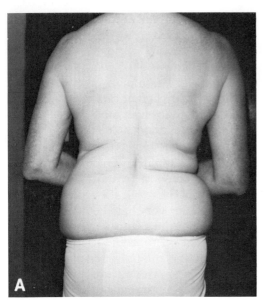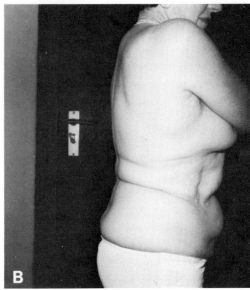

FIG. 6-13. Back and side views of a patient with spondylolisthesis. The transverse creases in the skin folds are obvious.

The rotation of the pelvis about its transverse axis may be so great that the thighs are not in a straight line with the trunk, even when the hips are fully extended. Hence the patient must stand with his trunk thrust forward if the legs are vertical, or with the knees and hips flexed if the trunk is held erect. The trunk is shortened by the downward displacement that accompanies the forward slip. Consequently the ribs approach or overlap the iliac crests, and transverse creases appear about the waist."

SIGNS AND SYMPTOMS

The signs and symptoms of stable and unstable spondylolisthesis also differ. The stable form produces symptoms because the muscles which control the lower back are working at a disadvantage. This subjects the back to added mechanical stress, and the symptoms are those of strain and early fatigue, with aching in the back and behind both thighs after standing and walking. Muscle tenderness is present on both sides of the lower spine and in both buttocks. Lower lumbar movements may be limited. Muscular and fit persons may carry a stable spondylolisthesis for years without disability and without more than occasional discomfort.

The unstable spondylolisthesis adds spasms of acute back—and sometimes root—pain to this picture. The spasms are precipitated by uncontrolled movements, chiefly flexion, or when the spine is jarred. Pain is often bilateral, though not necessarily of equal severity in both legs. Marked sensory or motor changes in the legs are a rare finding. More irritability is noticed on pressure over the L4 or L5 spinous process, whichever is affected, than in the stable variety.

The clinical diagnosis is confirmed roentgenographically. Lateral roentgenographs demonstrate the anterior displacement of the body on that of the vertebra below. Oblique views show the separation of the pars interarticularis. Lateral

FIG. 6-14. Lateral roentgen-ograph of the L5–S1 joint, showing the forward dis-placement that occurs in spondylolisthesis.

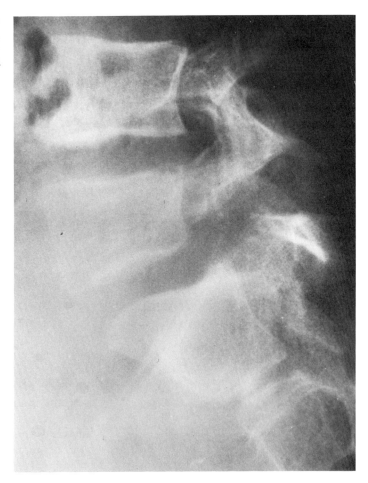

roentgenographs taken in flexion and ex-tension are necessary to determine whether the displacement is stable or un-stable (Fig. 6-14).

TREATMENT

Differences in the nature, the effects, and the degree of instability of these le-sions determine treatment, whether con-servative or surgical.

Stable spondylolisthesis may be treated by compensation for the mechanical weakness by increasing muscle power by exercise and, when indicated, the use of a short spinal support.

The unstable varieties present different problems. Posteroanterior glide must be prevented by arthrodesis or some form of bone-block by anterior transabdominal intervertebral body fusion according to the technique recommended by Cloward,[7] by any of a number of methods of poste-rior grafting between the laminae and spinous processes, or by posterolateral in-tertransverse process fusion. The poste-rior and posterolateral approaches are the simplest.

The patient may even recover function and comfort without solid fusion, pro-vided that the movement, limited though it may be, is stable and in the pattern normal for the joint, so that it moves syn-chronously with adjacent joints. Pain is felt when joint movement is aberrant and in conflict with that of its neighbors. Recovery of firm muscle control is also important.

Gill, Manning, and White asserted that removal of the loose posterior fragment relieves the pain of instability in most patients.[13] This is a simple operation with a minimum of immediate complications and is suitable for older patients. It has the advantage that, as the approach gives access to the disc and the lateral recesses, nerve root involvement, when present, may be relieved. On the other hand, increased postoperative slip and instability has been reported, and Gill found the operation unsuitable for adolescents because of complications with further growth. It is desirable, therefore, to reserve the procedure for older patients with unstable spondylolisthesis. It should be combined with posterolateral fusion.

Causes of Local Instability

Traumatic rupture of posterior ligaments, with or without fracture of the vertebrae.
Derangement of the intervertebral joint by osteoarthritis.
Ruptured intervertebral disc.
Derangement of an intervertebral joint following previous excision of the disc
Spondylolisthesis

Unless complicated by current painful disc pathology, most symptoms are relieved by bed-rest or an adequate brace. The brace should not be discarded until the patient has recovered and has normal posture with adequate muscle power and stamina. The appropriate exercise program should be instituted immediately. A spring brace is preferred, as it does not limit but aids postural exercises. Time and conservative treatment tend to heal and stabilize the complex and related structures of the spine, and this merits a counsel of patience for the patient.

Surgery is indicated when symptoms do not respond to simple treatment, when they recur with increasing frequency and severity, or when they are complicated by involvement of the cord or nerve roots. Greater stress is thrown on adjacent mobile joints after fusion. This is an important consideration when determining the level and number of joints to be fused. Roentgenographic examination, including stress views, is necessary to establish the type and extent of instability of an intervertebral segment, but clinical assessment is all-important in deciding the manner of management. The temptation to "treat the roentgenograph" must be resisted.

Where instability is mild, postural and muscular control may be sufficient, but however well compensated, the back remains vulnerable to unexpected stress and unguarded movements, leading to attacks of backache and sometimes pain in the legs. Should these symptoms persist or recur, especially if severe and complicated by leg pain, fusion is indicated.

Successful fusion depends on accurate diagnosis of the type and level of joint derangement and an accurate determination of the integrity of the adjacent joints. If unsound, they may be fused at the same time or may require protection by corset or brace after operation. Surgery must be gentle, adequate, and exact.

The authors prefer the technique of posterior interlaminar fusion, with or without metal fixation and compression, or posterolateral intertransverse fusion. The addition of transarticular screws has many advocates.[5] As an alternative to posterolateral fusion, the use of compression devices has advantages and is simple, comfortable and generally successful.[1,12,22]

Choice of Operation (Fig. 6-15)

For severe spondylolisthesis with displacement and instability, anterior, transperitoneal or retroperitoneal, fusion has been advocated by Sacks, Hodgson, and Freebody who report excellent results.[12,18,30] The posterolateral intertransverse fusion, preferably with compression, is safer, with fewer compli-

FIG. 6-15. Diagram of the methods of stabilization. *(A)* Posterior bone block. *(B)* Clamping the hinge for instability in flexion.

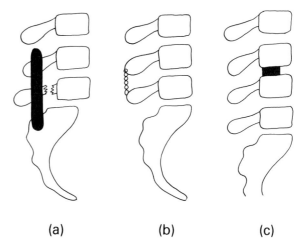

(a)   (b)   (c)

cations. After anterior fusion, retroperitoneal complications, including iliac vein thrombosis and damage to the hypogastric plexus leading to impotence, have been reported. It is technically difficult to approach the interspace between L5 and the first sacral vertebrae in spondylolisthesis if there is more than slight displacement.[16]

Taking the Graft

Autogenous bone is preferred to bank bone. In a personal series, bank bone did not always incorporate in the fusion mass but remained sequestered in heavy fibrous tissue.

The graft should be taken from the outer surface of the ilium. After dividing the fascia, the gluteal muscles are stripped from an adequate area of bone. Using an osteotome, a layer of the crest with the attached abdominal muscles is turned inward. This obviates the bleeding that cut muscles would entail. The cortical graft is taken with sufficient slivers of underlying cancellous bone. Care must be taken to remain anterior to the sacroiliac joint.

The lateral branches of the posterior primary divisions of the 1st, 2nd and 3rd lumbar nerves serve as cutaneous nerves of the buttock. They should be avoided as they cross the iliac crest. They emerge from the deep fascia covering the erector spinae muscles, to pass downward across the iliac crest into the buttock. When the graft is taken through a curved incision along the iliac crest, the nerves are damaged and neuromas may form, a painful complication, heralded by a causalgic reaction of moderate to severe pain and hypersensitivity over the donor site. The neuroma is locally tender, and Tinel's sign is present. An oblique incision across the iliac crest, parallel to the course of the dorsal branches of these lumbar nerves, should be used, to minimize the risk of injury.

In a series of 86 operations performed through curved incisions, five patients developed local pain referred into the buttock after operation, with signs of a neuroma. Three resolved after injection of local anesthetic and corticosteroid. Two required excision before relief was obtained.

Drainage

Suction drainage of both the spinal wound and the donor site is essential to prevent hematoma formation. It promotes postoperative comfort and reduces the risk of deep infection. In this series no patient developed more than superficial wound or stitch infection. After 48 hours, drainage is minimal and the tubes may be removed.

Blood Transfusion

Blood loss is measured during the operation and from the suction system postoperatively, and is replaced. Loss is somewhat greater with the posterolateral than with the posterior approaches.

After Operation

Diligent postoperative care and rehabilitation are required if the patient is to obtain the full benefit of the operation.

TECHNIQUES OF FUSION

In his lectures *On the Influence of Mechanical and Physiological Rest in the Treatment of Accidents and Surgical Diseases* (published in 1863, and later as *Rest and Pain*), John Hilton expressed his conviction that rest is the essential in the treatment of inflammation. Hugh Owen-Thomas interpreted this as prolonged, absolute, and uninterrupted rest, a tenet which became basic to medical teaching, and was observed to the letter. Gradually the practice of total rest has been abandoned, but as late as the 1940's it was customary after grafting for spinal fusion to immobilize the patient in bed and plaster for 4 to 6 months.

Although bony union occurs most satisfactorily and rapidly with complete fixity of the fractured bone ends, prolonged immobility of adjacent joints and muscles is a grave disadvantage, for recovery of motion is slow and often incomplete. Internal fixation of long-bone fractures, allowing early movement and isometric exercises, was a logical development. Undoubtedly the improvement in local circulation as a result of muscle activity promoted more rapid and more satisfactory repair.

Immobilization after operation for spinal fusion is a more difficult problem. As the spine is a powerful torsion bar it is unreasonable to expect a rigid tube-shaped brace or plaster jacket to provide firm fixation. Even in a snugly applied plaster jacket, movement takes place at the lumbosacral joint as the patient rises from a chair or sits down. This is one reason for the incidence of pseudarthrosis after fusion at this level.

Movement between the bone ends or graft, however slight, would delay or prevent union. This has fostered the development of internal fixation. Cortical bone grafts, or a metal plate, or both together, fixed by means of screws or bolts, have been more successful for treating fractures than for spinal fusion. Yet the Wilson plate and matching iliac bone graft[37] and articular facet fixation by dowel graft[28] or Boucher screw[27] are advocated.

The authors are convinced that bony fusion is most satisfactorily promoted by rigid internal fixation, using compression techniques such as that described by Charnley for arthrodesis of the knee or ankle,[6] or the methods of the AO Group of surgeons in Switzerland.[26] Contemporary techniques, developed primarily in Switzerland, have resulted in better treatment of some fractures.

The experience that delayed union and nonunion of fractures may be overcome by using bone grafts with compression plating has led, as a natural development, to a technique of fusion of the spine by bone grafting with compression fixation. The method has been applied successfully by Harrington, Knodt, Attenborough and others.[15] In 1963 Harrington reported the management of more than 200 cases of scoliosis, using his spinal instrumentation. Both Harrington and Knodt use metal rods for fixation, with compression applied on the thread-nut principle. Attenborough's device is simpler in design, less bulky, and easier to insert. It is composed of light stainless steel coil springs,

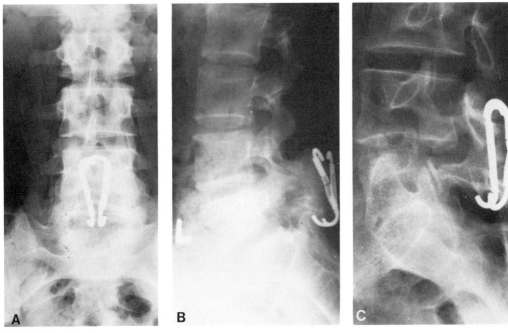

Fig. 6-16. Stabilization of L5 spondylolisthesis by fusion from L4 to the sacrum, using Attenborough springs. The advantage of compression is that a single joint may be fused.

which are measured to exert 13 to 15 pounds of compression. Fixation is obtained by small hooks screwed into the springs, which take purchase around the spinous processes or laminae of the vertebrae to be fused. A spring has the advantage over rigid fixation, for the torsional strains exerted by the spinal column tend to loosen plates and screws. At least for the period of graft fusion the springs absorb the strain, and fusion is usually quick and secure.

Firm fixation using a compression device also obviates the need to fuse more than the affected joint (Fig. 6-16). One of the virtures of this technique is that the patient seldom has much postoperative pain. Absolute recumbency is more for patients' comfort than strictly necessary. Within 24 hours most are comfortable and after 48 hours are turning themselves in bed. On the third or fourth day patients are allowed to sit out of bed, and they may walk the next day. Stitches are removed on the tenth day, and the patient is allowed to go home.

Because the springs clamp the spinous processes firmly, clinical tests for union and consolidation of the graft cannot be used, but tenderness has usually disappeared in 6 to 8 weeks, the roentgenograph showing the appearance of firm bone fusion within 12 weeks.

After operation the donor graft area in the ilium is often more troublesome, with tenderness and pain on movement, but

The Advantages of Compression

Fixation is more rigid

The gap to be bridged by new bone is narrowed

External immobilization required after surgery is reduced

Most patients are comfortable within 2 or 3 days of operation

Clinical and roentgenographic fusion is most frequently obtained

Lumbar joints may be stabilized singly, which improves the prognosis

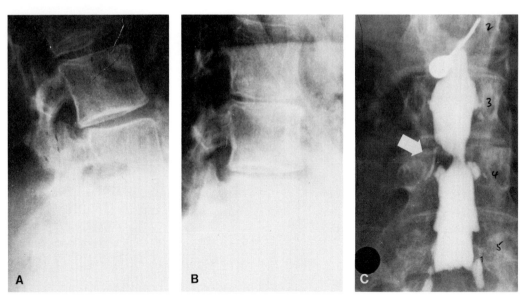

FIG. 6-17. *(A)* Lateral roentgenograph in a 58-year-old woman with L3–4 instability in extension. L3 is rotated on the L4, giving the appearance of retrospondylolisthesis. The double line of the posterior surface of the body of L4 can be seen clearly. *(B)* In flexion the retrospondylolisthesis is reduced. *(C)* Myelography demonstrates a large L3–4 disc prolapse.

the days of discomfort are suprisingly short.

Anterior body fusion, with its risk of intraabdominal and vascular complications and the technical difficulties, especially in spondylolisthesis, is hardly warranted when compared with this simple and comfortable method.

Posterior interbody fusion (Cloward) would be ideal, since the graft is inserted into the site of maximal instability, while the compression forces of gravity aid union, in theory. It is said to be simple to perform in a roomy space where the joint is lax and unstable after the removal of the disc. But in the authors' relatively limited experience, firm fusion was seldom achieved; flexion-extension lateral roentgenography sometimes shows union on one side of the graft but not on the other.

A system of postural exercises, as described by Goldthwait, is taught, preferably before operation. The patient must learn to turn and bend with a flat back, and to do so habitually. To stoop or to lift, one leg is put in front of the other with the knees slightly bent. Weight is taken by straightening the legs, thus transferring strain from the back to the muscles of the legs. The patient is allowed up in a dynamic spring brace or an adequate corset which has been made before surgery.

The spring brace was devised by Drs. C. Coplans and A. J. Helfet some 20 years ago (see Chap. 10) and has since been used consistently. It comprises a padded plate fitted to the small of the back. From the plate extend three twisted springs: one around the pelvis to fit the brace; the second along the crest of the ilium, which takes pressure on the anterior superior spines; and the third twisted upward to form pectoral pads. This brace has been found most effective in preventing lumbosacral movement, for the springs keep the back-plate stable and applied firmly to the contour of the patient's lower back during all movements. Efficiency is tested by asking the patient to sit down on and to stand up out of a chair. The plate should not move away from the patient. No rigid brace can do this (i.e., remain firmly applied during all movements).

One hundred and forty consecutive operations using this technique for local spinal fusion by grafting plus compression and dynamic bracing have been performed by one of the authors, (A. J. H.) between 5, and at least 1, year ago.

CASE 6-3. A stout, 58-year-old music teacher developed an acute attack of backache and leg pain after a fall. She gave a long history of recurrent back pain, although previously it had not been severe enough to affect her work. She also suffered from osteoarthritis of both knees.

Clinical and roentgen examination, including myelography, demonstrated changes in the lumbar spine. Principally there was an eroded, unstable intervertebral space between L3 and L4, with a large prolapse of the disc at this level to the right side (Fig. 6-17). Excision of the disc and fusion have relieved the spinal disability. Four years later, she continues to teach the piano, despite the fact that this entails long hours of sitting and playing.

CASE 6-4. A 46-year-old woman was seen in January, 1973. Fourteen years previously a heavy box had fallen onto her back while she was stooping. She felt immediate but transitory pain, and managed to return to work next day. Subsequently she suffered intermittent pain in the back after overactivity. For 7 months before she sought advice, her symptoms had become worse, especially when sitting, rising from the sitting position, or turning in bed. Occasional coughing caused a stab of pain, and at times she felt paresthesia in both legs. The pain was mid-lumbar in position, referred to the left buttock, but never lower.

Examination revealed tenderness at the level of the L2–3 interspace. Movements of the lumbar spine were excellent, except for pain at the extremes of flexion and extension. Rotation was free. The left knee jerk was diminished.

Roentgenographs (Figs. 6-18, a to d) demonstrated loss of the intervertebral space between the bodies of L2 and L3, with marked sclerosis and lipping (Fig. 6-18). Lateral views in flexion and extension revealed abnormal movement at this level.

Posterior fusion, using Attenborough springs, was performed in September, 1973. The patient was discharged from hospital in a spring brace 14 days later.

It is interesting to note that in time the marked bony sclerosis resolved. This is akin to the disappearance of sclerosis that occurs after osteotomy or fusion of the hip, and is the result of a profound metabolic reaction.

CASE 6-5. An 18-year-old female university student suffered a flexion injury to the L4–5 disc when she was involved in a rear-end automobile collision while wearing a lap safety belt. Following this, she had lumbar pain on weight bearing. Roentgenographs showed flexion tilting instability on the lateral views taken in flexion and extension (Fig. 6-19A, B).

Posterior spinal fusion was performed, with the insertion of two interspinous Attenborough springs. Lateral roentgenographs in flexion and extension, taken after fusion had occurred, show the solid mass of the bone graft (Fig. 6-19C, D). There is no residual movement between L4 and L5. The patient's backache disappeared.

CASE 6-6. A 37-year-old woman suffered attacks of backache and left sciatica for years. Manipulation had given temporary relief. She became worse, presenting the symptom of an unstable joint. Flexion/extension roentgenographs showed erosion of the L3–4 intervertebral space with sclerosis, osteophyte formation, instability, and rotational displacement.

Fusion was performed, using an H-graft and Attenborough compression springs (Fig. 6-20A). The patient was allowed up on the fourth day and wore a brace for 6 months. A roentgenograph 9 months after operation showed firm fusion (Fig. 6-20B). She has had no pain since.

TECHNIQUES OF SEGMENTAL FUSION

MacNab and Dall considered posterolateral fusion the technique of choice,[26] as did Kirkaldy-Willis and Wiltse. It is particularly useful after extensive posterior decompression, involving both laminectomy and foramenec-

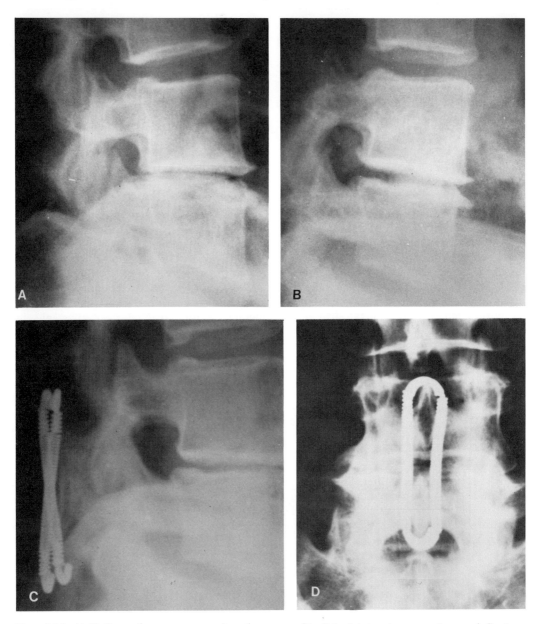

FIG. 6-18. *(A,B)* Lateral roentgenographs of an unstable L4–5 joint in extension and flexion. *(C,D)* Anteroposterior and lateral views after posterior fusion with fixation, using two Attenborough springs. *(Continued opposite).*

tomy, with removal of the posterior elements of the joints (Fig. 6-21).

The blood loss incurred in posterolateral fusion is a serious disadvantage. MacNab and Dall minimized this by using a Hastings frame, which avoids pressure on the abdomen, and an operative technique in which the constant muscular and articular branches of the lumbar arteries are displayed and coagulated by cautery (Fig. 6-22).

One of the possibly useful effects of the

the articular facets were included in the fusion. It was suggested that stenosis after posterior fusion is due to "shingling," which leads to thickening of the laminae and consequent decrease of the diameter of the spinal canal and spinal stenosis.[26] One of the authors, however, abrades the surface of the laminae to provide a satisfactory bed for union with the graft, rather than raising sturdy osteoperiosteal shingles, and has not experienced a significant incidence of spinal stenosis.

Callus forms where minor movement is possible at the site of a fracture or graft. It is possible that the absolute fixation afforded by the use of a compression spring allows primary union of the bony surfaces without the formation of exuberant callus, thus preventing spinal stenosis.

Technique of Posterolateral Fusion

Fusion is achieved by placing strip grafts and cancellous chips over the decorticated transverse processes, facets, and laminae of the segment to be stabilized and over the alae of the sacrum, if the lumbosacral joint is to be included (Fig. 6-23).

A mid-line incision with retraction of the sacrospinalis mass of muscles permits, when necessary, exploration of the spinal canal. To expose the transverse processes, the muscle stripping is continued over the posterior joints. This involves division of the intermediate layer of the lumbar fascia, which, as described by MacNab and Dall, is attached to the posterior border of the superior articular facets and the pars interarticularis. Behind the thin fascial layer lies the rich plexus of muscular and articular branches of the lumbar arteries. Their dissections confirmed that the main branches are remarkably constant in their anatomical distribution (Fig. 6-24). Careful incision of the fascia along the dorsal edge of one superior articular facet allows the superior and inferior articular branches to be identified and cauterized. After expos-

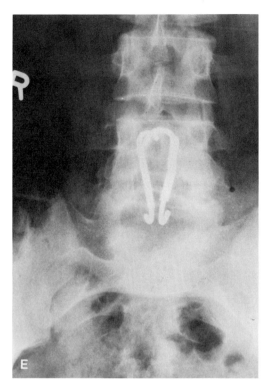

FIG. 6-18. *(Continued) (E)* Anteroposterior view shows that solid fusion has occurred.

posterolateral approach is section of the branches of the posterior primary nerve divisions or rhizolysis of the segmental nerves in their extradural course as they traverse or run around the intertransverse membrane.

Kirkaldy-Willis (Chap. 5) stated that anterior fusions had a 10 per cent success rate; posterior fusions 50 per cent, and posterolateral fusions were most successful. Anterior fusions, in his opinion, gave the highest rate of the complication of postoperative spinal stenosis. Posterior fusion also had an appreciable incidence, while posterolateral fusion gave rise to stenosis of the nerve root tunnel, not of the spinal canal. He found the latter to be an uncommon complication which occurred occasionally when the pedicles and

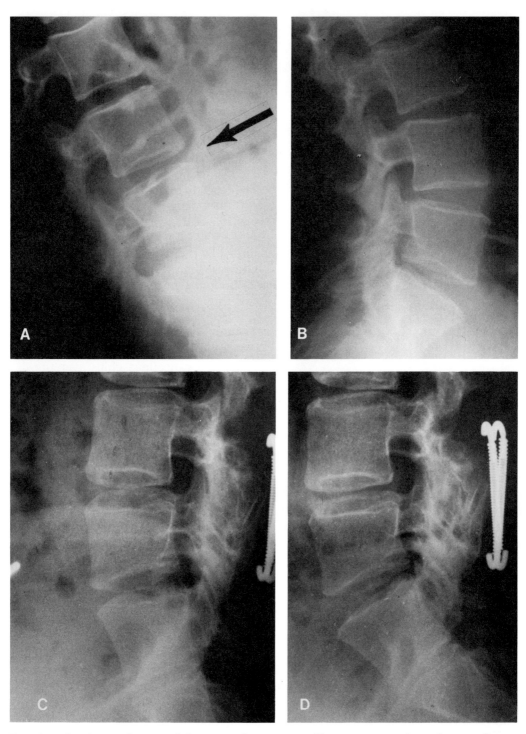

Fig. 6-19. *(A,B)* Lateral views of the spine of an 18-year-old university student, showing flexion instability at the L4–5 level. *(C,D)* Lateral views in extension and flexion after posterior spinal fusion with Attenborough springs. No residual instability is present.

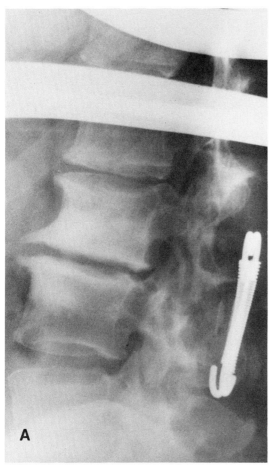 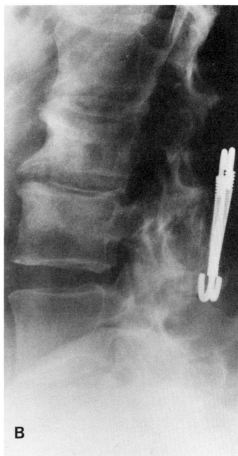

FIG. 6-20. *(A)* A lateral view of L3–4 collapse, with sclerosis and anterior lipping. This film was taken shortly after posterior H-graft fusion with Attenborough springs. *(B)* A similar view taken 9 months later shows fusion of the graft. Of interest is the loss of sclerosis.

ing the base of the transverse process with a periosteal elevator, the communicating artery and, immediately lateral to the pars interarticularis, the interarticular artery, are also identified and coagulated. Once this is done the whole transverse process can usually be stripped without further bleeding. The difficulty in controlling deep bleeding, which is the disadvantage of this posterolateral approach, is countered by this admirable, if meticulous, technique. The bone is roughened and grafts are inserted.

Suction drainage is instituted for both the spinal and the donor graft wounds and can usually be removed in 48 hours. Post-operatively, regimes vary. Usually the patient is allowed up in 3 or 4 days and discharged from hospital, wearing a firm corset, in 2 weeks. Some surgeons insist on 3 weeks' bed rest. On the whole, convalescence is comfortable and results are good, with solid fusion of the bone mass (Fig. 6-25). Nonunion is infrequent, although, on occasion, inexplicably, the graft may not take and is found lying as a loose body in the muscle bed.

Anterior Interbody Fusion

This operation carries hazards for surgeons who are not well-trained, experienced, or adept in the technique. Whether

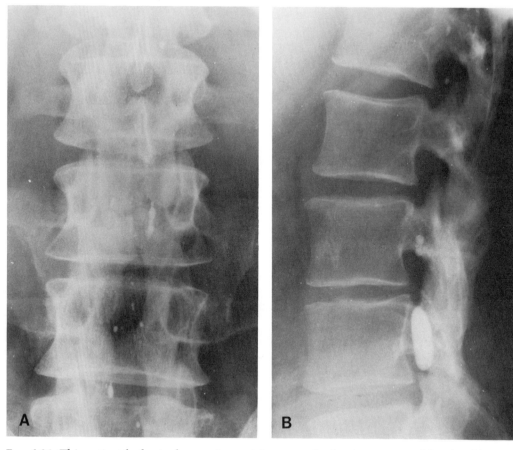

Fig. 6-21. This patient had spinal stenosis requiring extensive laminectomy and localized fusion. *(A)* An anteroposterior roentgenograph shows posterolateral fusion and loss of the laminae at several levels. *(B)* Lateral views show sound fusion of the graft (MacNab, I. and Dall, D.: J. Bone Joint Surg., *53B*:628, 1971)

performed transperitoneally or retroperitoneally, involvement of the iliac vessels or sympathetic nerves may cause serious complications. However, after posterior operations with extensive scarring of the dura and nerve roots, and especially after repeated operations, it has advantages, and both Sidney Sacks and Douglas Freebody have reported considerable success even when the approach is used routinely. The development of gentle microsurgical techniques in neurolysis and nerve repair will undoubtedly limit these indications.

In a personal communication, Sidney Sacks, who has considerable experience of anterior as well as posterior and lateral lumbar spinal fusion, writes that, "anterior interbody fusion for spondylolisthesis and other disabilities in the lower lumbar spine has some place in our surgical armamentarium. But, after becoming attracted to the *lateral* lumbar spinal fusion, I have found this method more satisfactory technically, with better results and fewer complications."

He believes that existing criticism of lumbar spinal fusion, and of anterior fusion in particular, is justified because: (1) lower lumbar spinal fusion is being done too frequently in patients who have been inadequately investigated; (2) the techni-

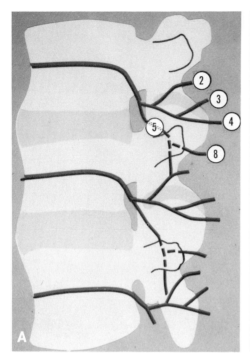 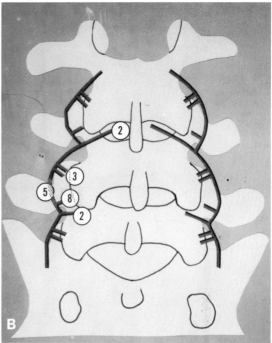

FIG. 6-22. *(A)* Diagram shows the disposition of the major muscular branches of the lumbar arteries. *(1)* Interarticular artery; *(2,3)* superior articular arteries; *(4)* communicating branch; *(5)* inferior articular artery. *(B)* Diagram shows the disposition of the muscular branches of the lumbar arteries in relation to the operative exposure. The interarticular artery *(1)* is found immediately lateral to the pars interarticularis. The two superior articular arteries *(2)* lie immediately lateral to the tip of the superior articular facet. The inferior articular artery *(5)* lies in the angle formed by the transverse process and the superior articular facet. The communicating artery *(4)* is a large vessel lying immediately lateral to the superior articular facet on the dorsal surface of the transverse process. (MacNab, I., and Dall, D.: J. Bone Joint Surg., *53B*:628, 1971)

cal aspects of the operations have not been strictly observed, and (3) postoperative rehabilitation has been neglected. When the indications for an anterior approach to the lumbar spine are present, he prefers the transperitoneal route. It requires less retraction, and other intraabdominal abnormalities can be dealt with at the same time.

"With the patient supine, the bladder is emptied by catheter, which is allowed to drain into a bag or perineal pad during the operation. The operating table should have a "kidney rest" which can be raised into a slight Trendelenburg position, which permits the viscera to be packed out of the way. The kidney rest is ele-

vated. The posterior parietal peritoneum over the sacrum is infiltrated with normal saline to demonstrate the presacral vessels, which are ligatured. Cautery is not used in this area, to avoid injury to the presacral nerves. The intervertebral disc is exposed by excising the anterior longitudinal ligament and the annulus. The disc material is removed entirely, as far as the posterior longitudinal ligament, with special attention to the posterolateral corners, where posterior herniation of the disc usually occurs. The adjacent endplates are scarified or excised, depending on the porosity of the vertebral bodies. Interbody grafts consisting of corticocancellous blocks, taken from the an-

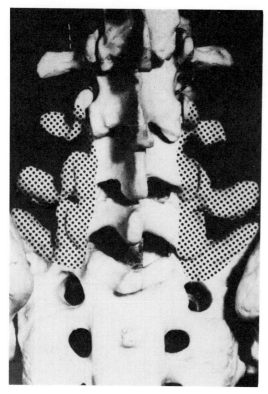

FIG. 6-23. The shaded zone demarcates the graft bed for an intertransverse fusion. Note that the graft bed extends further cephalad and includes the pars interarticularis of the most cephalad vertebra. (MacNab, I. and Dall, D.: J. Bone Joint Surg., *53B*:628, 1971)

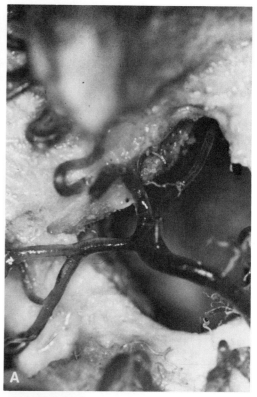

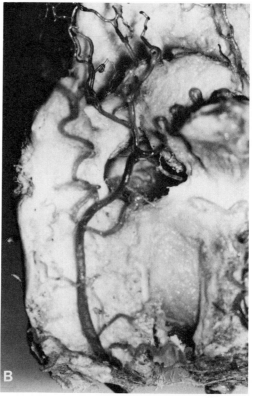

FIG. 6-24. *(A)* Enlarged photographs of an injected specimen showing disposition of the major muscular branches of a lumbar artery. *(B)* Injected specimen showing small, but constant, vessels entering the intervertebral foramen. (MacNab, I. and Dall, D.: J. Bone Joint surg., *53B:*628, 1971)

terior ilium, usually three in number, are inserted and tapped in firmly. Only autogenous grafts should be used. The kidney rest is lowered, the posterior peritoneum closed, the viscera allowed to fall back into position, and the abdomen closed in the usual manner."

After anterior interbody fusion the patient is allowed to sit in Fowler's position as soon as awake and is given nothing by mouth until bowel sounds are heard and flatus passed. Intravenous therapy should also be continued for that period.

The patient is allowed to sit out of bed on the third day, to walk on the fifth, and is usually out of hospital on the twelfth day. Depending on the number of levels fused and the indications for the operation, a spinal support is worn for about 4 months.

An interesting innovation in the use of the anterior approach has been introduced in patients with lumbar spinal instability at multiple levels, who have had previous unsuccessful posterior decompressions for their pain, with or without attempts at lateral spinal fusion. The anterior interbody fusion is reinforced and stabilized by the Dwyer screw-and-cable technique via the retroperitoneal route (Fig. 6-26).

Several complications which are not usually encountered by the posterior or lateral techniques may occur in the anterior approach (e.g., vascular injury, sterility, collapse of vertebral bodies, sympathectomy-syndrome affecting the legs, inaccuracy of fusion levels, and injury or adhesions to the ureter). With care, these can be avoided. Other complications are no more common with the anterior approach than with any intraabdominal operation.

Recurrence of symptoms should be mentioned, as it occurs more frequently with anterior interbody fusion than with lateral fusion. The time period is usually

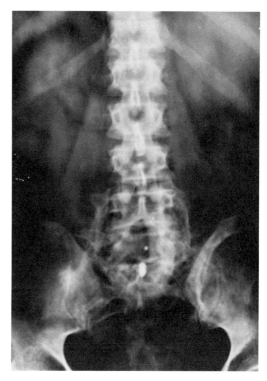

FIG. 6-25. Anteroposterior view following posterolateral fusion, showing an excellent fusion mass from L4 to the sacrum. (Courtesy D. Dall, M.D.)

7 years after operation and is due to disc degeneration at a level above the fusion, or a recurrence of instability at the same level from a pseudarthrosis which may develop after minor injury to the back. This usually occurs in patients who have a predisposition to generalized disc degeneration of the spine. Such an eventuality may require rest and corset immobilization or even a reinforcing lateral lumbar spinal fusion. Sidney Sacks concludes, "However, my present views are that when fusion is necessary for lumbar backache, lateral spine fusion is a more satisfactory primary procedure than anterior interbody fusion."

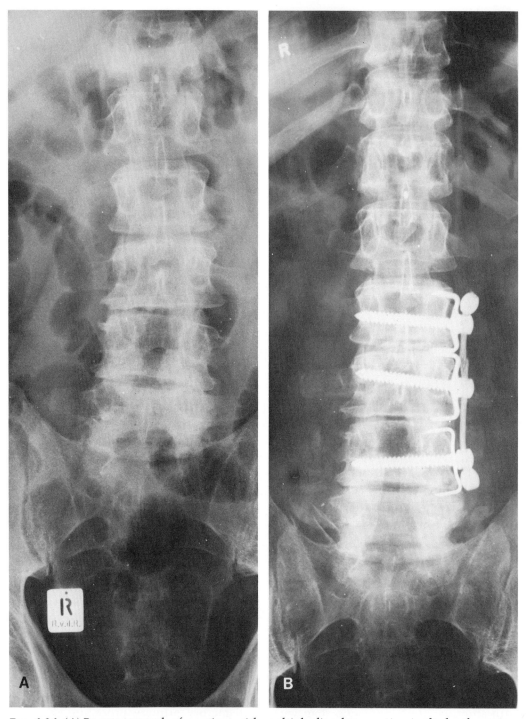

FIG. 6-26. (A) Roentgenograph of a patient with multiple disc degeneration in the lumbar spine. He had had wide laminectomy previously. (B) Postoperative film shows anterior fusion, reinforced by the Dwyer screw-and-cable technique. The L5–S1 disc was later fused by posterior intertransverse grafting, with excellent results. (Courtesy Mr. S. Sacks)

The only absolute indications for anterior interbody fusion in patients with low backache are listed below:

Failure of posterior and lateral fusion
In patients with previous laminectomy and small transverse processes
For developmental spondylolisthesis
For eradication of disease processes of vertebral bodies
When multiple lumbar levels are unstable and a Dwyer's screw-and-cable method can reinforce interbody fusion

---

Technique of Posterior Fusion

With the patient prone, the lumbar spine is flexed by raising the pelvis on blocks or on a frame. This leaves the abdomen free of pressure and minimizes bleeding. A mid-line incision exposes the spinous processes and the lumbar fascia covering the sacrospinalis muscles on either side. The fascia is split and, with knife or cutting diathermy or rugine, the mass of the sacrospinalis is separated and retracted from the spinous processes, laminae, and posterior surfaces of the facet joints. A self-retaining retractor maintains good exposure. The bone surfaces to be fused are thoroughly abraded by osteotome or bur, or thin osteoperiosteal flaps are raised from the spinous processes and laminae and neural arches of the sacrum, and the articular surfaces of the facet joints are guttered. The interspinous ligament is excised, and the adjacent bony surfaces are roughened. An H or "clothespin" graft is fashioned from the cortical surface of bone taken from the outer surface of the ilium and is jammed between the spinous processes. Alternatively, cortical strips are cut and laid alongside and between the spinous processes and on the roughened laminae. The cancellous bone chips are packed into the guttered intervertebral joints and around the cortical grafts.

To Apply Spring Compression

The back is straightened slightly. Two Attenborough springs of carefully measured length are hooked around the spinous processes. The length of each spring is calculated by plugging into a formula the distance (x) between the anchorage points: $3x - 6/5$. This allows for the lengths of the hooks, and the unstretched spring on the screw-ends of the hooks, and when applied exacts a 50 per cent increase in length to the spring, giving a tension of 6 kg. The firmness of fixation may be tested by holding the patient's legs and flexing the trunk to the left and to the right. No movement should be possible. Suction drainage is installed and the wounds are sutured (Figs. 6-8C, 6-19, 6-20).

Other methods of compression may be used in posterior fusion. The Knodt system is shown in Figure 6-27.

EXCISION OF A RUPTURED DISC AND FUSION

Opinions differ about whether fusion should be performed simultaneously with the removal of the disc. Excision of the disc alone is usually a simple procedure. The patient is up and about in a few days, and convalescence is not unduly taxing for the young patient with a short history. The surgeon's inclination is to avoid fusion, but in the experience of one of the authors (A.J.H.), more backs break down with each year after operation. The picture is worse after 20 years than 10, and worse after 30 than 20.

Since the long-term breakdown is rarely complicated by neurologic involvement, the operation at 10 years is no more difficult than initially. The complications, and in the past, the protracted nature of the postoperative care, discouraged immediate operation. But local fusion using a compression device keeps the patient in bed and hospital only a day or two longer—and posterolateral fusion, but little more—than the simple disc operation, so that when preoperative examination indicates a vulnerable intervertebral joint, the situation is explained, and most

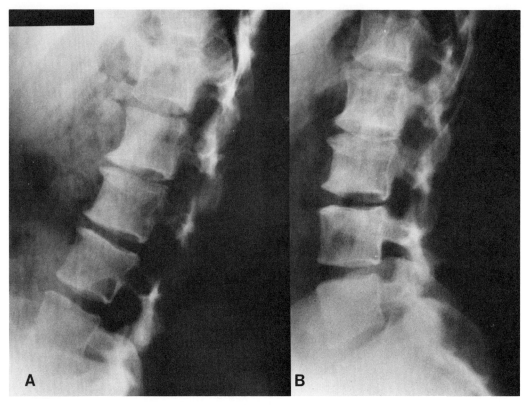

FIG. 6-27. *(A,B)* Lateral views, showing marked disc degeneration and instability on the L2–3 level, and, to a lesser extent, at L3–4 level in flexion and extension. *(Continued opposite)*

patients opt for immediate fusion. Marked instability or the presence of obvious osteoarthritic change is a positive indication. For mild instability, or retrospondylolisthesis with a long history of recurrent attacks with increasing pain, fusion is advised but not stressed.

Permission to fuse is requested preoperatively in case instability is detected. Where doubt exists, the use of a brace for a few weeks gives an indication of the benefit to be derived from fusion. At operation, after excision of the disc, the integrity of the interspinous ligaments and the stability of the segment are assessed by rocking the adjacent spinous processes, which are held in bone-holding forceps or Kocher's clamps. A prolapsed disc often locks the intervertebral segment, but after removal it may be quite lax.

A disadvantage of local fusion is the increased stress placed upon the mobile joints above and below it. Adequate rehabilitation, using postural exercises (Goldthwait), has minimized this complication.

Sometimes patients are comfortable in spite of unsound fusion. It would seem that sufficient stability may be achieved without complete fusion.

CASE 6-7. A middle-aged woman suffered significant disability only some years after a motor vehicle accident. Then she showed signs of an obvious mid-lumbar disc prolapse with some, but not marked, neurologic deficit. Her roentgenographs (Fig. 6-27) showed obvious instability and rotation of the intervertebral space between L2 and L3, as well as L3–L4. The myelogram showed evidence of a large disc protrusion between L3 and L4. At

FIG. 6-27. *(C)* Myelogram shows large prolapse at the L3–4 level. *(D,E)* Lateral and anteroposterior roentgenographs 6 months after excision of the disc and posterior fusion, using the Knodt compression devices.

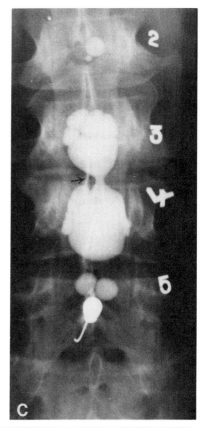

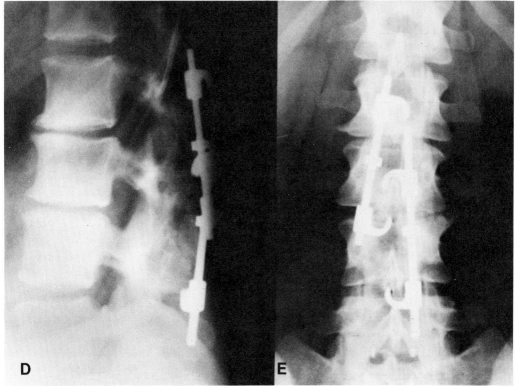

operation a hard, fibrous protruding disc was excised from the L2–3 space, and a softer disc was removed from the right side of L3–L4. The test for stability, by rocking the spinous processes, confirmed gross instability between L2 and L3 and between L3 and L4. Fusion was performed using H-grafts and cancellous slivers. Compression was applied by the Knodt device. Firm fusion resulted, and the patient had no more symptoms.

The Lateral Position for Disc Removal

One of the variants of the prone position (Mohammedan prayer position) for the patient is essential if disc removal is to be accompanied by posterior or posterolateral spinal fusion. It is not the only position suitable for excision of a lumbar disc.

The lateral position, as used by Mr. Young at St. George's Hospital, and Armstrong, has been used by one of the authors (D.G.L.) in a series of 67 consecutive cases. The technique used was that described by Jackson.[19] Some of the cases in Jackson's series were performed by the author but are not included in this series.

The rationale behind the use of this position is based on three considerations: gravity aids the drainage of extravasated blood from the incision; the surgeon can sit while he operates; and the 56 recorded cases of retroabdominal arteriovenous fistula occurred in patients being operated on in the prone position.

If the abdominal contents are inadvertently pressed against the posterior abdominal wall, it is possible that injury to one or more of the great vessels may occur if the surgeon does not realize that the jaws of his pituitary rongeur have penetrated the anterior fibers of the annulus and the anterior longitudinal ligament. There is no firm evidence for this, but it is thought that if the patient is in the lateral position the vessels and abdominal organs fall forward and downward, creating an actual (of what was merely a potential) space in the retroabdominal layers of tissue. After bladder catheterization, the patient, with intubation anesthesia, is placed in the lateral chin-on-knee (the lumbar puncture) position, with neck and spine fully flexed. The leg that had been subject to sciatica is placed upward, for ease of retracting the nerve root downward with a right-angled nerve-root retractor. Intravenous infusions are administered into the upper arm, to prevent the weight of the patient's body obstructing venous return and to prevent difficulty with transfusion of blood, should it be required.

Finally, before skin preparation, the table is broken at the level of the affected disc, or a renal pad is elevated, to straighten the lateral curve of the lumbar spine that is present when the patient lies in the lateral position.

The disadvantages of this position are few: the lights must be focused so that the beam is in an almost horizontal line; the surgeon must get used to operating with his hands held up in front of him, which can be tiring until he is accustomed to it; the use of an operating microscope is slightly more difficult.

COMPLICATIONS OF SPINAL FUSION

As with any other spinal operation, general complications, such as bleeding, infection, deep vein thrombosis with pulmonary embolism, and pulmonary infection, may occur. Careful preoperative assessment and assiduous nursing and physiotherapy after operation will reduce these to a minimum. Infection of the wound is directly related to meticulous technique for sterility in the operating room and gentle surgery, so that "prophylactic" antibiotics need seldom be used.

The two special complications of spinal fusion are inadequate choice of patients and failure of union of the graft. The former occurs when the surgeon fails to analyze the patient's symptoms in a satisfactory manner, choosing patients whose pain is caused not by instability but by a psychological problem, or in whom pain is referred from an unexpected source, such as an abdominal aortic aneurysm. Nonunion of the graft cannot always be prevented, although careful surgery and compression reduce this complication.

Pseudarthrosis

The grafts may not take at all or they may not unite at one or the other end, or, after fusion, they may break opposite the joint. Unsound ankylosis is more likely to occur at the lumbosacral joint, or at the L–5 joint, than higher up. It is also more likely if more than one segment is fused. Refusion for pseudarthrosis is somewhat more prone to failure. It is more difficult to achieve sound fusion for unstable spondylolisthesis than when instability is the result of disc degeneration or traumatic osteoarthrosis.

Inadequate fixation allowing recurrent movement, however slight, between graft and bone surfaces predisposes to delayed or nonunion. After the first 2 weeks any sudden, unguarded movement, especially a twist, is likely to cause a fracture. In the early weeks the reapplication of adequate splinting may, and often does, lead to union. As consolidation of the fragments proceeds, the bones become less vascular, so that union is less likely. In any event, a trial of further splinting is merited. Unsound ankylosis is not necessarily disabling. If the fibrous union is stable (i.e., movement is in the normal pattern even if not complete), the back is symptomless. Abnormal asymmetry of movement at the point of nonunion is painful.

MacNab and Dall reviewed the results obtained by the three techniques of two-segment (L4–S1) spinal fusion: anterior interbody, posterior, and posterolateral fusion for degenerative disc disease.[26] Table 6-1 shows their results.

Their figures are not strictly applicable when the operation is performed for spondylolisthesis, for gross displacement may deter attempts at anterior interbody fusion. Reports of the success of single-segment fusion from different orthopaedic units vary greatly but, as ex-

Table 6-1. Incidence of Pseudarthrosis in Two-Segment Fusions (L4–S1) for Degenerative Disc Disease

Type of Operation	Number of Cases	Pseudar-throsis	Per-centage
Anterior inter-body fusion	54	16	30
Posterior fusion	174	30	17
Intertransverse fusion	138	10	7

(MacNab, I. and Dall, D.: J. Bone Joint Surg., *53B*:628, 1971)

pected, are on the whole more favorable.

Nonunion cannot always be detected on straight roentgenographs, but lateral stress views usually show abnormal movement, even if it is not painful. The lack of fusion may be evident only when the graft is exposed at open operation.

As with fractures of long bones, fusion of the graft may be promoted by excision and regrafting, or by packing cancellous bone around the pseudarthrosis, or most simply and successfully by cancellous chips plus compression. In the appropriate circumstances any one of the three techniques may be chosen as the rescue operation.

Complications of the Attenborough Springs

The springs had to be removed or changed in nine patients. There were several reasons for this:

Fracture of both springs and grafts occurred in three cases. Regrafting, with the insertion of new springs, resulted in rapid consolidation again. Two case histories:

CASE 6-8. A 29-year-old woman had suffered from low back pain for 4 years, for which she had been treated by manipulation, etc. In June, 1971, she was involved in a motor accident, after which she developed sciatica down to the right ankle, with loss of sensation and weakness in the distribution of the 5th lumbar and 1st sciatic nerve roots. Roentgenographs suggested instability of the L4–5 interspace on flexion and retrospondylolisthesis of the lumbosacral joint on extension.

In January, 1972, a large protrusion of the L4 disc and osteophytes on the upper border of the

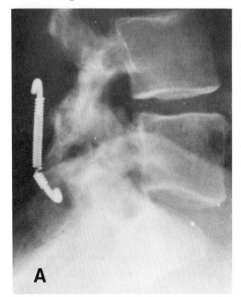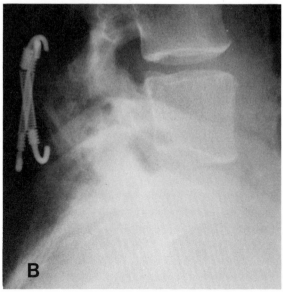

FIG. 6-28. *(A)* Lateral roentgenograph of the patient described in Case 6-8 taken after fracture of the Attenborough spring and graft. *(B)* Lateral view after the second operation for regrafting and the insertion of two Attenborough springs. Consolidation of the graft has occurred.

L5 lumbar disc were excised. The segment was fused, using a bone graft and a single Attenborough spring. The patient made a complete recovery, including full recovery of sensation and power.

In July, 1973, she was exercising her two Alsatian dogs on the beach, when one of the dogs tripped her and the other landed on her back. She fractured both the graft and the spring, with recurrence of pain and instability (Fig. 6-28A).

In August, 1973, the broken spring was removed, the graft was reinforced with cancellous bone, and a new pair of Attenborough springs were applied. Her convalescence was uncomplicated, and she recovered stability and comfort. Roentgenographs showed firm fusion, and she has had no disability since (Fig. 6-28B).

CASE 6-9. A boy of 14 was seen in 1971, suffering attacks of low backache for 1 year, due to an unstable spondylolisthesis. In January, 1972, fusion of the two lowest lumbar discs was performed, using one spring. The boy was able to return to school 6 weeks later and was comfortable in a spring brace. In September, 1972, he was stable, both clinically and roentgenographically (Fig. 6-29A, B).

Six months later he dived badly into the school swimming pool, snapping his back in extension and fracturing the graft and spring (Fig. 6-29C, D).

He underwent reoperation in April, 1973, when the broken spring was removed and new grafts were inserted. By September, 1973, fusion was clinically and roentgenographically sound. The oblique views taken at that time show fusion of the pars interarticularis on one side as well.

Nonunion of the graft occurred in one instance and led to stretching and angulation of the springs, with recurrence of instability of the segment (Fig. 6-30). Refusion with new springs had a successful result.

Metal Sensitivity. In five patients, comfort was obtained after fusion, but between 1 and 2 years after operation, the patients complained of aching and local tenderness over the springs, due to reaction to the metal. Removal of the device is simple, since it is relatively superficial, and it relieves these symptoms. There is no doubt that in some cases metal present in any situation in the body does, eventually, set up a local reaction and should be removed.

Superficial Sepsis. In four patients, superficial infection occurred in the midline or donor-graft incision, lasting for a few days. Fortunately no patient developed deep sepsis.

Neuromas. The occurrence of neuromas in the donor site has been described previously.

SOME CONTROVERSIAL TREATMENTS FOR BACK PAIN

From time to time new ideas have stimulated novel forms of therapy for the treatment of mechanical derangement of the lumbar spine. Without innovations we should be performing neither operative removal of the disc nor even spinal fusion. The concept of spinal stenosis has only gained acceptance in the past ten years and has added much to our understanding of symptomatology. In consequence, patients who would otherwise have remained incapacitated have been cured by simple decompression.

The objective assessment of such forms of therapy is made difficult by two facts. Firstly, statistical results of treatment are difficult to obtain because of the necessity of choosing adequate criteria for comparison.[21] There is a real dilemma for the surgeon. Should he allow the patient to be used in a controlled, double-blind trial of a new form of treatment when, for example, the consequences of denying the patient an operation may be permanent incapacity? This question has not yet been answered to the satisfaction of most clinicians. Secondly, there is a natural tendency toward recovery in mechanical conditions of the back. While this has enhanced the reputation of many a practitioner, both medical and lay, it does not aid the scientific observer. Before World War II, cases of sciatica were treated successfully by operative dissection of the sciatic nerve, because the prevailing theory was that the symptoms were caused by sciatic neuritis and would re-

spond to the stripping of adhesions. Many cases were undoubtedly "cured," but nobody now would advocate this treatment.

At present three controversial forms of treatment are under discussion. Mention of these will be made in this chapter. The authors have little firsthand knowledge of such treatments and are certainly not advocating their use. There is some value in considering them, however: on the one hand, they may represent a true advance in therapy; on the other, they may be merely fashionable.

Acupuncture

After broadcasts of several films on television in the United States and the United Kingdom which purported to show this simple treatment in use as a general anesthetic in surgical operations in China in 1975, considerable interest was shown in acupuncture by medical practitioners. The natural enthusiasm of many doctors has quickly waned, but the treatment remains popular with a large number of patients in Western countries. Dr. Hannington-Kiff mentions it (Chap. 8) within the framework of our present theoretical knowledge of the nervous system. The authors decided to allow a well-known practitioner of the art to speak for himself.

Dr. Yong Chai Siow, who practices in London, completed his study of medicine in Canton, China in 1957. He states the following:

Acupuncture has been practiced in China for more than 4,000 years. Its origins are lost in antiquity. Since the establishment of the Chinese People's Republic, it is studied by all medical students during their 6-year course. After qualifying, those doctors who wish to specialize in acupuncture must spend an extra 2 years studying the subject. Its popularity, even in China, is greater than ever before.

The indications for its use are mainly in conditions of disorder of the nerves, such as pain of various types. It can also help with many diseases of the internal organs by in-

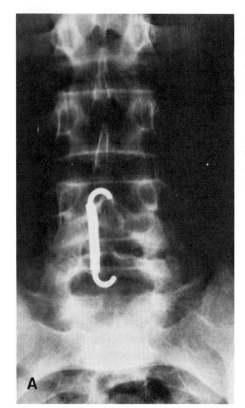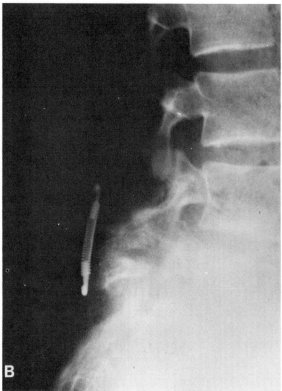

FIG. 6-29. *(A,B)* Anteroposterior and lateral views of the lumbar spine of a 14-year-old boy who had undergone posterior fusion with fixation by an Attenborough spring for spondylolisthesis. The graft is consolidated.

creasing the circulation in the affected organ and so aiding in the recovery of its function. It is also used in many nervous or mental diseases.

Dr. Yong continues by stating that the use of acupuncture as a general anesthetic is a new one and that he did not study this aspect of the treatment. He does not believe that acupuncture can give total anesthesia but thinks it may play a part in dulling sensation. He commented that Chinese people, like many other Asians, are able to withstand more pain than Westerners, because of their cultural traditions.

The treatment consists of placing needles into known "centers" of the body. Maps exist of these centers, that have been empirically discovered, and they have to be learned by the student. For example, there is a special acupuncture point on the vertex of the scalp, known as Governing Vessel 20, the stimulation of which aids recovery from psychological problems. Conditions such as neuralgia and arthritis of the cervical and lumbar spine can be improved in as many as 90 per cent of cases by a course of six treatments.

It is rare for one center to be stimulated alone. More commonly a minimum of 4 to 6 needles are inserted at the same time; sometimes there may be as many as 50 to 60. It is most important to reach the right spot on the right nerve. The needle is then rotated by rolling between finger and thumb to stimulate the center. Usually six treatments are given as a course. In acute conditions this may take place daily. In chronic disease the visits may be weekly or fortnightly. The needles are made of stainless steel, varying in length from ½ to 3 inches, depending on the depth to which they have to be inserted. This depth is critical if the centers are to be reached. The width of the needles is equivalent to the H-32 hypodermic

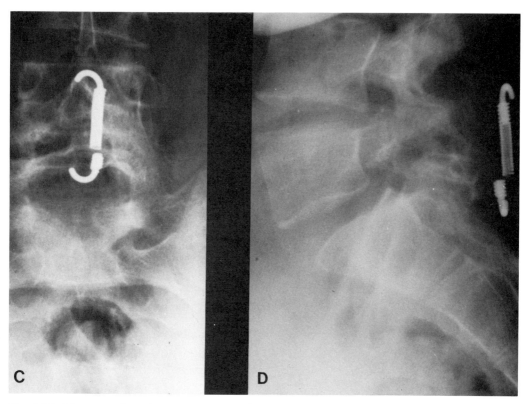

Fig. 6-29. (*Continued*)   (*C,D*) Two views of the same spine in 1973. Following a diving injury the spring had snapped, the graft had broken, and spondylolisthesis had recurred. After refusion, union again occurred.

needle. They are prepared by boiling and are then soaked in ethyl alcohol before use. Since they have no lumen they do not cause hepatitis.

Dr. Yong believes that about 25 per cent of cases that respond to his treatment do so because of a placebo effect. He points out that there are limitations to the effectiveness of the treatment. "Some mental troubles cannot be helped. Rheumatoid arthritis is rather difficult. There is no effect on cases of cancer. In fact, some patients with this condition may be made worse by the treatment."

The Operation of Multiple Bilateral Percutaneous Rhizolysis

Skyme Rees presented the thesis that the pain of intervertebral disc syndrome arises from the posterior intervertebral joints and not from the disc.[29] Whereas the pain pathway from the disc is via the sinuvertebral nerve, the intervertebral joints are supplied by branches of the posterior primary division of the segmental nerves. In their extradural course these run either through or around the edge of the intertransverse membrane, where they may be divided percutaneously.

The procedure is performed under epidural and local anesthesia. Through a stab wound 2 cm. lateral to the spinous processes and over the tender facet joints, a long, narrow-bladed knife sweeps across the intertransverse membrane, severing the nerve fibers. This is repeated bilaterally over each tender place.

Rees claims that out of every 100 patients with intractable backache, sciatica, neck pain, and chronic headache, 88 are relieved immediately. Hematoma was the

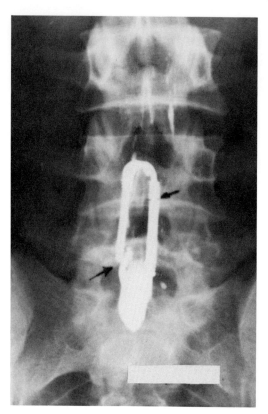

F‍ig. 6-30. Anteroposterior roentgenograph shows snapping of the Attenborough springs due to nonunion of the graft.

only complication. Two patients required laminectomy and excision of the disc. Subsequently Shealy and colleagues advocated radio frequency to block the nerve fibers, a technique that avoids the excessive bleeding.   They note that 25 per cent of patients with good results initially have recurrence of pain, usually within a week. Two-thirds of these are improved by a second procedure. These results are dramatic, and the success rate is unusually high for any form of therapy. Trials on smaller series of patients privately reported show the results to be less predictable.

Denervation of the apophyseal joints is the objective of this procedure, which is similar to the practice of denervation of the hip joint for osteoarthritis advised by Camitz and followed by Tavanier 30-odd years ago. After division of the branches of the obdurator nerve, 38 per cent of patients were relieved of pain. In other cases, total denervation of the hip was carried out by dividing the branches of the sciatic and femoral nerves also, and successful results were claimed in 90 per cent. It was feared that neurotrophic disorganization of the joint might follow. Instead, pain recurred and longer-term results were increasingly disappointing. It is, moreover, difficult to relate this procedure to symptoms such as motor weakness, especially in patients where the EMG demonstrates denervation action potentials. A further period of observation and follow-up is necessary to determine the true value of this procedure.

Chemonucleolysis

Of all the interesting suggestions for the treatment of the painful disc, that of the injection of proteolytic enzymes into the disc itself is the most logical. Since degenerate nuclear tissue probably undergoes chemical changes to become swollen, it is feasible that chemical means could be used to break down such tissue so that it could be replaced with fibrous tissue. In this way the natural process of involution could be hastened.

Nordby and Lucas advocated the use of such an enzyme, chymopapain, for this treatment, by intradiscal injection.[27a] Gibson, Dilke, and Grahame regarded this treatment as unproven and tried oral therapy with chymoral, a mixture of chymotrypsin and trypsin, both of which are proteolytic enzymes.[12a] They concluded that this treatment significantly improved straight-leg raising and reduced the necessity for analgesia, but had no effect on other parameters of the condition.

Since the placing of a needle into the affected disc has been greatly aided by the use of image intensification of roentgenographic screening, it seems certain that further advances will take place in enzyme therapy, as the drugs are improved.

The main theoretical danger is in cases of complete rupture of the annulus, in which the enzyme (or combined breakdown products) could be released into the extradural space with a consequent inflammatory reaction, or even fibrosis. Whether this disadvantage will prove to be a practical one, time will tell.

REFERENCES

1. Attenborough, C. G., and Reynolds, M. T.: Lumbar-sacral fusion with spring fixation. J, Bone Joint Surg., *57B:*283, 1975.
2. Barr, J. S.: Protruded discs and painful backs. J. Bone Joint Surg., *33B:*3, 1951.
3. Birkeland, I. W., Jr., and Taylor, P. K. F.: Major vascular injuries in lumbar disc surgery. J. Bone Joint Surg., *51B:*4, 1969.
4. Boucher, H. H.: A method of spinal fusion. J. Bone Joint Surg., *41B:*248, 1959.
5. ———: A method of spinal fusion. J. Bone Joint Surg., *41B:*628, 1971.
6. Charnley, J.: Compression Arthrodesis. Edinburgh, E. & S. Livingstone, 1961.
7. Cloward, R. B.: The treatment of ruptured lumbar intervertebral discs by vertebral body fusion. Neurosurg. *10:*154, 1953.
8. Coplans, C. W.: Lumbar disc herniation. S. Afr. Med. J., *25:*881, 1951.
9. ———: Lumbar intervertebral disc herniatus. S. Afr. Med. J., *27:*182, 1953.
10. Dommisse, G. F.: Report on symposium on spinal stenosis. S.I.C.O.T. 1975.
11. Dubue, F.: Knodt rod grafting. Clin. Orthop., *5:*283, 1955.
12. Freebody, D., Bendall, R., and Taylor, R. D.: Anterior transperitoneal lumbar fusion. J. Bone Joint Surg., *53B:*617, 1971.
12a.Gibson, T., Dilke, T. F., and Grahame, R.: Chymoral in the treatment of lumbar disc prolapse. Rheumatol. Rehabil., *14:*186, 1975.
13. Gill, G. G., Manning, J. G., and White, H. L.: Surgical treatment of spondylolisthesis without spinal fusion. J. Bone Joint Surg., *37A:*493, 1955.
14. Goldthwait, J. E.: Essentials of Body Mechanics in Health and Disease. Philadelphia, J. B. Lippincott, 1945.
15. Harrington, P. R.: Treatment of scoliosis. Correction and internal fixation by spine instrumentation. J. Bone Joint Surg., *44A:*591, 1962.
16. Harris, R. I.: *In* Nassim, R., and Burrows, H. J. (eds.): Modern Trends in Diseases of the Vertebral Column. New York, Appleton, 1967.
17. Hilton, J.: Rest and Pain. London, Bell & Daldy, 1863.
18. Hodgson, A. R., and Wong, S. K.: A description of a technique and evaluation of results in anterior spinal fusion for deranged intervertebral disc and spondylolisthesis. Clin. Orthop., *56:*133, 1968.
19. Jackson, R. K.: The long-term effects of wide laminectomy for lumbar disc excision. J. Bone Joint Surg., *53B:*609, 1971.
20. Junghans, H.: Spondylolisthesen ohne Spalt im Zwischengelenkstuck ("Pseudospondylolisthesen"). Arch. Orthop. Unfall-chir., *29:*118, 1930.
21. Kelsey, J.: An epidemiological study of acute herniated lumbar intervertebral discs. Rheum. Rehab., *14:*144, 1975.
22. Knodt, H. M. D., and Larrick, R. B.: Distraction fusion of the spine. Ohio State Med. J., *60:*1140, 1964.
23. Knutsson, F.: The instability associated with disc degeneration in the lumbar spine. Acta Radiol. *25:*593, 1944.
24. Morgan, F. P., and King, T.: J. Bone Joint Surg., *39B:*6, 1957.
25. Muller, M. A., Allgower, M., and Willinger, H.: Manual of Internal Fixation. Berlin, Springer Verlag, 1970.
26. McNab, I., and Dall, D.: The blood supply of the lumbar spine and its application to the technique of intertransverse lumbar fusion. J. Bone Joint Surg., *53B:*628, 1971.
27. Newman, P. H.: Surgical treatment for derangement of the lumbar spine. J. Bone Joint Surg., *55B:*7, 1973.
27a. Nordby, E. J., and Lucas, G. L.: A comparative analysis of lumbar disc disease treated by laminectomy or chemonucleolysis. Clin. Orthop., *90:*119, 1973.
28. Overton, L. M.: Lumbosacral arthrodesis: an evaluation of its present status. Am. Surgeon, *25:*771, 1959.
29. Rees, S.: The Treatment of Pain as a Major Disability. Sydney, Visual Abstracts (Australia) Pty. Ltd., 1946.
30. Sacks, S.: Anterior interbody fusion of the lumbar spine. J. Bone Joint Surg., *47B:*211, 1965.
31. ———: Anterior interbody fusion of the lumbar spine. Indication and results in 200 cases. Clin. Orthop., *44:*163, 1966.
32. Steindler, A.: Kinesiology of the Human Body. Springfield, Charles C Thomas, 1955.
33. Watkins, M. B.: Posterolateral fusion of the lumbar and lumbo-sacral spine. J. Bone Joint Surg., *35A:*1014, 1953.
34. Watkins, M. B.: Posterolateral bone grafting for fusion of lumbar and lumbosacral spine. J. Bone Joint Surg., *41A:*388, 1959.
35. Watson-Jones, R.: Fractures and Joint Injuries. Edinburgh, E. & S. Livingstone, 1955.
36. Wilse, L.: A.A.O.S. Symposium on Spine. St. Louis, C. V. Mosby, 1969.
37. Wilson, P. D., and Straub, L. R.: A.A.O.S. Instructional Course Lectures. 9:1952.
38. Wiltsie, L. L., Bateman, J. G., Hutchison, R. H., and Nelson, W. E.: Paraspinal sacrospinalis-splitting approach to the lumbar spine. J. Bone Joint Surg., *50A:*919, 1968.

7 The Significance of the Signs and Symptoms of Lumbar Spinal Disorders

In this chapter an attempt will be made to delineate the patterns of clinical signs and symptoms of disc and other lumbar spinal pathology.

TAKING A HISTORY

Of all the events that influence the outcome of an acute or chronic attack of lumbar pain, the taking of an adequate history is the most important. The orthopaedic surgeon must allow his patient to tell the story of his problem in his own way. A past history of trauma, a story of psychological stress, or repeated attacks of increasing pain, may be critical to the understanding of the patient's problem. If the doctor interrupts, or if he leads the patient away from the relevant points, the wrong conclusion may be reached. Incorrect initial diagnosis is probably the most important reason for failure of treatment.

Onset. Attention should be directed not only to the onset, type, and severity of the pain in the back, but also to its exact position. Mid-line or bilateral pain suggests disc collapse or swelling, while unilateral pain is indicative of root pressure on one side, or even extravertebral derangement.

Referred Pain. The exact reference of the pain is next sought by careful questioning, after which sensory and motor symptoms in the leg are elicited.

Disability. The level of disability must be defined in detail: What is the patient's work? Is he able to carry it out fully or must he be protected by his colleagues or superiors? Is only light work possible?

Domestic Problems. The patient is asked about his home circumstances and the family commitment. He should feel able to confide in the doctor any worries that may arise during the course of the treatment.

Hobbies and Sports. The patient's hobbies are discussed so that an assessment can be made of the level of activity to be regained. Similarly, the patient is questioned about his sports.

Bladder Function. A careful history of the bladder function is taken. It is often found that there is some loss of muscular sphincter control, as well as the sense of fullness the patient feels. Questions may have to be asked about the patient's sexual function.

Systemic History. A systemic history of the heart, lungs, bowel function, and central nervous activity is taken. In some cases it may be necessary to question the patient about endocrine function.

Past Illnesses. A full knowledge of previous illnesses and operations is necessary to assess their part in the present disorder.

In most cases it will be found that after

a proper history is taken a presumptive diagnosis can be made and a plan drawn up for the management of the patient. If the doctor finds himself unable to reach an adequate conclusion at this stage, he is probably wiser to return to the patient's story. He will usually find that somewhere during the course of the consultation he has made an unwise assumption and so lost the thread of the patient's history. On occasion, the author has had to repeat the questioning of the patient, months after the treatment has begun, before he has understood the nature of the problem.

EXAMINATION

When the patient's symptoms are understood, the examination may begin. The purpose is to confirm the provisional diagnosis.

It is conventional to describe the examination of the patient under the headings of inspection, palpation, percussion, and auscultation. Many textbooks include clear descriptions of the examination. Hoppenfeld presented an admirable chapter on the subject, and his illustrations, in particular, are entertaining as well as helpful.[3] Apley, as always, is precise and systematic, while the addition of photographs to his book has added greatly to the reader's understanding.[1] Armstrong is authoritative, as one would expect from a man with such a wide experience of treating the lumbar spine.[2]

The author would prefer not to spoil the reader's pleasure in these three authors by repeating the details of examination. Instead, it will be approached, including those special investigations required to confirm the clinical diagnosis, from the viewpoint of some questions which require answers if the management of the patient is to be carried out.

These questions are:

Is the patient suffering from a sinister disease?

If not, is the patient suffering from mechanical derangement of one or more of the elements of the spine?

Can such derangement be classified according to one of the categories discussed in this book—*They are:* locking or swelling of a degenerate disc; prolapse of a disc, with nerve root involvement; intervertebral instability; spinal stenosis; or problems apart from disc disease?

The answer to these questions will usually give enough information to start nonoperative treatment. If conservative therapy fails and surgery is contemplated, the following further questions must be answered.

If disc prolapse has occurred, what is the level or levels of the lesion? Is prolapse central or lateral?

If the problem is one of vertebral instability, is it present at one or more intervertebral spaces? Is the instability one of forward or backward slide, tilting, or rotation?

If spinal stenosis is the cause of the trouble, what is the extent of compression? The answer to these questions will be discussed in turn.

The Signs of Sinister Disease

The possibility of neoplastic disease, either secondary or occurring primarily in the spine, always exists. Its rarity should cause the doctor to take more care in looking for it. Infections of the spine are still found, usually staphylococcal rather than tuberculous, while rare diseases such as hyperparathyroidism occasionally present.

Spasm is usually present in all planes of movement, unlike the patterns of mechanical derangement. In all such conditions local bone tenderness is obvious, in contradistinction to mechanical derangement, in which the tenderness is in the soft tissues between the bones.

Careful palpation of the breasts is essential, since carcinoma of the breast is probably the most common tumor presenting with metastases in the spine. All women over the age of 35 must have such an examination, even if they have no secondaries in the back. The occasional primary tumor will be found in this way.

Similarly, the abdomen and thyroid must be palpated adequately. Rectal and vaginal examination, when necessary, must not be forgotten.

All cases must have a full blood count and erythrocyte sedimentation rate at the first interview. The ESR has been found the most accurate screening test to exclude sinister pathology, especially in a busy clinic, provided the test is performed within a short time of the taking of the specimen. In two cases seen by the author, a condition of hyperparathyroidism was discovered as a result of persistently raised sedimentation rates, despite normal calcium levels at first.

Although 30 per cent of spinal metastases are not visible on routine roentgenography of the spinal bones, most cases of primary and secondary tumors will be discovered early.

Intervertebral Disc Prolapse

Posture. Inspection of the patient's standing posture will reveal most cases of lower lumbar disc prolapse.

Segmental kyphosis and spasm of the back muscles in the region of the affected joint usually suggest the lesion. Sciatic scoliosis with a tilt to "port" or starboard" makes the diagnosis almost certain. Alternating scoliosis, in which the patient adopts a unilateral sciatic tilt with spasm but can be persuaded by the examiner to straighten the tilt, with increasing difficulty until the back suddenly tilts to the opposite side, is pathognomonic. This deformity is probably due to incarceration of a nerve root on one side. As the back is extended, the prolapsed portion of the disc squeezes the nerve root ever tighter until the root suddenly slips over the fibrous lump and ends on the other side.

Figure 7-1 shows a patient with typical sciatic kyphoscoliosis as well as spasm of the muscles of the back, especially on the left. Three other features are obvious: the patient's pain is evident in his face; his flexed knees are an extreme form of loss of straight-leg raising, and his severe disability is revealed by his total dependence on a walking-stick to remain upright at all.

Movement. Few healthy people realize the disability that results when someone loses his normal easy gait because of reflex muscle spasm. The energy used in such a situation is probably 10 times as great as normal. The patient tires very quickly. If he is asked to walk, this is soon obvious.

The significant feature of lumbar spinal movement in disc prolapse is that some arcs of movement are normal, whereas others are markedly reduced. This confirms the mechanical nature of the condition. Usually the flexion-extension arc is grossly reduced, while lateral flexion to each side often takes place at different levels, but always well above the affected intervertebral space. Rotation is normal in at least one direction. The patient is then asked to lie supine so the legs can be examined.

Straight-Leg Raising. This can be tested firstly. Unilateral loss signifies prolapse lateral to the nerve root. Bilateral loss suggests more central prolapse in which the nerve roots to both legs are compressed.

Cross-leg pain is significant for two reasons. First it is thought to indicate "axillary" prolapse, in which the projecting portion of the prolapsed disc is caught in the axilla of the nerve root, which is stretched laterally over it.[2] Since the origin of the nerve root is in contact with the prolapse, the dural sheath is involved, and pain and spasm are severe. Such a sign may suggest slow resolution and, therefore, a greater likelihood of the case end-

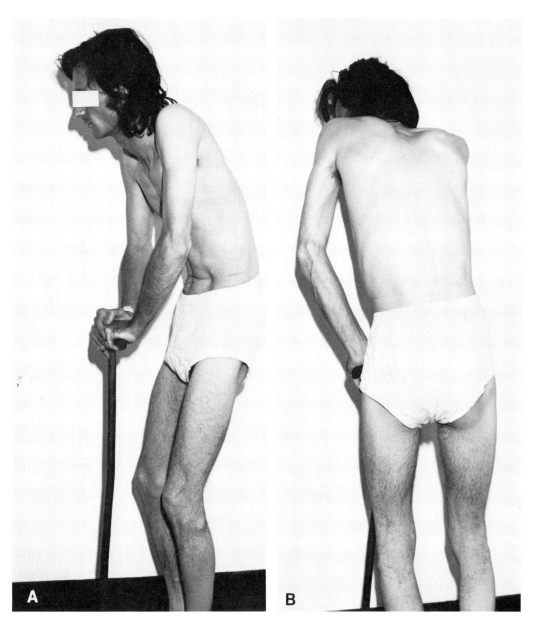

FIG. 7-1. Photographs of a 32-year-old man with severe disc prolapse. Signs included bilateral loss of straight-leg raising, cross-leg pain, and no ankle jerk on the left. The patient recovered well after removal of a large L5–S1 disc prolapse.

ing in operation. Secondly, cross-leg pain is pathognomonic of severe disc prolapse, while the distribution of the pain is usually so precise that the level of the prolapse can be diagnosed with confidence.

Nerve Root Signs. Altered sensation, loss of motor power, and reflex changes confirm the diagnosis of nerve root compression. Each root presents a different syndrome of functional loss: the 4th lumbar causes loss of the knee jerk, weakness of the tibialis anterior muscle and paresthesia on the medial side of the ankle and big toe; the 5th lumbar causes weakness of the extensor hallucis longus muscle and sensory changes on the dorsum of the foot; 1st sacral nerve root loss causes weakness of the peroneus longus and brevis muscles, absent ankle jerk, and altered sensation on the lateral side of the ankle, foot, and fifth toe.

The problem is, however, that nerve roots at more than one level may be implicated by a single prolapse. It is not a practical difficulty. Ninety per cent of disc prolapses occur at the L5–S1 level, while most of the rest are at both the L4–5 and L5–S1 levels. If both levels are routinely explored at operation, mistakes will not occur. Provided the ankle jerk is lost, there is sensory change in the little toe, and the extensor hallucis longus muscle power is reduced significantly on one side, not only has the diagnosis been made, but the levels of operation are confirmed. Myelography, with its attendant dangers, is unnecessary.

Mid-lumbar prolapse is much more rare and, if suspected, requires myelography before operation. Probably the most common presentation is loss of a knee jerk associated with a weak bladder.

Palpation of the Back. The importance of careful palpation of the anatomical features of the lumbar spine and pelvis cannot be overemphasized. The level of disc prolapse can be confidently predicted

Other Mechanical Derangements

The shape, posture, and deformity of the spine will aid diagnosis. There may be multiple lesions, so that diagnosis depends on a precise analysis of several deformities. Palpation of the spine and pelvis in a systematic, anatomical manner is a great help if there is no loss of straight-leg raising or nerve root signs.

Intervertebral instability can be diagnosed, as can such conditions as sacroiliac tenderness, especially if combined with pelvic stress pain. Coccygeal pain, trochanteric or ischial bursitis, or even muscle injuries, can be differentiated. Roentgenographs confirm the diagnosis.

Spinal Stenosis

Diagnosis can often be made by the appearance of increasing back or leg signs and symptoms on standing or walking. The effort tolerance can be measured accurately. Final diagnosis of spinal stenosis depends always on myelography, since a knowledge of the exact extent of the lesion is essential.

FACTORS AFFECTING PROGNOSIS IN DISC PROLAPSE

Mathews[4] has described a simple diagram which is very useful in assessing the seriousness of disc prolapse and consequently the prognosis of the condition.[4]

A modified diagram illustrates this (Fig. 7-2). It shows, in an abstract manner, that increasingly severe prolapse (represented by the three central arrows in the figure) is associated with greater injury to the annulus (represented by the dotted line). There are two significant features about the figure. First, it can be seen that as the prolapse increases in severity the patient's clinical signs change from mainly symptoms to mainly signs. This fact is of great help in determining prognosis. It can be seen that the signs and symptoms are

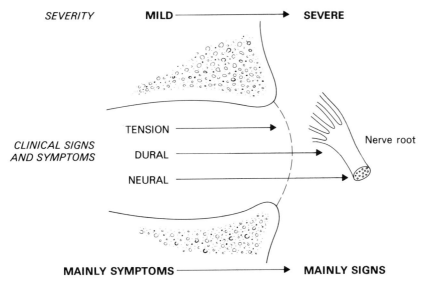

Fig. 7-2. The relation between signs and symptoms, their cause, and the severity of the syndrome. (Adapted from Matthews, J. A.: Symposium on lumbar intervertebral disc lesions. I. A rheumatologist's point of view. Rheumatol. Rehab., *14*:160, 1975.)

of three orders of severity, depending on their anatomical basis. The least serious may be called *articular* signs, arising as they do from the stretched and inflamed annulus. They consist of pain and spasm in the back and buttock. At the next level of severity the signs are *dural,* that is, they are caused by stretching and irritation of the dural sheath. In the most severe cases, the signs and symptoms are *neural* in origin, caused by stretching or compression of the nerve roots.

Gauging Response to Treatment

There are three other ways that the surgeon can estimate the patient's response to treatment. Only the first is objective, but all three are surprisingly accurate as prognosticators:

Straight-Leg Raising. This test is not only of great value in diagnosis of nerve root compression, but since it can be measured accurately by means of a goniometer, is a very useful indicator of the state of the nerve root and, therefore, of the extent of the prolapse and how it is shrinking.

Cough Pain. The severity of the pain on coughing should be estimated and recorded—both the strength of the cough required to cause pain and the severity of the response as elicited from the patient.

"Disability Percentage." Some patients, if asked to estimate their percentage of disability, will be able to arrive at a subjective figure that can be of much help to the doctor. Records of repeated estimates by the patient often reveal a very smooth natural curve in the graph of their recovery.

CASE 7-1. There may be multiple lesions, not even confined to the back, so that a precise analysis depends upon the careful consideration of many deformities. Figure 7-3 shows a 64-year-old woman who complained of severe back pain. She was found to be suffering from

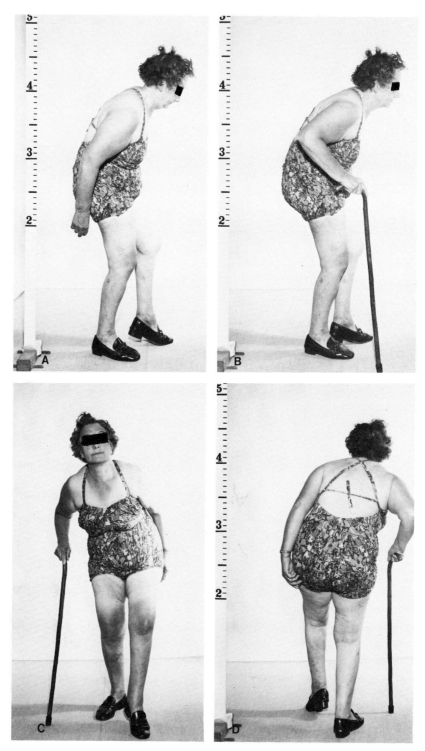

FIG. 7-3. Gross lumbar instability due to flexion deformity of hips following osteomalacia. Right total hip replacement was performed.

severe generalized lumbar spondylosis with instability at several levels. Further questioning revealed that in 1942 she was widowed soon after the birth of her only child and suffered severe malnutrition for a year. As a result she developed osteomalacia, and her pelvis collapsed until the acetabula had migrated almost into the pelvic brim. The resultant fixed flexion deformity was more marked on the left. With the gradual superimposition of osteoarthritis of the hips, unstable collapse of the lumbar spine occurred. Right total hip replacement allowed her to adopt a posture sufficiently erect to prevent further spinal collapse. Two years later the condition of her back is unchanged.

REFERENCES

1. Apley, A. G.: A system of Orthopeadics and Fractures ed. 3. London, Butterworth, 1968.
2. Armstrong, J. R.: Lumbar Disc Lesions. Edinburgh, E. &. S. Livingstone, 1965.
3. Hoppenfeld, S.: Physical Examination of the Spine and Extremities. New York, Appleton-Century-Crofts, 1976.
4. Mathews, J. A.: Symposium on lumbar intervertebral disc lesions. A rheumatologist's point of view. Rheumatol. Rehab., *14*:160, 1975.

8 The Modulation of Pain

J. Hannington-Kiff

The relief of chronic pain remains a relatively underdeveloped area, largely because it has not received the attention that it merits. While it is reasonable to view pain as only the symptom of an underlying disease process in conditions which are amenable to medical or surgical cure, it is unhelpful when the cause of the pain is ill-understood or incurable. In this case the relief of pain must become the center of our attention, rather as a discipline in its own right. The majority of patients with chronic backache require conservative treatment, and no single specific measure will cure them of pain. Treatment in these cases is directed to finding a suitable plan of medication and other maneuvers that will relieve or modulate pain—a strategy that often will be based on trial and error. The main objectives of this chapter are to promote the better understanding of pain in general and to discuss the wide array of methods available to ease chronic pain.

THE NATURE OF PAIN

The highly subjective nature of pain makes it hard for us to communicate about it. Both clinical and scientific discussions are complicated by the words we use in reference to pain, which reflect personal, cultural, educational, emotional, and other values. Aristotle believed that pain should not be included with vision, hearing, smell, taste, and touch as a primary sensation but should be considered rather as an agony of the mind. Certainly there is no one-to-one relationship between a potentially painful stimulus and the pain felt by the individual. For example, a severely injured man in a car crash made no complaint of pain but worried instead only about the members of his family who were still trapped in the wreckage. Some days later in hospital, when he was fully aware that his family had survived the crash, he was full of complaints about pain from this and that source, all of which were quite minor compared with the initial injuries. Evidently, the mental state can greatly influence whether or not the patient feels pain, and this must be taken into consideration when he is being treated.

THEORIES OF PAIN

There are three principal theories of pain, which may be called, for convenience, specificity theory, pattern theory, and modulation theory. A more detailed account is given elsewhere.[1]

Specificity Theory

The specificity theory is the classical view that proposes that there are specific receptors for pain (as there are for other

120

sensory modalities), with specific connections in the central nervous system which process information relating to pain only. These pain receptors are thought to be the free nerve endings of unmyelinated and finely myelinated nerve fibers. There is modern evidence that a small proportion of unmyelinated nerve fibers have exceptionally high thresholds, but these cannot be called pain fibers. There is also evidence of specificity among unmyelinated fibers—to cold for instance—but this seems to be the exception rather than the rule. A disadvantage of the specificity theory is that it proposes to separate the central nervous system into a multiple channel system in which the possibilities of integration are limited.

Pattern Theory

This questions the classical view that there are separate receptors and pathways for various cutaneous sensory modalities, such as light touch, deep touch, vibration, pain, warmth, and cold. It is a failing of language that we refer to nervous pathways and centers in the nervous system in terms of these modalities; and the pattern theory strives to correct this by postulating that different sensations are the result of the interpretation by the central nervous system of spatiotemporal patterns of a great variety of nerve impulses. In these circumstances, pain is considered to be the result of patterns set up in the central nervous system by intense stimulation of nonspecific receptors. However, the pattern theory is an oversimplification and does not sufficiently take into account the known physiological and anatomical specialization of certain receptors. An advantage of the pattern theory is that it emphasizes that the central nervous system acts as a coordinated whole at all levels.

Modulation Theory

The correct hypothesis probably lies somewhere between the specificity and pattern theories. For the working of a system as complex as the central nervous system, which must revise its activity in keeping with current events, neither theory is sufficiently comprehensive. Inescapably, theories about the function of the central nervous system will evolve from the model of a telephone exchange, with fixed terminals and relatively limited patterns of wires, to the sophisticated models of systems engineering. One of the first requirements in any system that is subjected to a continuous barrage of information is the reduction in the input of this information by selection at its source. So great is the input of information from all regions of the body that the central nervous system could not work purposefully unless input were heavily selected at the periphery. The clinical application of this principle of input control has become the basis of new methods of modulating the central nervous system to relieve pain. This will be discussed later.

One of the first references to input control was made at the turn of the century by Head and Rivers, to explain their clinical findings during the regeneration of a cutaneous nerve in Head's forearm.[2] They found that the return of sensation to the denervated region was in two stages. Firstly, after a few weeks, crude sensation returned to the area. Light touch was not felt, and pain was not readily aroused, but when it did occur it was of a particularly nasty, diffuse type. They called this type of sensation "protopathic." Secondly, after a further delay of several months, normal sensitivity returned to the area. Light touch could be felt, and pain of the expected intensity was normally aroused. The discriminating sensation which was necessary to restore the normal state of affairs was called "epicritic sensation." Head and Rivers made the interesting suggestion that the epicritic innervation had a controlling effect on the protopathic sensation. Their choice of terms shows how much they were influenced by ideas of evolution at the time: protopathic sensation was considered the primitive condition and epicritic sensation was, phylogenetically, a later addition. Had these workers been given the advantage of modern physiological knowledge, they might well have concluded that epicritic sensation is subserved by thick, myelinated nerve fibers and protopathic by thin, myelinated and unmyelinated nerve fibers. Thereby they would have anticipated the more recently introduced concept that activity in thick, myelinated nerve fibers can suppress that in thin myelinated and unmyelinated nerve fibers which are closely involved with the experience of pain.[4] Noordenbos has shown that there is a relative deficit of thick, myelinated nerve fibers in the in-

tercostal nerve affected by postherpetic neuralgia. He suggested that the reason that stimulation of the affected skin gives rise to abnormal sensations, including nasty diffuse (protopathic) pain, in this condition is that the thin, myelinated and unmyelinated nerve fibers have readier access to the central nervous system. Consequently, even light stimulation may give rise to pain.

The site of this peripheral input control, exerted by the larger myelinated nerve fibers over the thin, myelinated and unmyelinated nerve fibers is probably in the dorsal horn of the spinal grey matter. Melzack and Wall have suggested that the cells of the substantia gelatinosa act as a gate that controls the afferent impulses as they pass through to the more deeply

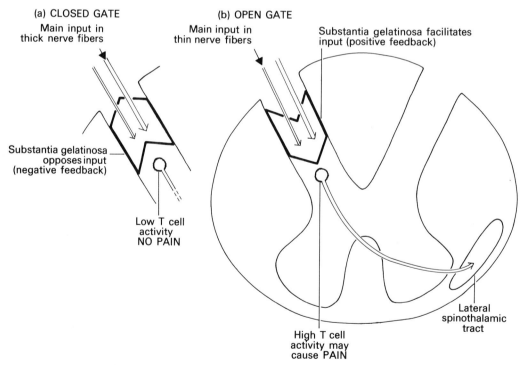

FIG. 8-1. *(a)* Closed gate: Significant afferent activity in the thick, myelinated nerve fibers causes a build-up of negative feedback in the substantia gelatinosa, which then inhibits the passage of further impulses to the T-cells in any type of nerve fiber. *(b)* Open gate: Afferent activity, mainly in the thin, myelinated and the unmyelinated nerve fibers, induces a positive feedback in the substantia gelatinosa that facilitates the passage of all neural traffic to the T-cells, the consequence of which may be pain.

placed first transmission cells (T cells) that give rise to the lateral spinothalamic tract, the classical ascending pain pathway (Fig. 8-1).[3] The arrival of sufficient impulses in the thick, myelinated nerve fibers as part of the physiological barrage normally entering the dorsal horn tends to activate a negative feedback in the substantia gelatinosa, which has the effect of closing the gate to all further input. (Fig. 8-1A). Thus the afferent impulses caused by a mild to moderate stimulus, while first stimulating the T cells, soon become ineffective. The gating mechanism can be overcome by an intense stimulus that activates a lot of thin, myelinated and unmyelinated nerve fibers, which have a higher threshold, because these fibers cause positive feedback in the substantia gelatinosa. In this way the gate is opened to allow the free access of all afferent input to the T cells, the high activity of which may be interpreted as pain by the brain (Fig. 8-1B). Since thick, myelinated nerve fibers adapt more quickly than thin, myelinated or unmyelinated nerve fibers (unless the nature of the stimulation is an intermittent one such as vibration), a prolonged, even stimulus of lesser intensity can also produce the conditions which give rise to pain. This may partly explain why physiotherapy with simple mechanical vibrators can temporarily ease the pain of rheumatism, chronic backache, and other types of moderate pain. The above arguments also help to explain why rubbing or tapping around an injured area can alleviate pain.

The peripheral gate control is itself under the overall control of descending influences from the higher centers, and it is therefore possible to envisage how a subject can consciously or unconsciously modulate the very input which subserves pain. While these ideas are not fully substantiated and accepted, they provide a very powerful theory to guide our thoughts until more is known. For instance, a corollary of the gate control theory is that any stimulation that selectively activates the thicker myelinated nerve fibers will close the gate in the dorsal horn and inhibit pain. This has proved to be the case in practice and has led to the introduction of simple electrical apparatus which has successfully relieved pain in selected patients. This sort of argument may also explain the mode of action of acupuncture in the relief of pain.

BIOCHEMICAL MEDIATION OF PAIN

The preceding neurophysiological theories of pain fail to take into account the known substances which are released by tissue damage and are capable of sensitizing or stimulating nerve endings to cause pain. This tissue mediation of pain can be the result of ionic changes in the extracellular fluid, as when potassium ions are released from damaged cells or when anaerobic tissue metabolism raises the hydrogen ion level locally. There is also some evidence that a raised level of ionized calcium can increase the sensitivity of nerve endings to pain.

It is likely that a key role will be found for prostaglandins, which are universally released by injured tissues. Prostaglandins sensitize nerve endings to a variety of other substances, such as bradykinin, histamine, and 5-hydroxytryptamine, which are also released during inflammation of tissues and are capable of stimulating nerve endings to cause pain. Aspirin and related antiinflammatory agents are known to suppress the synthesis of prostaglandin and to block the action of bradykinin, which probably accounts for their efficacy in the treatment of chronic inflammatory conditions like rheumatoid arthritis.

The free nerve endings of unmyelinated and thin, myelinated nerves are directly exposed to many tissue mediators, and high activity in such nerve fibers would tend to open the dorsal horn gate and signal pain.

NEURAL INTEGRATION OF PAIN

In the past there has been a tendency to consider the spinal cord largely as a conduit to the brain, but now it is known that it can modulate the input of information, as discussed in the previous section. Our knowledge of the spinal white and grey matter is still rather limited. The principal "pain pathway" relays in the base of the dorsal horn, crosses the midline in the anterior white commissure and ascends in the anterolateral quadrant (ALQ) of the white matter of the opposite side of the spinal cord in the so-called lateral spinothalamic tract. This is a misnomer, as the spinothalamic tract carries relatively few fibers directly to the thalamus and is a composite tract, comprising at least spinotectal, spinoreticular, spinorubral, and spinovestibular pathways. In addition to these ascending fibers in the anterolateral quadrants of the spinal white matter, some information about pain is also carried in the exteroceptive nerve fibers of the dorsal columns. The nerve fibers in the ALQ carry information in a well organized, uninterrupted manner to the brain stem nuclei and neothalamus, whence it is relayed to the cerebral cortex. They are relatively fast-conducting and serve to identify and localize the noxious stimuli. The selective destruction of the ALQ fibers, at open operation or percutaneously with electrodes, is an effective method of relieving severe pain in suitable patients.

Exteroceptive nerve fibers in the dorsal columns provide another fast, uninterrupted, ascending path. Having a particularly well organized somatotopical mapping onto the neothalamus and thence to the postcentral gyrus, they are capable of giving a rapid, accurately-located assessment of potentially painful stimuli. Antidromic stimulation of these dorsal column fibers by implanted electrodes has been used successfully to relieve chronic pain. The ALQ and dorsal column fibers are collectively called the oligosynaptic ascending system (OAS).

In addition to these long, uninterrupted paths to the thalamus and brainstem nuclei, there exist multisynaptic chains of neurones around the grey matter of the cord, which are also thought to subserve pain. These slow conducting paths, which constitute the multisynaptic ascending system (MAS), lack a somatotopical organization and probably contribute to the diffuse, persistent quality of pain. Information in these multisynaptic paths probably projects to the paleothalamus, and the subsequent radiation to the limbic system would account for the profound emotional effects of pain. The principal action of the opiates is on this multisynaptic path and its central connections.

THE CLINICAL EVALUATION OF PAIN

In the first instance a doctor has only the patient's history to guide him in the diagnosis of pain, and much of diagnostic value can be learned from carefully noting the actual words used by the patient to describe his pain. With a little prompting, the doctor should be able to establish the following features of the pain: location, quality, intensity, time-relations, modifying factors, and associated physiological changes. It is important to record relevant negative, as well as positive, findings.

If a feature associated with the pain is measurable, then measure it, remembering that in many instances when pain is unilateral individual variation can be overcome by using the opposite side of the body as a control. Repeatable measurements can be invaluable in the assessment of progress in chronic pain. Quantification of the feeling of pain by the patient is difficult, but a simple method is to ask the patient to mark off on a 10-centimeter line his estimate of the degree of his pain, knowing that the beginning of the line represents no pain and the other end the worst imaginable pain. Such measurements are of most value when repeated over a long period, when trends in relation to various trials of therapy may be compared.

THE MANAGEMENT OF PAIN BY OBJECTIVES

It is helpful in treatment to consider that pain is a complex feeling with physical, emotional, rational, and social components (Fig. 8-2). This view not only emphasizes that the successful relief of pain requires the sympathetic handling of the whole patient but also supplies the basic objectives for our management of protracted pain.

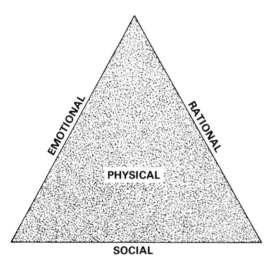

FIG. 8-2. The Pain Triangle: a representation of the four interacting attributes of pain, each of which requires attention in the successful management of the agonized patient. As a basis for argument, it may be envisaged that the reduction of one or more of the triangle's boundaries, comprising three of the attributes, will diminish the physical component of pain, which corresponds to the area of the triangle. Conversely, it may be seen that the greater the physical component of the pain, the greater will be the dimensions of the three associated attributes.

THE PHYSICAL COMPONENT

The physical component of pain may be reduced by either removing the underlying noxious stimuli or preventing the neural integration of the pain.

Removal of Noxious Stimuli

Removing noxious stimuli is the immediate aim of both patient and doctor. A patient in severe pain from nerve root pressure caused by acute prolapse of a lumbar intervertebral disc will usually take to his bed to reduce the load on the spine and thus the protrusion of the disc. The surgeon may decide to remove the offending intervertebral disc at laminectomy. The greatest difficulty in the relief of pain arises when no such clear diagnosis or solution is possible. This is all too common in chronic low-key backache. Recourse must then be had to methods of modulating the pain as much as possible.

Prevention of Neural Integration of Pain

Natural Defenses. Pain may be the result of disproportionately raised activity in thin nerve fibers and can sometimes be inhibited by raising the level of activity in thick nerve fibers. It is common experience that rubbing and other counterirritation in the area of an injury can ease pain by diversifying the regional neural traffic following the stimulation of larger nerve fibers. Thick, myelinated nerve fibers are readily stimulated, but they adapt with similar ease, unless the stimulation is varied and intermittent: the objective of the physiotherapist (and the acupuncturist) is usually to apply mild, intermittent stimulation by manipulation or with the aid of apparatus.

Analgesics. Antipyretic analgesics, of which aspirin is the most commonly used, have their main effect by inhibiting the synthesis of prostaglandins and blocking the action of bradykinin, as described above. These substances probably account for the hyperalgesia associated with inflammation and explain why antipyretic analgesics are so effective in inflammatory diseases such as rheumatoid arthritis. Thus the action of antipyretic analgesics is likely to be almost entirely peripheral, whereas the opiates act more centrally at synapses. Morphine particularly affects the multisynaptic ascending system and its diffuse paleothalamic projections to the general cortex and limbic system, so that its administration causes profound central nervous effects like euphoria and detachment as well as analgesia.

Local anesthetics can be used to block the conduction of nerve impulses in the peripheral nerves and the spinal cord. Unmyelinated and thin, myelinated nerve fibers have a large surface area in relation to their volume and are therefore more susceptible to local anesthetics than thick, myelinated nerve fibers. Consequently, a weak concentration of a local anesthetic agent can be found which will block selectively the fine nerve fibers that subserve pain without causing general sensory loss and motor weakness. A single injection, or a course of injections, of a local anesthetic can produce relief of chronic pain, especially when it involves the musculoskeletal system, which long outlasts the duration of pharmacological action of the drug and, occasionally, the relief is permanent. Local anesthetic blocks are often done for diagnostic and prognostic reasons in patients with intractable cancer pain, but even then there occurs the exceptional case of prolonged pain relief. These instances demonstrate that pain is sometimes a self-perpetuating functional disorder, the cycle of which can be interrupted.

Drastic Measures. In some cancer patients there may be indications for drastic measures which permanently interrupt the regional pathway subserving intractable pain. These measures comprise the selective destruction of the nervous system with neurolytic agents such as alcohol and phenol, high frequency electrical currents, radiation, and neurosurgery. Less drastic procedures, such as barbotage of the spinal column with its own cerebrospinal fluid, hypertonic saline, or ice-cold saline, can sometimes give a relatively prolonged period of pain relief, but they are usually less effective than those procedures which divide central nervous pathways.

THE EMOTIONAL COMPONENT

The emotional component grows in proportion to the severity, the duration, and the significance of the pain. Its contribution to chronic pain may be reduced in a number of ways.

Psychological Support

Chronic pain causes much anxiety, especially when a patient knows that no cure can be expected and that he must learn to live with at least some degree of pain for the rest of his life. In these circumstances a good doctor-patient relationship is of inestimable value. If the patient is given an unhurried explanation of the cause of his pain and the opportunity to discuss the outlook for the future in words which he can really understand, he may be able to come to terms with his pain. We all have the power consciously to control our emotions to a degree, and, with practice and psychological support from a confident person, we can improve this ability. This power of inner control is epitomized by the transcendental state, and it is interesting to speculate whether suitable subjects could be taught to attain at least a degree of the transcendental state by the technique of biofeedback and so learn to alleviate their pain.

Drug Therapy

Much of the relief afforded by the opiates in chronic pain is the result of synaptic depression in the diffuse connections between the paleothalamus, the limbic lobe, the temporal lobe, the prefrontal lobe, and the hypothalamus, which form the neural basis of the emotional attribute of pain. Drugs have now been synthesized which have a more specific and selective effect on these parts of the brain: for instance, diazepam acts mainly on the limbic lobe and selectively affects the underlying amygdala. This minor tranquilizer is a most useful adjuvant in the relief of chronic pain and can be used to supplement a mild analgesic like aspirin to match more closely the effect of a narcotic analgesic, the administration of which can thereby be postponed or even avoided.

In the relief of severe pain, a major tranquilizer such as chlorpromazine can be used to potentiate a narcotic analgesic, the dosage of which can then be kept to a minimum. The effects of chlorpromazine in the central nervous system are more diffuse than those of diazepam and probably result from widespread inhibition of the brain stem reticular formation and suppression of hypothalamic activity. However, chronic pain can cause depression, and, when this is suspected, the patient's mental condition and reaction to pain can sometimes be improved by elevating the mood with an antidepressant like imipramine. Sometimes electroconvulsive therapy is helpful in this form of reactive depression. The placebo effect of drugs and other forms of therapy should not be forgotten, and occasionally this effect can be put to good use in the management of the emotional component of pain.

Psychosurgery

In extreme cases prefrontal leukotomy has been employed to produce psychological indifference to intractable pain. This procedure was first introduced in an attempt to alter for the better the personality of psychotic patients, but occasional disastrous results have limited its use. To relieve the effects of severe pain the operation has to be more extensive, and the risk of wrecking the personality is so great that it is questionable whether this operation should continue to be used for this purpose. More selective operations on the limbic system, such as cingulotomy, are preferable; but any decision to undertake psychosurgery for the relief of pain should be considered most carefully.

THE RATIONAL COMPONENT

To some degree all patients can obtain relief of pain, in a sense, by accepting their pain and learning to live with it. This personal compromise can be promoted in a number of ways.

Doctor-Patient Relationship

A good relationship between doctor and patient can be most rewarding by giving the patient the best opportunity of evaluating his pain against the background of accurate full information. It is extraordinary but understandable that patients often have irrational fears based on half-truths that they have picked up from well-meaning friends and relatives about their "condition." A patient may suspect that his pain is due to cancer and be afraid to ask the doctor directly about it, in a way not wishing to know the worst. He may suspect that everyone knows and that either nobody has the courage to mention it or that his family is trying to protect him from this knowledge. These tortuous thoughts can be banished in the right circumstances by a sympathetic discussion with the family doctor, who knows the patient's background. The patient may have cancer yet have a good prognosis and will be pleasantly surprised to be told this by his doctor. Cancer is still generally regarded as a rapidly progressive condition and a death sentence to be particularly feared as a terrible ending to life.

Occupational Therapy

Distraction will often reduce the feeling of pain, and a good way of promoting this effect is the involvement of the patient in an interesting hobby which requires dexterity rather than mental concentration. Consequently, occupational therapy can be very useful in the management of some patients with chronic pain. The value of such therapy may be acknowledged by the patient only in retrospect when it is pointed out to him that several hours have passed without his having been troubled by pain. It is possible that distraction works by keeping parts of the brain busy which would otherwise be involved in the neural integration of pain, for the central nervous system can only deal consciously or unconsciously with a certain number of "bits" of information at any one time.

Group Therapy

I have found that a form of group therapy in which patients with similar pains are encouraged to meet and swap experiences can lead to an increase in their morale and some alleviation of their suffering. Such groups can be "seeded" with at least one happy extrovert who will encourage the others. It is so easy for a patient who is relatively isolated by chronic pain to lose sight of the fact that others may be similarly blighted; and it is human nature to take courage from the afflictions of others. In this way a patient can often get his pain into perspective and learn to live with the fact that he will have to put up with some degree of pain, perhaps for the rest of his life.

THE SOCIAL COMPONENT

Our personal and communal reactions to the problems of chronic pain are strongly influenced by the conventions of the society in which we live. The word pain is derived from the Greek for penalty, which in itself reveals the mental association of pain with punishment and retribution in a spiritual sense. A glimpse of this attitude is provided by the religious and moral opposition which greeted the inception of obstetric analgesia in our society in the middle of the 19th century. How much of this type of prejudice remains today in relation to terminal pain? The social attribute of pain will be discussed here under two main headings: the family and the community.

The Family

Individual reaction to pain depends to some extent on behavioral patterns that are laid down in infancy and childhood. An anxious mother may teach a youngster to overact to the slightest injury, and this type of response will then be typical of that individual as an adult. The opposite, of course, will be true of the child with a stoical upbringing. Some families seem to be predisposed to pain, which may be due not only to acquired behavior patterns but to inherited conditions that are not completely understood.

The Community

Cultural pressures from infancy, exerted through the family from the community, probably account for the characteristic attitudes adopted by different races toward pain. This is perhaps the main reason that acupuncture analgesia is much more successful in the Far East than in the West. In many primitive societies initiation ceremonies involve the infliction of pain which must be tolerated bravely. It is possible that the strong motivation in these circumstances actively dulls the perception of pain and alters its meaning, so that the initiates do not have to tolerate what appears to the onlooker to be such a high degree of pain. Overcoming pain in this way can instill confidence and help to build character for the adult life to come.

To the misery of chronic pain can be added that of isolation from the community, which can arise for a number of reasons: the individual may be confined in his activities and unintentionally unsociable because of his continued pain; and the patient who is on large doses of drugs will inevitably be either withdrawn or odd in his behavior. In turn, the community may choose to shun patients in chronic pain from a sense of helplessness as much as indifference. Backache is the most common way in which individuals misuse the complaint of pain to retaliate against a society that has made welfare payments comparable with earned income.

THE USE OF ANALGESICS

The proper use of analgesics is, regrettably, not part of the undergraduate curriculum and only exceptionally do newly

Classification of Analgesics

Antipyretic Analgesics
   Salicylic acid derivatives
      aspirin
      Paracetamol
   Aniline derivatives
      Phenacetin*†
   Pyrazole derivatives
      Phenylbutazone
      Oxyphenbutazone
   Indole derivatives
      Indomethacin
   Anthranillic acid derivatives
      Mefenamic acid
      Flufenamic acid
Narcotic Analgesics
   Morphine group
      Natural derivatives
         Papaveretum*
         Morphine
         Codeine*
      Synthetic derivatives
         Diamorphine
         Phenazocine
         Oxycodone
         Levorphanol
         Pentazocine*
         Dihydrocodeine*
   Meperidine group
      Pethidine
      (Demerol)
      Fentanyl
      Phenoperidine
      Ethoheptazine*
   Methadone group
      Methadone
      Dipipanone
      Dextromoramide
      Dextropropoxyphene*

*Often used in mixtures with aspirin or paracetamol
†Phenacetin is no longer recommended because of the high risk of renal damage associated with its use.

qualified doctors obtain experience of the handling of analgesics other than for premedication or postoperative care. In other words, they will have some knowledge of the effects of analgesics in acute pain, but this is quite inappropriate to the needs of patients with chronic pain.

It behooves the doctor who has to care for patients with chronic severe pain to get to know a few drugs very well and to be aware of the best routes and the correct timings for their administration. For example, should an oral narcotic analgesic be required in the treatment of chronic severe pain it is quite common for meperidine (Demerol) to be prescribed. It is a poor choice, as this drug is unreliable by mouth and is short-acting. Injection of meperidine is quite painful, can cause hypotension, and tends to produce dysphoria rather than euphoria. These are some of the disadvantages that rule out this drug in the treatment of chronic pain.

The comments which follow are intended to highlight the salient features of the progressive management of patients with increasingly severe chronic pain. A simple classification of analgesics is given below.

Antipyretic Analgesics

Aspirin and Paracetamol. The analgesic effects of aspirin, which is probably the most widely used panacea, should not be underrated. It can be effective in all types of pain and should be thought of as the first line of analgesic therapy, although its effect is greatest in somatic pain and least in visceral pain. Slightly greater analgesia can be obtained by increasing the standard dose from 600 mg. (two tablets, B.P.) to 900 mg. (three tablets, B.P.) at 4-hourly intervals; above this dosage side effects become troublesome, with little or no increase in analgesia. A good-quality soluble preparation of aspirin should be prescribed, and sensible proprietary preparations should not be looked upon with disdain: many patients who cannot tolerate cheap aspirin preparations have no difficulty with the prolonged administration of the better products. Aspirin is best given with meals, to avoid gastric irritation, and the risk of gastrointestinal bleeding should be borne in mind during prolonged administration. Paracetamol, the dose of which is 1,000 mg. (two tablets, B.P.), is a useful alternative to aspirin; it is preferred by those who claim it has a lesser incidence of gastric irritation than aspirin.

Fortified Aspirin and Paracetamol Preparations. Analgesic action of aspirin and paracetamol can be fortified by the addition of codeine, dihydrocodeine, propoxyphene, or pentazocine. Again it is emphasized that good-quality soluble preparations should be used for prolonged administration, although the mobile patient may wish to keep a few insoluble (noneffervescent) tablets in pocket or handbag for those occasions when soluble tablets are inconvenient.

There is often indecision about replacing these fortified aspirin or paracetamol mixtures with narcotic analgesics when something stronger is required. This decision-gap may be bridged by the use of higher doses of codeine, dihydrocodeine, propoxyphene or pentazocine; but the results of this can be disappointing, and the unwanted effects of these drugs can often offset the moderate increase in analgesia. Alternately, a minor tranquilizer of the benzodiazepine group (such as chlordiazepoxide, diazepam, medazepam, and oxazepam) may be added to the established nonnarcotic analgesic regimen.

Narcotic Analgesics

Although it is better to postpone the use of these powerful drugs, because of the mental clouding and psychological and physical dependence which they produce, their administration should not be withheld needlessly. This crucial decision must be made according to the circumstances and should not be prejudiced by irrational fears of addiction. It is not sufficiently realized by doctors in general that psychological dependence on narcotics is less of a problem in agonized patients than in the population as a whole: most patients who are being treated for chronic pain with an opiate readily accept a reduction in the dosage if, for any reason, the pain is much reduced. For instance, if an amenable pain is successfully stopped by percutaneous cordotomy, the patient can nearly always be weaned off the previously high doses of a narcotic analgesic without trouble. The patient is often keen to do this himself once his pain has been relieved; for example, a patient who was an avid reader could not stop taking narcotic analgesics quickly enough because these drugs had affected his vision and taken away his greatest delight in life. Of course, in terminal patients the risk of addiction is a relatively unimportant consideration, and even here any craving of the patient for his next dose of narcotic can be minimized by a flexible and regular regimen of administration.

Morphine is still the most commonly used analgesic in the treatment of severe pain and is the standard against which all other analgesics are tested. Pharmacologically, it produces an interesting combination of depression and excitation in the central nervous system. Its depressant action promotes analgesia, tranquilization, sleep, respiratory depression, and suppression of cough. Its excitatory action can cause vomiting by stimulation of chemoreceptors in the medullary vomiting center, and stimulation of other parts of the brain may cause anxiety and restlessness. Morphine has a direct effect on the bowel, increasing the tone of sphincters and decreasing peristalsis, so that constipation can be a troublesome effect of repeated administration. The most serious complication in the general use of morphine is, of course, the risk of addiction.

Papaveretum, B.P., an injectable aqueous extract of opium, owes its analgesic action mainly to its morphine content, although it contains codeine and other alkaloids. About 20 mg. of papaveretum are equivalent to 10 mg. of morphine in analgesic potency. It is popular with British anesthetists for premedication and postoperative analgesia. A useful oral preparation for the control of chronic and terminal pain contains 10 mg. of paraveretum with 500 mg. of soluble aspirin per tablet in an effervescent base. The usual dose is two tablets dissolved in water, which can be flavored with domestic fruit drinks.

Diamorphine (heroin), which is simply prepared by the double acetylation of morphine, is the best of all for easing the terminal stages of malignant disease. It is a more powerful analgesic than morphine and provides a high degree of euphoria without as much sedation. It also causes less nausea and vomiting than morphine. The lower incidence of unpleasant effects and the high degree of euphoria with a relatively clear mind make it a very considerable addiction risk, for which reason its sale and manufacture are prohibited in the United States of America. However, the bad reputation of this drug compared with morphine may be due more to its unfortunate history than to its high potential for addiction. Diamorphine causes more suppression of the cough reflex than morphine and is consequently very useful for treating intractable cough in patients with malignancy affecting the respiratory tract. Like morphine it causes constipation. A disadvantage in some circumstances is that diamorphine is relatively short-acting, lasting about 2 hours, as opposed to about 4 hours for morphine. A more serious disadvantage is that, unlike morphine, diamorphine is unstable in solution: solutions for injection are best prepared from freeze-dried powder in the ampule before use, and solutions for oral administration should not be kept for more than a few days.

Other Narcotic Analgesics. Although of interest, the array of synthetic potent analgesics which are now available will not be discussed here. However it is worth making one or two comments. Should a patient being treated for severe chronic pain particularly require a clear mind, methadone may be the drug of choice. Diamorphine, as has been mentioned, produces little clouding of consciousness, but the doctor may prefer to keep this drug for terminal cases. Methadone has less risk of addiction than morphine and diamorphine, which is an important consideration when a long period of analgesic treatment is required in an ambulatory patient with good life expectancy. Addiction to morphine can be treated by the gradual substitution of high doses of methadone: when the craving for morphine has waned, the methadone dosage can be progressively decreased without causing such unpleasant withdrawal symptoms as those associated with morphine (or diamorphine). Other members of the methadone group of analgesics are dextramoramide, dipipanone, and propoxyphene, all of which are effective by mouth and have a place in the treatment of chronic pain.

ADMINISTRATION OF ANALGESICS

Dosage

Small doses of drugs give less unwanted effects than large doses, and more frequent administration of a reduced dose is often better and more effective than full dosage at 4- to 6-hour intervals. It is sometimes feared that a patient will have no confidence in a newly prescribed drug if it is given in hardly effective doses but the doctor must explain to the patient the importance of measured progress with potent drugs: we are, after all, dealing with the complex interaction of a pharmacologic agent and an individual, and feedback is necessary to establish the best dose, which will not be supplied by a book or a schedule.

The dose of a narcotic analgesic can often be kept to a minimum by the concomitant use of a major transquilizer like chlorpromazine, which potentiates its effect. However, the mixing of drugs can lead to complications; for example, a mistake to avoid in narcotic analgesic therapy is the administration of pentazocine (Fortral, Talwin) which, aside from being an analgesic, is a weak morphine antagonist and may therefore counteract the effects of concurrent opiate analgesic therapy. Pentazocine can even precipitate withdrawal symptoms in a patient on opiate therapy.

Route Selection

Whenever possible the oral route should be used, both for logistical reasons and comfort of the patient. An alternative method of administration which avoids the need for injection is the rectal route: it is most appropriate in bed-ridden patients or for ambulatory patients at night. Several analgesics are available commercially in suppository form, and it is always possible to get other drugs made up into suppositories by a pharmacist. The value of the rectal route is better appreciated on the continent of Europe than in the United Kingdom. Oxycodone pectinate, a sustained-release compound of a potent analgesic, is particularly useful in suppository form and can provide 8 to 14 hours of analgesia—ideal for tiding the patient with intractable pain over the night without disturbing him to administer the usual 4-hourly dose of opiate or other drug. It should not be forgotten that short periods of intense analgesia, to cover physiotherapy or the movement of the patient in bed, can be provided by the inhalation of Entonox (an equal mixture of nitrous oxide and oxygen from one cylinder) or trichloroethylene. A suitable narcotic analgesic can be given by the intravenous route, either as a bolus injection from a syringe to give immediate potent action or as a slow infusion of a dilute solution to give a relatively prolonged, controllable effect for a day or two.

Time Relations

Timing of the administration of drugs is also very important in the relief of chronic severe pain. Doctors in training learn the management of pain in the postoperative care of patients whose pain is getting less as their wounds heal. In these circumstances it is perhaps reasonable, but by no means ideal, to prescribe drugs p.r.n. 4- to 6-hourly. This sort of schedule is definitely to be avoided in the relief of chronic pain, when the patient's need for analgesia must be anticipated. The patient cannot be expected to withstand peaks of pain to give the staff a guide to the absence of respiratory depression and other signs of possible cumulative effects of the drugs. Furthermore, the patient will lose confidence and the alerting effect of the recrudescense of pain will most likely increase the dose of analgesic needed to suppress it compared with that required to keep the pain in abeyance.

It is emphasized that analgesic escalation, from aspirin alone to aspirin and codeine, then to aspirin, codeine, and diazepam, and finally to morphine and chlorpromazine, should be regarded as cumulative in the sense that the earlier drugs are also continued when morphine is started. Consequently, a patient may be taking several agents, with the weaker and stronger drugs strategically used at different times of the day and night. For instance, a patient may require the opiate only on rising in the morning and going to bed at night, whereas in the day the aspirin mixture with the supplement of a tranquilizer may suffice. The important thing is for the patient to know that, by further manipulation of the combinations and the timing of his drugs, pain relief can be adjusted as necessary on a day-to-day basis.

Finally, the patient can be assured that a sudden deterioration in his condition can be alleviated by the use of a powerful analgesic cocktail and, if necessary, the injection of larger doses of a potent analgesic agent. Successful analgesic cocktails contain either morphine or diamorphine (sometimes both) in a selected amount with 10 mg. of cocaine made up to a 10-ml. dose with sweetened spirits. Diamorphine is more appropriate if the patient wishes to be relatively alert, but it has the disadvantage of being shorter-acting than morphine, which produces more sedation and may be preferred at night when its longer action will also be helpful. The initial dose of morphine is usually 10 to 15 mg. but may have to be increased to 30 mg. or more. The initial dose of diamorphine is usually 5 mg., and this too may have to be increased. In a patient who has been carefully managed it may be possible to begin with smaller doses of morphine or diamorphine than those suggested above, and in some cases the doses of narcotic analgesic can be reduced later, when pain relief has been firmly established. In refractory cases the addition of a steroid drug, such as prednisone, will increase pain relief, owing perhaps, to one or more of the following: an antiinflammatory effect, an unrecognized pharmacologic effect, or a euphoric effect.

SURFACE METHODS OF PAIN RELIEF

Counterstimulation of the body surface over and around the site of pain can be most effective in the relief of musculoskeletal pain; and occasionally it can be helpful when applied to the site of pain referred from visceral pathology. Suitable types of stimulation may be classified as follows:

Mechanical—manipulation, mechanical vibration and acupuncture

Thermal—warm and cold immersion, cold sprays

Electrical—Surface and transcutaneous electrodes

Chemical—counterirritants

The mode of action of these various forms of counterstimulation may be related to the following considerations:

Pain Modulation

The gate control theory predicts that pain may be relieved by preferential stimulation of thick, myelinated sensory nerve fibers in which high activity is able to close the gate in the dorsal horn of the spinal cord to the ingress of neural traffic in the thin, myelinated and unmyelinated nerve fibers that subserve pain. It is easy to envisage how mechanical vibration and certain other stimuli, which are capable of keeping the thick, myelinated nerve fibers busy, may act: but how are thermal stimuli, which affect mainly thin, myelinated and unmyelinated fibers, so effective? Perhaps any type of extra stimulation can compete with pain stimuli for ingress to the central nervous system which can deal effectively only with a certain amount ("bits," in computer language) of information at a given time.

Modality Switching

There is evidence from animal physiology that first-transmission neurones in the dorsal horn can switch their activity from proprioception to exteroception—in other words from muscle to skin monitoring. Since neural circuits can be shared in this way, is it possible that first-transmission cells can alter their activity from pain to cutaneous or proprioceptive by suitable counterstimulation?

Novel Pattern

It is possible that any change in the stereotyped input pattern associated with chronic pain can break a self-perpetuating cycle of neural activity and therefore produce pain relief. Sometimes patients find that changing the nature of a pain makes it more tolerable—even changing its location can help.

Reduction of Noxious Stimuli

Pain caused by the mechanical effect of sustained muscle spasm may be eased by physical measures such as massage, which promote muscle relaxation. However, part of the effect may be due to improvement of the local circulation, and consequently the dilution or dispersal of tissue mediators of pain such as bradykinin, 5-hydroxytryptamine, prostaglandins, ionic imbalance, and pH changes.

Brain Stem Intensity Monitor

An important function of the brain stem reticular formation is the inhibition and cutting short of excessive nervous activity after sensory input. It is possible that the persistent, stereotyped, low-key neural activity associated with chronic niggling pain, of the neuromuscular sort in particular, may fail to swing the bias of the brain stem reticular formation against its continuation. In these circumstances a burst of counterstimulation may activate the bias and cut short the chronic pain. The central siting of this biasing mechanism would also explain why counterstimulation remote from the actual site of a pain may nevertheless alleviate the pain. This is a common state of affairs in acupuncture, in which needling in the wrist or ear, for example, may be used to relieve pains in a wide variety of locations in the body. It is worth noting that acupuncture must itself usually produce a degree of pain locally to be effective, and that infiltration of a local anesthetic agent at the site of the needling may abolish the effects of acupuncture. That there may be ill-understood links between certain acupuncture points and the activity of the central nervous system

is undeniable, but the now familiar meridian charts of classical acupuncture therapy are not an integral part of modern acupuncture analgesia for surgical procedures, although they may still act as a guide in the treatment of chronic pain.

Mental Factors

The general mental distraction and the placebo effects of counterstimulation contribute significantly to its effectiveness in relieving chronic pain. Many lonely, elderly people use complaints about the natural aches and pains of old age as a means of calling attention to their despair and the social bonhomie of the physiotherapy department is undoubtedly a factor in the success of physical measures in the treatment of chronic pain.

LOCAL ANESTHETIC BLOCKS

Attention has already been drawn to the way in which local anesthetic injections can relieve pain, especially myofascial pain. Occasionally, the relief of pain after one or more injections greatly outlasts the direct pharmacologic action of the local anesthetic agent; and relief may even be permanent. This suggests that some cyclic neural activity which subserved the pain has been interrupted. Clearly, any injection that can obviate the effects of prolonged analgesic therapy is worth a trial.

Minor Local Anesthetic Blocks

The value of the injection of trigger areas and tender spots in the relief of musculoskeletal pain is well known. A local anesthetic is usually given mixed with a steroid preparation which produces an antiinflammatory effect. A particular problem is that acutely tender areas are far too painful to be injected adequately in conscious patients, yet a general anesthetic will preclude the cooperation of the patient when it is necessary to locate the most tender area with the point of the needle to maximize the chances of success. The solution is to give the patient sufficient intravenous sedation to reduce the pain of the injection to a bearable level while retaining the patient's cooperation. This can be achieved by an experienced anesthetist. Over the years, Mr. Gruebel-Lee and I have found that the success rate of minor injections of lignocaine and methylprednisolone has been greatly improved by careful attention to the fine control of intravenous sedation. I favor Althesin in light doses, because this agent does not damage small veins and recovery is rapid. Moreover, since Althesin is metabolized quickly, there is no hangover, which is an important consideration in patients who are discharged from hospital within hours of the injection. A second choice is diazepam, which has the disadvantages of being relatively slow-acting and associated with a slower, relapsing recovery. Injections of diazepam must be given into a large vein, since small veins are readily damaged by this agent.

A bonus from the intravenous sedation of these patients is that the patients are in an amenable state for mental reinforcement by the surgeon and anesthetist about the successful outcome of the injection. In other words, a judicious hypnopsychological influence can be achieved simultaneously with the local anesthetic block in selected cases.

Major Local Anesthetic Blocks

Major procedures, such as epidural and paravertebral blocks, require specialized knowledge and should only be carried out in places where adequate facilities are available to ensure the safety of the patient. The treatment of intractable sciatic pain by the sacral epidural injection of up to 40 ml. (15 ml. if the lumbar route is used) of a dilute solution of local anesthetic agent mixed with a steroid preparation is advocated by some specialists, but the results are equivocal. In selected cases

this procedure may be followed by gentle manipulation and straight-leg raising, in the hope that any fine adhesions around the affected nerve roots will be broken down.

Paravertebral block is easier to perform and is relatively free from complications, except in the thoracic region, where pneumothorax is a risk. It is particularly useful in unilateral sciatic pain. I have used these blocks to facilitate the initiation of continuous traction for very painful prolapsed intervertebral discs. In this way the patients have been spared the side-effects of potent analgesics, not least of which is the discomfort of constipation—an unhappy predicament for the patient confined to bed in traction.

THE PAIN CLINIC

The successful management of pain is best served by the organization of an interdisciplinary pain clinic. It is usual in district general hospitals for a pain clinic to be run by a consultant anesthetist who has an interdisciplinary role in clinical practice and special knowledge of pain relief. In a teaching hospital or a regional center, a neurosurgeon may also play a leading part. There are advantages in forming a pain clinic team with representatives from hospital specialties and family medicine. The precise constitution of the team will depend upon local requirements.

The types of patient treated at a pain clinic in a district general hospital are shown in Table 8-1. Back problems represent a significant group, despite the fact that the majority of such patients are referred either to the orthopaedic or the physical medicine department. Plans are now in hand to organize a back problem clinic under the combined supervision of an orthopaedic surgeon, a physical medicine consultant, and an anesthetist.

It is a matter for concern that, on the whole, analgesics are not used rationally.

Table 8-1. Conditions Affecting 100 Consecutive Patients at a Pain Clinic

Complaint	Incidence
Postherpetic neuralgia	24
Cancer	19
Ischemic feet	15
Sympathetic dystrophy syndrome	9
Back problems	9
Raynaud's disease	6
Trapped nerves	4
Amputation stump pain	4
Causalgia	4
Trigeminal neuralgia	1
Phantom limb pain	1
Migraine	1
Brachial neuritis	1
Coccygodynia	1
Postsympathectomy pain	1
Total	100

Some doctors prescribe analgesics haphazardly and fail to consider other maneuvers to relieve pain. Patients themselves buy large quantities of weak analgesics without prescription to treat mild or moderate pain, and consequently are at risk from side-effects such as gastrointestinal bleeding, blood disorders, and kidney damage. These patients are understandably dissatisfied when the family doctor prescribes another weak analgesic. Patients in chronic pain require more than anything else *time* for discussion with the doctor. A doctor in a pain clinic should be able to spend more time than can a busy practitioner.

Patients in hospital fare badly when analgesics are prescribed p.r.n., because this method of prescription puts the onus on the nursing staff to decide when the next dose should be given. When drugs are written "4–6 hourly p.r.n.," the patient will almost certainly have periods when pain relief is inadequate. One of the objectives of the pain clinic team must be to supervise the more flexible administration of analgesics, to anticipate each patient's needs. No patient should be allowed to suffer unnecessary pain as the consequence of a rigid system, which in the first place was the result of expediency. In the treatment of severe chronic pain "p.r.n." stands for "pain relief neglected."

The pain clinic should aim not only to raise the standards of diagnostic acumen in problem cases but to promote the better understanding of pain relief in general by hospital doctors, family doctors, nurses, and paramedical staff. Last but not least, the patient also deserves a full explanation of the significance of his pain.

REFERENCES

1. Hannington-Kiff, J. G.: *Pain Relief.* London, William Heinemann, 1974.
2. Head, H.: *Studies in Neurology.* 2 vols. London, Oxford Medical Publications, 1920.
3. Melzak, R., and Wall, P. D.: Pain mechanisms: a new theory. *Science, 150:*971, 1965.
4. Noordenbos, W.: Pain. Amsterdam, Elsevier, 1959.

9 Management of the Patient

A survey of the management of the patient as a whole must include a consideration of the clinical problems associated with the patient's history, with some comments on the psychological aspects; his understanding of his condition; his expectations; the patient-doctor relationship, and, finally, the indications for operation.

SOME PROBLEMS OF COMMUNICATION

Precise diagnosis of the various syndromes causing back pain is possible by a careful consideration of the details of the patient's story and the manner of his telling it. This is not always easy. The doctor must evaluate as objectively as he can the patient's account of his symptoms, since signs are few and, by their nature, easily overlooked.

The patient who is garrulous may succeed in confusing the doctor or misdirecting his questions. Worse, it may cause him, in the midst of some busy clinic, to lose interest. Since the lack of attention is instinctively felt and resented, the doctor may well be saddled with the problem of the patient's failure to recover. Even more difficult to assess is the patient who says little, or expresses his symptoms in an unusual manner. The doctor's powers of divination are unequal to the patient's expectations where there is a belief in the physician's ability to discover and deal with the cause of suffering without recourse to a detailed and accurate history of the condition. The doctor may be led to reach the wrong conclusions, and even to to act on them.

The Patient's Motivation

What must be decided first is the reason for the patient's having sought the doctor's help. This motive may seem obvious, but it is by no means always so.

In many cases the patient simply seeks an explanation for his symptoms. When he understands them, he is prepared to put up with them. What he wants is the reassurance of knowing that he is not suffering from some sinister disease. There is no greater help the doctor can give than to allay the patient's fears. Unless the doctor realizes this he may easily consign the patient to frequent return visits to the orthopaedic clinic.

A knowledge of the impending medicolegal consequences of a back injury is vital, because, where there is litigation, the patient has every motive for exaggerating the severity of his symptoms. His emotions become involved; he seeks to

137

justify himself. There is little likelihood that the complaints will subside fully before the case is settled.

Some patients are attention-seekers, who move from one specialist to the next, either because they wish to make boring lives seem extraordinary or because, sadly, they suffer from loneliness. And then there are the malingerers. Surgery in such cases can be catastrophic.

Sexual problems, usually of male impotence, have brought many a patient complaining of back pain to the orthopaedic surgeon. The patient is seldom prepared to discuss the real difficulty openly, unless he is carefully led to the subject. Since impotence usually does not have a physical basis, a short, open discussion will often help.

In the case of women's sexual problems, in a changing social climate it is often they themselves who bring the discussion around to the subject. Their difficulties are more complex and may require specialist advice which is outside the competence of most orthopaedic surgeons, unless all the patient requires is a platform to air her grievances.[1] Since the trouble is usually due to her partner, and most women maintain an objective and even humorous attitude to the act of intercourse, this is often therapeutic.

Psychological Syndromes

It must be recognized that the most neurotic patient may undergo lumbar disc prolapse. Provided the nature of his neurotic illness is understood by the doctor, its contribution to the patient's symptoms can be assessed and need not interfere with the treatment. The psychotic, either in an active phase of the disease or in a normal mental condition, is equally liable to develop back trouble. His description of his symptoms may be bizarre or confused, but with the help of a psychiatrist who knows the case, adequate diagnosis is possible.

There are three specific psychological syndromes that may present with back or leg symptoms of sufficient severity to bring the patient to the orthopaedic clinic.

Hysteria, more properly called a psychological conversion syndrome, is one in which it is thought that some mental complex in the patient's subconscious mind is converted to a physical symptom. Patients may complain of paralysis of a limb, difficulty in swallowing, or of back pain and disability. The condition is more common in women, hence the derivation of the name, hysteria (wandering uterus).

There is great danger to the patient if a neurotic conversion syndrome is not recognized, since the symptoms do not subside readily on conservative treatment, and the patient drifts gradually toward the operating theater. There is little likelihood of improvement after surgery. If the symptoms are relieved, the patient's inner conflict merely manifests itself by a different set of symptoms, and she changes over the years from one specialist to another. Since the only way to cure the condition is by giving the patient insight into her major psychological problem, surgeons are ill-suited to the task. The patient should be referred for psychiatric help as soon as the condition is diagnosed. Probably deep psychoanalytical methods hold the best chance of success.

What makes the doctor suspect hysteria? The presence of a large load of case-notes is always suspicious, especially if they contain a history of symptoms wandering from one organ to another. Often there is a record of many operations; laparotomies, hysterectomy, prolapse, laminectomy, follow each other over the years. (Patients with the so-called Münchausen syndrome, who are probably psychotic and seeking immediate gratification by operation, seldom ask orthopaedic advice for back pain, because few spinal operations are performed as an emergency, unless there is obvious cause.

Two other features suggest hysteria. Both are difficult to define, but with experience can soon be recognized by the doctor. The first is that the patient seems to take no notice of the doctor's explanation and advice, returning, during the consultation, to the symptoms which brought her to the clinic. Just when the doctor thinks he has made progress with the patient, he will find himself on a well-worn path of repetition of pain, weakness, and the like. This often takes the form of circular questions, repeated again and again; there is no true communication. Perhaps this is an indication of the subconscious, and therefore the nonlogical, motives that drive the sufferer on.

The final indicator of conversion hysteria is the patient's emotional state. What strikes the disinterested observer is an element of pleasure that seems to exist in the patient's suffering. It is this unexpected emotional overtone that led Freud to his original theory of hysteria: that it is infantile (noncivilized, if you like) pleasure, demanding immediate gratification. A strong "censor" represses these drives into the subconscious but is unable to prevent them from reaching conscious level, where they are distorted (converted) into physical, instead of mental, feelings, producing pain instead of pleasure.

Agoraphobia. It seems unlikely that a patient suffering from an irrational fear should be referred to an orthopaedic surgeon, yet in 118 consecutive cases reaching the clinic of one of the authors, three patients were diagnosed as suffering from this condition.

It happens in the following way: many people who are undergoing psychological stress develop illogical fears. Such phobias are common in normal children and many adults. Their development is more common in women than men (85% of cases) whereas most doctors are men, and so, unfortunately, there has been little sympathy from doctors for these patients.

Phobic reactions are explicable if the fears seem reasonable; for example, many people are afraid of spiders or elevators. Who fears shoes? Yet the patient can develop fears of the most unlikely object or place. Fear of open spaces (agoraphobia) is one of the most common phobias.

It begins in the not unreasonable shyness in public that many introverted people feel. To stay at home seems preferable. Soon the patient develops panic when away from home. This panic reaction is the basis of the syndrome, for when the patient panics she has an acute adrenaline reaction (the "fight or flight" reaction). This is so severe that she develops tachycardia and pounding of the heart, a dry mouth, peripheral vasoconstriction, vertigo, and even a most unpleasant sensation of impending doom.

These unpleasant feelings cause a further panic reaction, and the cycle is perpetuated; she suffers wave after wave, each more frightening than the last. They occur so quickly that the patient has difficulty in analyzing the deluge of sensations to which she is subjected and assumes that she is suffering from some serious illness. She becomes depressed and loses confidence in herself. What is more natural than for her to seek to avoid the situations that give rise to her symptoms?

To the agoraphobe, home represents an escape, the only safe place in the epicenter of an area of increasing psychic pain. When the radius has collapsed sufficiently the patient finds herself unable to leave her house. From time to time the newspapers report such a case of a woman who has not left her home for years, or even decades.

Many patients are denied this ultimate sanctuary, either because of a husband who will not allow them to remain at home, or because the circumstances of their life prevent them from doing so. Each day they must brave the torments inflicted by their autonomic nervous system. They regard life as a struggle, and it is not difficult to understand why they complain of increasing weakness in the legs.

This is the critical phase. If the general practitioner misunderstands the nature of the patient's weakness, the stage is set for a diagnosis of back trouble with associated leg weakness. Such patients end up in the orthopaedic clinic and may undergo special investigations and even laminectomy. They seldom recover full health.

Provided the doctor makes the diagnosis in good time, the condition is eminently treatable. The phobic reaction is best treated at the conscious level. Patients can be taught to break the vicious circle of panic reactions by understanding its physiological basis, realizing that they are not near collapse or death, and so regaining control of the autonomic nervous system. One patient described it thus: "It is like holding a candle into the darkness. The shadows fly away before it." The patients who have learned to control their reactions have a feeling of elation, almost of triumph. Each success makes the next attack easier to cope with.

Psychoanalytic techniques have not proved useful; electroconvulsive therapy and tranquilizers merely insulate the patient from reality. Behavioral techniques, group therapy, and even simple supportive therapy, on the other hand, are often helpful, especially if combined with the use of β-blocking agents, which can be highly successful in preventing the secondary autonomic symptoms. The best form of treatment is usually to admit the patient to an orthopaedic center for a concerted physical rehabilitation program. Provided the physiotherapists are aware of the cause of the weakness, and sympathetic, the treatment is generally highly successful. The patient's basic character is not changed: for the rest of her life, at times of physical illness or psychological stress, she will be vulnerable to further attacks.

Depression. This word has become so fashionable as to be almost universally used. Often people say they are depressed when they mean they are run-down, tired, or merely bored. Many people have a cyclothymic personality, with periods of elation alternating with depression. Usually they are aware of their trouble and come to terms with it.

People who have not suffered psychological problems before may develop depression, either endogenous or from some external cause. Diagnosis depends on the presence of the following features:

A feeling of depression and lack of energy

Insomnia, which may be severe and is of a specific type, manifesting in an inability to sleep, with the worries of the day being turned over in the patient's mind. Finally, in the early hours of the morning the patient falls into a deep, troubled sleep, to awake unrefreshed.

Loss of appetite

Reduced libido

Lowered threshold to pain

It is this last syndrome, of lowered threshold to pain, that brings the patient to the orthopaedic surgeon. The complaint is of pain so severe that it does not respond to analgesics, even in large doses.

The normal threshold to pain fluctuates during the 24-hour cycle, being lowest in most people in the early hours of the morning. Little is known about its mechanism, but then little is known about the cerebral function we call consciousness. In some ways it is a process of exclusion by the nervous system. If we did not maintain thresholds to sensory input, we should be drowned by our sensations. The process of maintaining a barrier against extraneous stimuli is a physical one. This is why physical processes, such as pyrexia, may lower the barrier. We are all aware of the direct relationship between a rise in temperature, for example during an attack of influenza, and a lowered threshold to pain. In the end, a touch, a loud noise, or even a cold wind blowing on one's neck, may cause pain.

It is this state that patients are trying to communicate when they use words like "agonizing" or "numbing," to describe their pain. Some even have a lowered threshold to touch and may complain of symptoms such as aching in the legs or even formication (a feeling of ants crawling on the skin).

The significance of the low-threshold pain syndrome to the orthopaedic surgeon is that it magnifies symptoms out of proportion to the cause. Unless this is clearly understood, the surgeon may choose an inappropriate form of treatment. Manipulations, injections, and even operations may be undertaken. Not only may they be unnecessary but, in their turn, will cause exaggerated pain and delayed recovery. If painful treatment is required, it should be delayed until the pain threshold has returned to normal.

Treatment of depression consists essentially in the use of antidepressant drugs to alleviate the symptoms. A simple explanation to the patient and a confident assurance that the condition will settle spontaneously, even without treatment, because that is its natural history, is often a great comfort.

It must be emphasized that it is not the author's intention, in this chapter, to suggest that trouble in the back, whether inflammatory or mechanical, has some special link with psychological problems. Apart from a suggested association with psychosomatic stress in the "executive disc syndrome" (Chap. 2) there is no reason to assume this. Most of the observations in this chapter could apply equally to any other region of the body.

The Doctor-Patient Relationship

As the doctor has climbed down from the pedestal upon which he was placed by the rest of the community and has come to be regarded merely as another expert in a society of experts, his role has had to be redefined. He is no longer regarded as the voice of authority in health matters, and has to justify his decisions to the patient.

Much has been written in recent years about the doctor-patient relationship, but nothing clearer than Freud's original invention of the concept of transference. Freud was a dedicated determinist, believing that everything the patient said or did (even his dreams and mistakes in grammar) had a reason. When he noticed that his patients, very soon after beginning treatment, developed an unexpected emotional attachment to himself, he did not assume, as many of us would, that there was something special in himself. He realized that he had discovered a universal effect of the relationship between the doctor and his patient. To this unexpected psychological dependence he gave the name "transference." Perhaps Freud's greatest achievement was to understand that transference was essential to the therapeutic effect of analysis. He noticed, in the later stages of his treatment, that the patient began to react against the analyst, becoming late for appointments, arguing with him, and so on. He called this "negative transference," and understood that it was a stage in the recovery of the patient, who was asserting his independence.

Freud's observations were of neurotic women in Vienna at the end of the 19th century. Surprisingly, they apply equally to patients with an attack of physical disability, and even more to those undergoing major operations. If used wisely, positive and negative transference can assist greatly in helping a patient recover. Ignored, they may lead to disaster.

People vary in the depth of their emotional reactions, but any patient who has decided to undergo a major operation puts his "trust" in the surgeon. This emotional attachment means that he listens closely to the surgeon's instructions, as well as to those of the surgeon's "helpers," the nurses and physiotherapists. His "faith" in the doctor implies that he will do what is necessary to get himself back on his feet.

There is danger in this positive transference. If the surgeon accepts unnecessary gifts, or even if he refuses reasonable presents; if he loses interest in the patient, or especially if, misjudging the patient's interest in questioning him, he becomes evasive; or, most dangerous of all, if he misunderstands the patient's emotional reaction and becomes emotionally involved himself, he will lose the patient's trust. The result may well be failure of recovery and can even end in charges of unethical conduct.

Negative transference is also essential to recovery from a major operation. The surgeon should look forward to the first signs of independence from the patient. He should not be dismayed by trivial complaints about the food, the nursing, or the physiotherapy. He should recognize them as a further step on the road to recovery. He must remain cheerful and optimistic, knowing that when the patient has recovered fully the emotional reaction will have disappeared. If the surgeon becomes defensive or emotional, negative transference will never be overcome. This is one of the main causes of malpractice allegations.

The Patient's Understanding and Expectations

No condition is more liable to be misunderstood by the layman than prolapse of an intervertebral disc. The lesion is usually pictured in the patient's mind as a joint or bone out of place. Some osteopaths and chiropractors use such explanations. There are two reasons why such explanations are disadvantageous to the patient if he believes them. If he thinks of a prolapsed disc as a hard object that is out of place, he will not be satisfied unless something active is done to put it back or remove it. This is unfortunate,

unless the patient requires manipulation or operation.

Secondly, there is nothing in the concept to make the patient understand that the natural outcome in most cases of disc prolapse is spontaneous recovery. Of course, the intelligent, educated patient will understand the cause of his trouble and what he must expect, provided the surgeon does not use technical language or jargon. For the others, it is worthwhile to invent some simple simile to explain the condition, for example: The disc is like a rubber grape. It can become squashed and stretch the skin, which causes pain in the back. If the skin tears, some of the material is squeezed out and pinches the nerves. This causes pain in the leg, as well as loss of feeling and weakness. Don't worry, because usually it will shrivel up, in time, like a raisin, and the symptoms will disappear.

Orthopaedic Bidding

The doctor's responsibility to explain what is happening does not end when the patient understands something about the pathology of disc prolapse. If he can be made to appreciate that the doctor's response is a logical one, depending upon the severity of the signs and symptoms he describes, the patient will understand the rational basis of the treatment he is being offered. During the course of his illness he can tell if he is improving by the changes in treatment.

A useful metaphor is the bidding in a card game. The patient is told that the doctor, having listened carefully to the patient's problem, as though it were a bid, will reply with an appropriate response. Provided the improvement is maintained, the doctor will not change his bid.

Figure 9-1 gives some idea of usual bids and the increasing response. In all cases, laminectomy is best regarded as "trumping the hand" and so ending the "game." The table does not imply that the patient

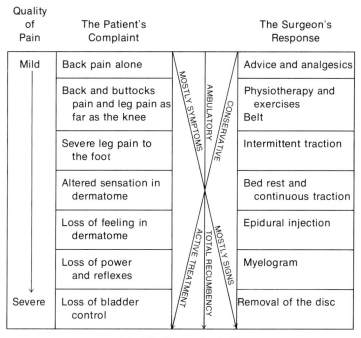

Quality of Pain	The Patient's Complaint				The Surgeon's Response
Mild	Back pain alone				Advice and analgesics
	Back and buttocks pain and leg pain as far as the knee				Physiotherapy and exercises Belt
	Severe leg pain to the foot				Intermittent traction
	Altered sensation in dermatome				Bed rest and continuous traction
	Loss of feeling in dermatome				Epidural injection
	Loss of power and reflexes				Myelogram
Severe	Loss of bladder control				Removal of the disc

Fig. 9-1. "Orthopaedic bidding."

always improves or deteriorates in the order of symptoms given, nor that the occurrence of each new symptom means the loss of those above. It does imply that the doctor moves from one form of treatment to the next in his attempt to control the disease.

INDICATIONS FOR SURGICAL REMOVAL OF THE DISC

There is no place for excision of a lumbar disc for pain alone. The only absolute indication is *disability* that cannot be overcome. This implies not only an assessment of what a patient is prepared to suffer, but also of the patient's feelings about undergoing an operation. The financial problems associated with ill health must also be considered.

The only justification for emergency operation is complete loss of bladder control and sensation (acute central prolapse).

Surgery is then an emergency because of the possibility of permanent incontinence. In all other cases the reasons are relative, operation being performed when the patient is convinced that the time is right. Some people reach this conclusion early; others may cope with their problem for many months first.

Some patients in the last category sol-

A Descending Scale of Indications for Surgery

Bladder incontinence
Inability of the patient to be mobilized from a hospital bed
Recurrent episodes, resulting in repeated returns to recumbency
Inability to return to work
Chronic pain and disability, which do not prevent the patient working but gradually cause a physical deterioration because of pain

dier on for many months before finally giving in and deciding on surgery. The surgeon has the difficult task of persuading the patient to undergo operation before matters have deteriorated too far, while taking care that he intimates that not all patients are satisfied after operation.

Myelography

Most patients are keen to undergo myelography, despite the discomfort of the procedure, because they feel that they want their lesion to be defined precisely. In those centers in which modern techniques are available, (see Chap. 11) it is reasonable to use these special procedures routinely for diagnosis. In most hospitals where myelography with an oil-soluble medium only is possible, it is wiser to use the investigation only when the possibility of some other space-occupying lesion exists, or when the surgeon cannot decide, on clinical grounds, which level is involved, and then only once the decision to operate has been made. This is not only because of the development of later dural adhesions, but because a false negative result complicates the decision to operate.

REFERENCE

1. Masters, W., and Johnson, V.: Human Sexual Response. Boston, Little, Brown, 1966.

10 The Conservative Treatment of Low Back Pain

Carl W. Coplans

The history of low back pain is as old as the stresses created by man. The invention of the wheel and the discovery of the lever did much to reduce these, and protect the vulnerable mutating human lumbar spine. Traditionally, treatment has been empirical; even after the introduction of roentgenography this is still true, despite the desire of physicians and surgeons to treat patients more scientifically. The literature relating to low back pain reveals the interest shown by the practitioners of many different specialties concerned in its treatment.

Conservative treatment of the lumbosacral spine would be simpler if the linkage of vertebrae to each other and to the pelvis by means of the intervertebral disc was straightforward. Unfortunately, asymmetry of development exists, while the natural tendency toward mechanical failure of the lumbar spine is increased by the acceleration forces man has devised and which have rapidly outstripped his ability to protect himself.

Since the advent of bioengineering as a science, the full dimension of the problem has become apparent. Low back pain and sciatica are the dominant symptoms that have pursued man through his adoption of the orthograde posture. They still present considerable therapeutic and diagnostic problems. Mechanical failure is not confined to the vertical spine of man. Nature's alternative concept, the horizontal spine, particularly in "long" dogs such as the dachshund, is also subject to breakdown. This vulnerability to disc herniation is familiar to veterinary surgeons.

The function of the lumbar spine may be likened to that of a torsion bar, since few of its movements do not contain an element of torsion.[5] Because of the relative fixity of the inferior part of the lumbar spine to the pelvis, and the mobility of its upper junction to the dorsal spine, the lumbar segment of the spinal column suffers most easily from trauma during athletic activity. It is also subject to the gradual, degenerative changes of aging.

Conservative treatment is directed mainly to the linkage system rather than the bones themselves (i.e., to the discs, joint capsules, ligaments and muscles). A joint is capable of being moved through its full range by the associated muscles and is limited at the extremes of range by its ligaments. Unguarded passive movement of a joint may take place too rapidly for protective reflex contraction of the muscles to occur, and the full force is then borne by the ligaments alone, so that they are stretched or torn.

The essential integrity of the spine depends on the discs and ligaments. Even when it is stripped of its musculature, it

145

maintains its shape and will not collapse. Thus, the intrinsic equilibrium of the spine consists of a balance of two forces: the pressure exerted by the turgor of the discs, counteracted by the tension of the ligaments. Steindler compared this to the wires maintaining a vertical pole in position.

When the anterior pier of the intervertebral joint is diminished in height, either by frank herniation of the disc or by degeneration and fragmentation within the intervertebral space, the vertebral bodies are approximated. As a result the adjacent spinous processes separate and ultimately an increase in tension of the supraspinous and interspinous ligaments takes places. This increased tension is continuous, leading in time to stretching of the ligaments. The abnormal force is borne mainly by the apophyseal joints, which undergo osteoarthritic changes. The capsules of three joints in turn become stretched and lax, permitting abnormal movement and so increasing the stresses on the intervertebral joint, which becomes unstable.

Floyd and Silver pointed out that, in the final stage of full flexion of the lumbar spine, the erector muscles of the spine relax.[9] As further flexion takes place, the tension on the intervertebral ligaments increases until they bear the full weight of the trunk. Stretching can occur. The intervertebral joint reaches the stage of full instability when these two elements are present: failure of the anterior supporting pier and loss of the posterior limiting ligaments. The result is an uncontrolled rocking movement of the spinal joints on flexion and extension, the fulcrum being the apophyseal joints at the affected level.

Limitation of extension of the lumbosacral joint is assisted by the impingement of the spinous process of L5 against the sacrum; but in flexion the final check is ligamentous: supraspinous, interspinous, and ligamentum flavum, in that order.

During laminectomy for intervertebral disc herniation, the interspinous ligament may be observed to be slack, scarred, and torn. Kohler developed a method of visualizing these ligaments by the injection of a radiopaque contrast medium. His roentgenographs demonstrated tears due to rupture of the fibers.

When this instability is present at the 4th and 5th lumbar intervertebral levels, the iliolumbar ligament is subject to abnormal stress. These ligaments are a checking mechanism against the shearing force produced by the forward inclination of the sacrum at the lumbosacral joint; but they are only a partial check, since the control of this force is vested in the whole ligamentous apparatus at the lumbosacral level. This includes the intervertebral disc, damage to which diminishes its efficiency.

Movement of the sacroiliac joints is restricted by the massive sacroiliac ligaments, as well as the iliolumbar, sacrospinous and sacrotuberous ligaments. Although these joints have no visible movement, they are particularly prone to injury by vertical and torsional forces. Vertical thrust occurs as a result of landing on the extended legs when jumping from a height or falling onto the buttocks in a sitting position. The force is first buffered by the lumbosacral joint, but mechanical failure of this joint causes transmission of the force to the sacroiliac joint. The lumbar spine possesses a small range of rotary movement, and the lumbosacral excursion is the smallest component of this total.[4] Consequently, when this joint suffers mechanical breakdown, the force is transmitted through the sacrum to the sacroiliac joints.

Rotational movements of the trunk are not controlled by the same efficient motor system as are the movements of flexion and extension. If rotational forces are not dissipated in free motion, damage occurs to the ligamentous apparatus, commonly the long and short posterior sacroiliac ligaments. This accounts for the sacroiliac strain that is associated so frequently with lumbosacral disc break-down, and for the localization of pain by the patient over the posterior superior spine, to which the long posterior sac-roiliac and sacrotuberous ligaments are massively attached.

Conservative treatment has increased in importance since the recent apprecia-tion of the limits of surgery, which re-lieves some 9 out of 10 patients with sci-atica, but only 5 out of 10 patients with low back pain. On the other hand, com-plete relief of local and peripheral pain due to intervertebral disc herniation by operation may require laminectomy and fusion.

The armamentarium of conservative treatment consists of rest, traction, mobilization, manipulation, injection, exercise, and bracing. Each will be dis-cussed in turn.

REST

Non-weight-bearing rest is as instinc-tive to the patient suffering from low back pain as is the rubbing of an injured area. Rest bears a direct relationship to the cause of the pain. Particularly in interver-tebral disc herniation with root compres-sion, rest in one position may increase discomfort.

Bed Rest

The position adopted by the patient at rest is often the first pointer to diagnosis, since the posture adopted is influenced by the relationship of a herniated disc to the compressed root. In a similar way, the pa-tient with an acute interspinous lig-amentous tear will adopt an instinctive posture to diminish the pain. Resting pat-terns are specific to the lesion and its situation, and only after precise diagnosis can the correct pattern of rest compe-tently be advised.

The problem with bed rest, whatever its

virtue as a form of therapy, is its eco-nomic disadvantage to the patient, his family, and the community at large, which may not only be losing his pro-ductivity but in many cases may be bear-ing part of the cost of his long period of confinement in hospital. To this is added the impatience of the patient and his fam-ily, who may be worried by the inertia of the treatment and the imponderable out-come.

When the family breadwinner is dis-abled, the ill-advised drive to search for some rapid and successful treatment, however bizarre, is strong. In his desire to return to employment the patient will readily submit to any treatment that is dramatic and brief. Inevitably, it com-prises some form of mobilization, whether orthodox or unorthodox.

The Resting Surface

A firm mattress of reasonable thick-ness, supported by a rigid board, is ideal; but should a deformity such as kyphosis exist, this must be comfortably housed by the supporting surface. The essential fea-ture is a non-sagging, but comfortable, surface. The patient will soon find a posi-tion of optimal rest and will resent dis-turbance.

Where the lumbar spine has retained its normal anatomical relationships, the supine position is sufficient; the patient rolling from side to side, intermittently, to relieve inertial fatigue. In the lateral position the lumbar spine sags between the pillars of the shoulders and pelvis, and support of the loin by a pillow is indi-cated.

Conduct During Rest

If the duration of rest is prolonged, or the patient elderly, the following ac-tivities should be instituted:

Respiratory drill

Static leg exercises to prevent venous thrombosis

Care of the bowels. Feces should be

kept soft, so that a bedpan can be used without the patient sitting erect. Otherwise a commode is more comfortable and physiologically superior.

Isometric exercises, which must be carried out short of pain and without disturbing the fundamental rest. A planned program of exercises is essential to combat the effect of prolonged bed rest on general health.

Rest, without more active treatment, is generally resented by the patient, who regards it with a lack of confidence and becomes impatient. Sedation is an important therapeutic factor and should be of sufficient dosage to keep the patient relaxed, with a blunted awareness of his surroundings, so that he is insulated from minor but irritating stimuli.

TRACTION

Traction is an ancient remedy for the treatment of low back pain. A form of violent, intermittent traction was carefully described by Hippocrates, the very employment of which, in that era of priest-doctor medicine, suggesting more than a primitive understanding of its effects. The patient was fastened firmly in an inverted position to a ladderlike frame, which was repeatedly dropped from a gallows to the ground, producing axial stress on the lumbar spine brought about by the patient's relatively free trunk and head. This was known as *succussion.*

The Purpose of Traction

A multiplicity of benefits are claimed for this simple form of treatment. Its value has been proven in the treatment of fractures where, not only is the limb kept at rest, but the fracture is reduced, and painful muscle spasm overcome. There is no doubt that the benefit of rest is increased by continuous traction, since the patient is discouraged from moving by its application. Where root compression exists, traction efficiently applied will often cause decompression and permit the

swollen, inflamed root to become reduced in size and, therefore, more mobile. Even if the condition is of long standing, with ligamentous shortening and capsular contracture, it will improve. If "binding" of a roughened osteoarthritic facet joint occurs, particularly when the relationship of the opposing surfaces has been altered, due to disc attrition, mobilization may be accomplished, with reduction of a bulging intervertebral disc. The combination of rest and traction possibly produces sufficient vertebral separation to allow sequestered material and the spinal root to occupy a slightly increased space. In this way pressure on the nerve root is gradually diminished as inspissation of the sequestered fragment occurs.

Continuous Traction

The purpose of continuous traction is two-fold: the patient is encouraged to rest and his peripheral pain is relieved. The patient is confined to bed on a firm mattress supported by a board. The pelvis and legs are flexed sufficiently to overcome lumbar lordosis, so that traction can be direct and axial. A short corset is then applied to the pelvis and is connected to two lateral cords, which are attached to a spreader bar. From the center of this bar a cord runs over a pulley at the bottom of the bed to a suitable hanging weight. This method of traction avoids the danger of thrombosis in the leg veins, caused by the immobilizing effect of Buck's plaster, and permits essential movements of the legs. Opinions differ considerably as to the optimal pull required to produce a therapeutic effect. My experience of 30 years indicates that 10 per cent of the patient's total weight is optimal.

The common indication for lumbar traction is peripheral pain due to root compression, and the time required for effective treatment is variable, ranging from a few days to 2 weeks. The last period seems to be the ultimate, beyond which little improvement may be expected.

Traction should be accompanied by

suitable sedation and antiinflammatory analgesics. When traction is completed, the patient should be provided with a well-fitting corset containing a Goldthwait plate before being permitted to bear weight.

When root pain is persistent, the effects of continuous traction may be assisted by paravertebral root blocks, which reduce discomfort by diminishing the irritable condition of the nerve root and overcome reflex muscle spasm.

Intermittent Traction

Intermittent traction (Fig. 10-1) is given on a traction table, where the pull is controlled and carried out by a motor which produces a rhythmic extension, usually at the rate of 12 per minute. The rhythm may be varied. Most patients readily submit to a 30- to 40-kg. intermittent pull for 10 minutes. Knees and hips are supported in flexion, in order to abolish lordosis and thus increase the efficiency of traction.

The Windlass Table

This method is much the same as the previous one, except that traction is gradually increased to a desired peak and then equally slowly diminished, since if it be loosened too rapidly, the patient may suffer a violent and painful muscle spasm. Opinion varies in the estimate of the weight required. Cyriax has maintained

that loads up to 91 kg. are useful. In the author's experience, however, this has proved an intolerable weight and is generally resented by patients, even for very short periods. Intermittent rhythmic traction of 30 to 60 kg., after a paravertebral block of the affected lumbar root, is a useful addition to both these types of traction. An overpulled or overstretched spine constitutes a more difficult problem than the original dysfunction and often leads to a stiff back with chronic irremediable pain. One cannot stress too emphatically the long-term traumatic effect of a "pulled" back.

MOBILIZATION

Gravity-Free Mobilization

The type of mobilization suitable for a painful low back must be carefully selected. Where the condition is acute and weight bearing itself is a pain-producing factor, movement in suspension is the method of choice. The advantages are clear. Gravity is eliminated, and weight-free movement in a fixed plane gained. Painful structures are relieved of the forces of gravity and weight bearing, with consequent reflex muscle spasm, and painless movement becomes possible. What is more important, essential movements of the lumbar spine, such as flexion and extension with the patient in the side-lying position, and lateral flexion

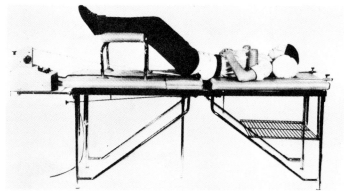

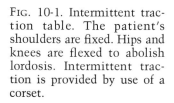

FIG. 10-1. Intermittent traction table. The patient's shoulders are fixed. Hips and knees are flexed to abolish lordosis. Intermittent traction is provided by use of a corset.

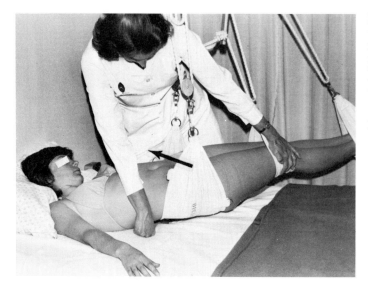

FIG. 10-2. Mobilizations of the lumbar spine in gravity-free suspension. (The Guthrie Smith system of slings.) The physiotherapist's right knee and right arm stabilize the patient's thorax while the lumbar spine is flexed laterally to the left.

with the trunk supine, with its combination of rotation, may be performed accurately with minimal distress to the patient. The apparatus employed is the Guthrie Smith system of slings (Figs. 10-2–10-4). A series of slings bears the weight of the patient's pelvis and legs, the shoulders resting on the plinth. The point of suspension of all the slings must be situated directly above the area to be mobilized. Movements, active or passive, are initially of small amplitude, and limited in range and area by the physiotherapist. This type of apparatus may be suspended conveniently from a Balkan beam fixed to the patient's bed. Exercises become more vigorous, until the patient is ready for early weight bearing. Mobili-

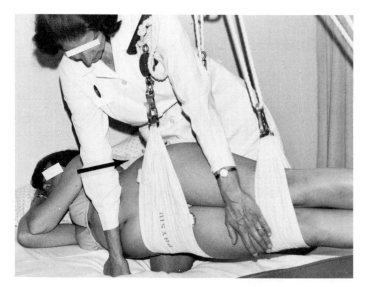

FIG. 10-3. Mobilization of the lumbar spine in gravity-free suspension. The patient is placed in a side-lying position. The physiotherapist's right arm and right leg stabilize the thorax and dorsal spine while her left arm controls and swings the lumbar spine into controlled extension.

FIG. 10-4. Mobilization of the lumbar spine in gravity-free suspension. The patient's thorax is controlled as in Figure 10-3, and the physiotherapist's left arm forces the suspended pelvis and legs forward, so that the lumbar spine is flexed.

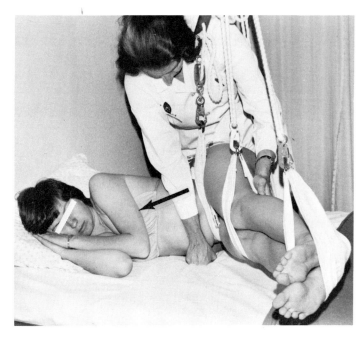

zation in suspension should be an accurately prescribed form of both resisted and assisted exercises. As active, neutral movement becomes painless, the point of suspension of the slings is moved anteriorly or posteriorly, vis-a-vis the patient, so that greater muscle effort is required. Conversely, the point of suspension may be altered to assist movement. This is a valuable and painless method of mobilizing the lumbar spine in which active movements against gravity are painful. It has the added advantage of simplicity and low cost.

A therapeutic pool permits gravity-free movement, but has the disadvantages of expense and also of difficulty in controlling the patient's plane of movement, as well as the resistance engendered by the water.

Passive Movement

Passive movements of the lumbar spine are carried out as a prelude to manipulation without anesthesia and are employed either for individual intervertebral joints or for the lumbar spine as a whole. The movements are of small excursion and carried out repetitively and with minimal force. They are: extension, rotation in extension, rotation, and lateral flexion. Forced flexion is undesirable and dangerous. Each passive movement will be described in turn.

Extension. The patient is placed prone upon a surface which is both firm and comfortable. The physiotherapist places the pisiform bone of her right hand, with elbow extended, over the lumbosacral joint, while reinforcing the pressure with the left hand (Fig. 10-5). A series of gentle springing movements are commenced, using a definite rhythm which diminishes in response to evidence of pain from the patient. The hands move up and down the spine until adequate painless movement is achieved. During this procedure the most painful level is located, and mobility should first be gained above and below this level. This is an ancient method of treatment and was used by early Far Eastern and Indian practitioners. A barefoot

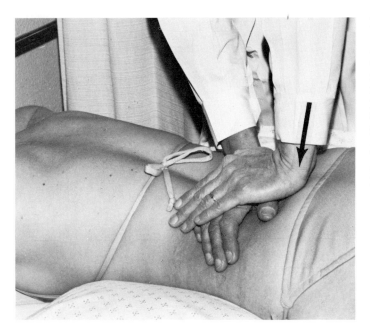

Fig. 10-5. Manipulation of the lumbar spine in extension. The right hand is placed over the joint to be mobilized, so that the thrust may be delivered by the pisiform bone. The left hand reinforces the thrust which is given in a vertical and slightly lateral direction. This manipulation is carried out at different levels in the lumbar spine.

child or lightly built woman walked gently up and down the spine of the patient.

Rotation in Extension. The patient is positioned in the same way, but the fulcrum of movement is shifted laterally over the transverse processes (Fig. 10-6). The rhythmic gentle movements are continued on either side of the spine.

Rotation. However bulky the patient may be, the use of the flexed leg as a long lever will permit gentle, graduated, rotary

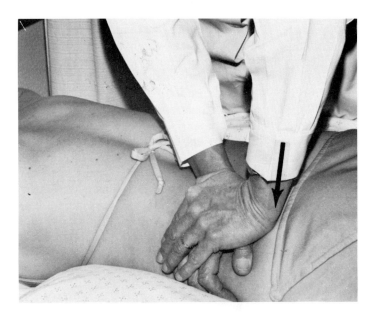

Fig. 10-6. Manipulation of lumbar spine in extension and rotation. The manipulator's right hand is placed so that the pisiform bone is thrust over the transverse process of the vertebra to be manipulated. The left hand covers the right and adds its thrust in a vertical and lateral direction.

movements to be carried out to right and left (see Fig. 10-13). The patient lies supine, and if rotation is desired from left to right, the operator stands on the right side of the patient. The left hip and knee are flexed, and the left fore-foot hooked under the right knee. The operator's right arm is threaded through the flexed limb, so that the dorsum of the hand faces the left side of the couch. The left shoulder is firmly fixed against the couch by the operator's extended left arm, and the operator's forearm is used to force the lever constituted by the patient's flexed left leg downward and toward him. The amount of force which may be employed in this manner is surprising and the movement should be carefully initiated.

Lateral Flexion. The patient lies supine, and both hips and knees are flexed. The flexed limbs are used as levers (Fig. 10-7), and the lumbar spine is easily and smoothly moved in a combination of lateral flexion and rotation.

Provided that the passive movements described are carried out carefully with minimal discomfort to the patient, not only has a fair degree of mobilization been gained therapeutically or as a preparation for manipulation; but these movements assist in the location of the painful structure. Both patient and physician are familiar with stories of accidental minor movements which may result in dramatic relief of the patient's symptoms. Some of these tales are apocryphal, but experience has demonstrated the value and effectiveness of these gentle, passive, repetitive movements of small amplitude, which do not require the dexterity demanded by manipulation without anesthesia.

MANIPULATION

Manipulation is a vague term which simply denotes a form of passive movement, but which in no way describes the particular method used. It is as imprecise as the titles "medicine" and "surgery,"

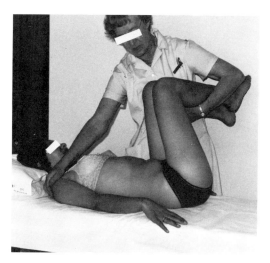

FIG. 10-7. Passive lateral flexion of the lumbar spine. The patient's hips and knees are flexed at right angles, and the physiotherapist's right hand stabilizes the right shoulder of the supine patient. The therapist holds the flexed legs firmly and rotates them toward herself, thus laterally flexing at the same time rotating the lumbar spine. The position of the physiotherapist is then reversed, and the same procedure is carried out on the opposite side.

which describe the simple origins of the multiple specialties which have sprung from the parent skills. In the past, manipulation has been the stormy petrel of the treatment of joint, tendon, and ligament pathology. The skill with which it has been exhibited was largely denied, its value derided, and its practitioners often vilified. With notable exceptions, the medical profession has failed to play its part in the scientific development of this skill. It was left to the heterodox practitioners to evolve a method of manipulation which has now largely been adopted by the medical profession and which forms the groundwork of the practice of manipulation.

Manipulation under anesthesia attained more easily a degree of respectability, since it could, and may, only be performed by a medical practitioner. We must accept that there are a number of groups of medically unqualified practitioners who teach manipulation without anesthesia and who treat large numbers of patients suffering from backache. Despite this, the systematic teaching of manipulation without anesthesia is barely carried out in our medical schools. Students of the paramedical profession of physiotherapy are, however, in some schools, carefully instructed in this skill; but it is important that it should be practiced as well by both the general practitioner and the specialist who deals with locomotor disabilities.

It is not the province of the physiotherapist to diagnose, and it remains the responsibility of the doctor to provide precise prescriptions for manipulation as well as diagnosis. In some hospitals an unrewarding and unsatisfactory relationship has grown up between the medical profession and the physiotherapist. Vague prescriptions, such as "low back pain; please treat," are uninformative and unfair to the therapist.

Manipulation without anesthesia has much to commend it. The risk attendant upon the use of anesthesia is avoided, and the manipulations may be carried out in stages. What has been gained may be maintained by simple mobilizing exercises. It is more difficult than manipulation under anesthesia because a patient tends to resist what he fears may be a painful maneuver. The basis of joint manipulation is an ability to move the joint authoritatively to its maximum range. The "slack" of muscle and ligament is taken up until the joint will not move any farther, the manipulation is firmly and fluently carried out through a determined range before the patient is aware that it has been completed, otherwise the involuntary resistance of the patient will result in therapeutic failure and, possibly, trauma.

Manipulation of the Lumbar Spine

Manipulation of any kind is, of course, contraindicated in the presence of inflammatory change, malignancy, osteoporosis both generalized and due to local disease, disuse, or neurologic deficit. Manipulation of children and the aged should be regarded with circumspection. Mobilization is more difficult to achieve in the lumbar spine, because of its heavy musculature and general limitation of movement except in extension, than in other areas of the body. It is easier to carry this out under general anesthesia, which, however, is not always readily available.

Manipulation of the lumbar spine is indicated in a variety of conditions. In chronic conditions of a minor character, the spine may be stretched effectively and gently by maneuvers employing the legs alternately as levers. This is not a manipulation, since no final, decisive thrust is made; but in conditions in which there is soft-tissue-, joint-, and capsular contracture, this type of movement is an excellent preparation for manipulation.

Since the lumbar spine is a chain of five vertebrae linked by apophyseal joints and ligaments, it is essential that the mobilizing force be focused on the link to be freed, preventing as far as possible an overflow of force. The direction of the force may be controlled by fixing the apophyseal joints below the level as follows:

Basic Technique of Mobilization. The patient is placed in the lateral position and hip and knee on the affected side are flexed. The degree of flexion determines the level at which fixing of the apophyseal joint takes place. The flexed leg is allowed to hang over the edge of the couch. The left shoulder is steadied by the manipulator's right arm, and the left forearm is placed over the left buttock. The buttock is rotated gently until movement ceases, and the manipulator's weight is transferred through the flexed right arm, so that a short, sharp thrust with a follow-through is delivered by the right arm. It is essential that the movement of mobilization is performed firmly and effectively, since failure to effect this

FIG. 10-8. Manipulation of the lumbar spine in rotation. This manipulation is a fundamental procedure and is the most commonly used manipulation in the treatment of the lumbar spine. The manipulator steadies the patient's left shoulder with his left arm and rolls the patient's pelvis toward him, the right leg being held in extension, the left leg hanging over the side of the plinth. The manipulator's right hand is placed over the patient's left buttock and with the "slack" taken up, a final sharp controlled thrust is given in a lateral and downward direction.

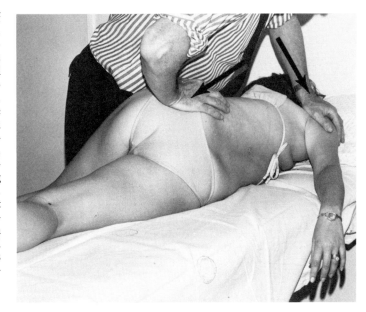

will result in forfeiture of the patient's confidence and painful failure of the maneuver (Fig. 10-8).

A variation is for the manipulator to place the anterior surface of the pronated left arm, with the elbow flexed firmly, on the patient's left shoulder; the right forearm similarly on the patient's left buttock, thus giving the advantage of freedom of both hands, so that movement at the essential levels may be palpated and identified (Fig. 10-9).

When the patient is heavy and muscular, the thigh may be used as a long lever to increase the mobilizing force. The patient's left foot is placed below her right knee, and the manipulator's left arm is introduced as demonstrated in Figure

FIG. 10-9. Manipulation of the lumbar spine in rotation. This is a variation of the previous manipulation (illustrated in Figure 10-8) in which the elbows and forearms of the manipulator are used to procure movement, freeing the hands so that they are able to palpate and determine the level at which movement takes place in the lumbar spine.

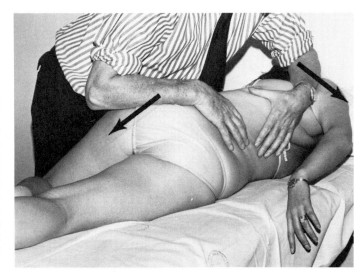

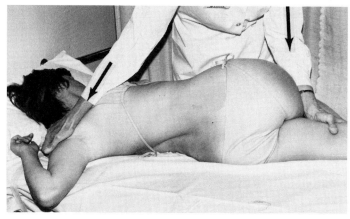

FIG. 10-10. Passive movement of the lumbar spine in rotation. The physiotherapist's right hand stabilizes the patient's right shoulder. The patient's right foot is hooked under her left calf, and the physiotherapist's left hand is placed so that her fingers lie over the anterior aspect of the right thigh, and the thumb over the posterior aspect. This permits her to use her right forearm effectively against the left thigh, which is then forced laterally and inferiorly, the right leg being used as a powerful lever. This maneuver permits a lightly built physiotherapist to exert a powerful torque on the lumbar spine.

10-10. Where loss of mobility is recent, the freeing of the affected structure is often sufficient.

A further variation of manipulation for rotation is carried out by the manipulator immobilizing the patient's left shoulder with his right hand, thrusting the patient's left buttock with his extended left arm. It is important that body weight increases the power of the straight-arm thrust from the manipulator's position behind the patient (Fig. 10-11).

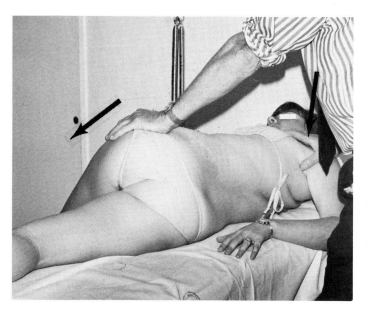

FIG. 10-11. Manipulation of the lumbar spine in rotation. A further variation of a rotational manipulation of the lumbar spine. The manipulator stands behind the patient who lies on the right side with the right leg extended and the left leg flexed at the hip and hanging over the edge of the plinth. The manipulator's right hand fixes the left shoulder, and his extended left hand thrusts the left buttock in a lateral and downward direction.

FIG. 10-12. Manipulation of the lumbosacral joint in extension. The patient lies prone with a pillow under the pelvis. Both legs are lifted by the manipulator's left arm, while the right hand thrusts against the lumbosacral joint. The "pisiform thrust" is again utilized directly downward over the joint.

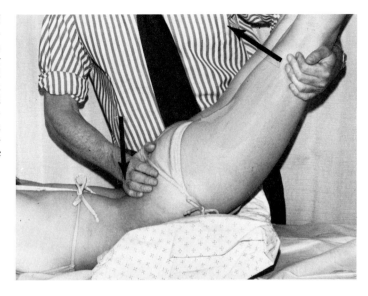

Manipulation in Extension. The patient is held prone, the manipulator's right arm is placed so that the pisiform rests against the intervertebral level to be manipulated, the left arm extends the hip joints and pelvis to approximately 45 degrees, and then a sharp thrust is delivered by the right hand and arm (Fig. 10-12).

Rotation of the Lumbar Spine Posteriorly. The patient clasps the back of her head with her entwined fingers and places them over her left ear. The manipulator thrusts his left arm through the flexed left arm of the patient, fixing the shoulder girdle to the couch. The right arm then delivers a backward and downward thrust over the anterior superior spine on the left side (Fig. 10-13).

Succussion. This manipulation is particularly valuable in loss of mobility of

FIG. 10-13. Manipulation of the lumbar spine in posterior rotation. The patient lies supine with the hands clasped behind the head and then moved over the left ear. The manipulator "threads" his left arm through the flexed arms of the patient and stabilizes his arm by holding the free edge of the plinth. The shoulders will consequently rotate toward the manipulator, whose right hand is then placed over the left anterior superior iliac spine, which is thrust posteriorly until all "slack" is taken up, the final thrust is then delivered.

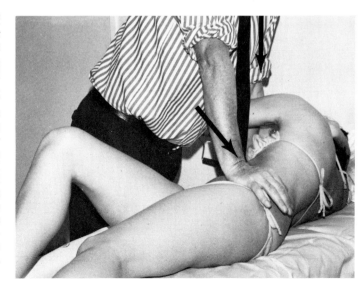

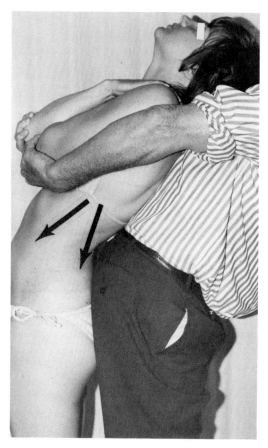

Fig. 10-14. Manipulation of the lumbar spine in extension with added traction. This manipulation is known as succussion. The manipulator and patient stand back-to-back. The patient crosses her arms and holds on firmly to the contralateral shoulders. The manipulator takes the patient's elbows in his hands and flexes his spine forward, extending the patient's lumbar spine across his buttocks. When the patient's feet are felt to be off the ground, the manipulator raises his heels and flexes his knees. He then thrusts them hard against the floor, at the same time extending his knees. This produces a force which extends and applies axial traction on the lumbar spine. It is one of the oldest known forms of manipulation.

the lumbosacral apophyseal joints. The patient stands with arms across her chest and hands grasping the contralateral shoulders. The manipulator stands back

to back, grasping her elbows with both hands. He flexes his hips, lifting the patient's feet off the ground and plantar-flexing his own feet. His heels are then slapped rapidly against the floor while the patient is held firmly. The lumbosacral joint is submitted to a downward and extension force (Fig. 10-14).

Where there is any degree of chronicity, it is essential that the manipulation be followed by precise mobilizing exercises, so that the contracted ligaments and joint capsules may be stretched and the recovered mobility retained. This important addition to manipulation is too often neglected, and failure to achieve relief is consequently blamed on the mechanical maneuver which, at best, is only a preparation for active mobilizing exercises.

The patterns of movements that injure the lumbar spine are those which are obstructed by the bony and ligamentous architecture (i.e., flexion, rotation, lateral flexion, and compressive forces acting in the longitudinal axis). The disability which results from extension injuries rarely requires manipulation. Manipulation used in the lumbar spine differs little from that in the rest of the spine apart from the cervical region, where the accessibility of the apophyseal joints makes manipulation more precise.

INDICATIONS FOR MANIPULATION OF THE LUMBAR SPINE

The Intervertebral Disc

It must be accepted that manipulation in the lumbar spine cannot be expected to have a precise and selective effect because of the robust nature and strength of the lumbar musculature and ligamentous apparatus, as well as the diminution of movement other than extension which occurs in the lower lumbar spine as it approaches its mooring to the semi-rigid pelvis. The nucleus pulposus of the aging disc loses its fluid content, with consequent impairment of the turgor of the whole structure, both nucleus and annulus. The nucleus becomes fibrosed and diminished in size, so that its area of movement within the annulus increases in response to stress. At the same time, the detachment of the contracted nucleus contributes to the vulnerability of the annulus, which itself has now to deal with forces that it is not competent to mediate. The aging lumbar disc may, apart from incursion of the nucleus into the body of the adjacent vertebra, break down in two ways: there may be extrusion of the nucleus posteriorly or posterolaterally, or the annulus itself may undergo change. Despite the anatomical apposition of the apophyseal facets, there is little doubt that rotation takes place in these joints, mainly due to the laxity of apophyseal capsules. Robbed of their youthful ability to cope with stress, the aging annular lamellae undergo structural changes. It is during its slow destruction between the upper and lower millstones of the adjacent vertebrae, with consequent mobility and instability of the intervertebral joint, that the misshapen annulus may act in the same mechanical fashion as the cartilages of the knee; the back may become "locked." It is this type of disc herniation which responds best to manipulation.

Root Pain

When the posterolateral aspect of the annulus has undergone degenerative changes, the nucleus pulposus may be forced posterolaterally and may cause the annulus to bulge until the protruding knuckle is jammed between two adjacent vertebrae. Reflex muscle spasm may produce incarceration and locking of the intervertebral level. Presumably this type of early herniation may be reduced by manipulation; but it does tend to recur, and final rupture of the annulus and lamellae allows the nuclear material to escape and form a sequestrum. Intrusion into the intervertebral foramen and pressure on the

nerve root may then produce peripheral symptoms with the appearance of limited straight-leg raising, although this may be caused by other factors. Any sensitive structure in the lumbar spine which is compressed by extension of the spine will produce this clinical sign; particularly an injured interspinous ligament.

Sacroiliac Strain

Injuries to the sacroiliac joint and strain of this joint are discussed in Chapter 3. Alteration of mechanical integrity affecting the mass of sacroiliac ligaments may occur in the pelvic tilting of pregnancy; and particularly, the failure of involution which follows the postpartum period. An analysis of maneuvers carried out in manipulation of the sacroiliac joints demonstrates conclusively that most of these passive movements embody an element of torsion, which must affect the lumbar spine mechanically. In any case, it cannot be overemphasized that manipulation in the lumbar area is imprecise.

MUSCLE INJURIES

Primary injury to the massive musculature of the lumbar spine is uncommon and when present is readily detected by the presence of local pain, swelling, and tenderness, and often by the appearance of hematomas. Treatment is by rest at first, progressing to gentle gravity-free exercises and the application of ultrasound over the injured area. The dosage of ultrasound (in watts/cm^2) should rarely be more than 0.5 watts/cm.^{2}, particularly for superficial injuries, and should be applied no longer than 15 minutes.

LIGAMENT INJURIES

The integrity of the spine depends upon the mechanical interrelationship of the discs and ligaments (see Chap. 3). Because it represents the final link with the relatively immovable sacrum, the lumbosacral intervertebral joint, including the intervertebral disc and all ancillary ligaments as well as the apophyseal joints, represents the commonest locus of breakdown. It is important to accept that failure of any of its component structures may initiate disability at this level; and the crowded anatomy of the lumbar spine, with its chain reaction of protective reflex mechanisms, does not make the acute clinical problem easier of solution. This is true, but to a lesser degree, of the higher levels of the lumbar spine.

It has been claimed that 40 per cent of all lumbosacral joints may lack a complete supraspinous ligament, with consequent additional stress borne by the ligamentous residuum at this level. Degenerative changes take place in the interspinous ligament with the appearance of small hiatuses, fissures, and the formation of small islands of cartilage, with consequent formation of an area of potential weakness. It may undergo repetitive disruption, which should be regarded as a cause of stress on the disc. Hackett describes the ligaments of the intervertebral joints as well as related ligaments of the sacroiliac joints, particularly the long and short sacroiliac ligaments, as undergoing structural failure, or "relaxation," at the ligamentous-osseous junctions (see Sclerosant Therapy below).*

The whole lumbar spine possesses a small range of rotation, but the lumbosacral joint has the least. When this joint breaks down, force is transmitted through the sacrum to the mass of ligaments of the sacroiliac joint, with production of local pain and tenderness commonly sited at the lateral aspect of the posterior superior spine. It may later be referred peripherally in a somatic pattern. This is distinguished from root pain by the absence of paresthesia, alteration of sensation, or motor power.

---

*Hackett, G. S.: Personal communication.

ACUTE LUMBOSACRAL INTERSPINOUS LIGAMENT INJURIES

A triangle, whose superior angle is formed by the lumbosacral joint and whose two base angles are formed by the posterior superior iliac spines, constitutes one of the most familiar patterns of pain in the low back. Acute disc herniation without peripheral reference and acute failure of the lumbosacral interspinous ligament, whether due to a tear or acute strain, present similar and confusing clinical patterns. Both incidents usually cause massive muscle spasm of the extensors of the spine with loss of lumbar lordosis, probably due to the spinal erector muscles acting in segmental compression rather than as a bowstring. At a later stage, localizing signs will distinguish the two entities; but it is helpful to make a clinical and therapeutic distinction in the acute phase. A patient suffering from lumbosacral or L4–5 ligamentous disability particularly resents extension of the affected level, since this movement compresses an already acutely tender and edematous interspinous ligament between the spinous process of the sacrum and that of L5. The intervertebral space is acutely tender, but flexion of the lumbar spine in the prone position gives temporary relief, since the injured ligament is relieved of compression. The introduction of a 22-gauge, 3-cm. needle and the injection of 4 ml. of 2-per-cent procaine and 1 ml. of soluble steroid will give dramatic relief.

Technique of Injection. The injection is given as the needle is withdrawn, thus minimizing the chance of an accidental epidural injection. It is interesting to note how often, in this type of ligamentous disability, the needle appears to "fall" into the ligament, the stream of fluid meeting little or no resistance.

Following injection, the patient is placed side-lying, in slings, with the shoulders supported by the table and the legs and pelvis supported by slings. Gentle, non-weight-bearing flexion mobilizing exercises of the joint are begun and carried out to the level of pain, followed by ultrasound to the interspinous ligament. Friction is given across the direction of the long and short sacroiliac ligaments, and the patient is provided with antiinflammatory analgesics for a week.

The lumbosacral pain is primary and commonly due to ligamentous damage. The pain at the posterior superior spine is secondary, since the stress of the mechanically incompetent lumbosacral joint is accepted by the long and short sacroiliac ligaments. Once the interspinous ligament becomes vulnerable in the manner described, recurrent episodes tend to occur and the patient should be instructed carefully in the simple kinetic handling of weights, with the correct method of diminishing stress on this part of the spine. In the author's experience, tears or acute strains of the interspinous ligament of the lumbosacral joint are responsible for a substantial portion of acute low back pain, so commonly diagnosed as acute disc trauma, and which may be so easily distinguished and treated by the method described above.

Acute Apophyseal Joint Strain

The occurrence of asymmetry of the apophyseal joints of the cervical spine must be continued, to some degree, throughout the spine, particularly since one is aware of the commonly occurring tropism of the lumbosacral apophyseal joints.[24] Diminished mechanical efficiency makes these joints vulnerable to stress. The condition is readily diagnosed by painful limitation of passive rotation of the lumbar spine; a condition which is uncommon in disc or ligamentous pathology and may be readily relieved by simple manipulation without anesthesia. It requires a strong and skilled manipulator, however, to carry it out successfully; otherwise the intravenous injection of 10 mg. of diazepam or the use of

pentothal may be necessary. The introduction of local anesthetic or steroid into these joints is not difficult and will increase both the ease of manipulation and speed of recovery.

Epidural injection may be a useful adjunct. Mobilization and maintenance of integrity of joint capsules and ancillary ligaments should be carried out by non-weight-bearing exercises.

THE USE OF LOCAL ANESTHESIA

Control of local pain in the low back and peripheral pain in the form of sciatica may be reduced by epidural blocks, both lumbar and caudal, and by paravertebral injections in and around the affected nerve root. The materials used are low concentrations of suitable local anesthetic agents and the corticosteroid of personal preference.

Sacral Epidural Block

Sacral epidural block enjoys several advantages. The technique is easier than intervertebral block. It is not a "spinal" injection, and consequently the patient is less fearful of it. It may be given prone, so that movement of the lumbar spine is eliminated and there is also less likelihood of dural puncture with its attendant complications.

A 5-per-cent variation in the structure and shape of the sacral hiatus exists and may complicate, or even prevent, the procedure. By the time the patient is submitted to this type of block, however, the lumbar spine and sacrum should have been visualized roentgenographically. Local anesthetic solution, with or without corticosteroid, is introduced through the sacral hiatus and ascends superiorly and epidurally, reaching a level which depends upon the amount of fluid used and on the force of the injections (Fig. 10-15).

Indications for sacral epidural block are intractable backache, which has not responded to rest or which is of such mag-

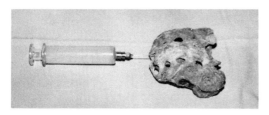

FIG. 10-15. The placement of the needle into the sacral hiatus is illustrated. This is the position in which injection is carried out. The needle is inserted at an angle of 45 degrees, and the syringe is then lowered into the position illustrated.

nitude that traction and manipulation are not possible, and intractable root pain. This is a time-honored and reasonably safe method of dealing with acute pain in the back and lower extremities.

Technique. The sacral hiatus is identified by the two bony prominences which lie at the inferior end of its lateral margins, covered by the prolongation of the supraspinous ligament. The dural tube usually ends at the superior border of the first sacral segment, but may be found at lower levels, and this variation should be remembered in selecting needle length. The patient is placed prone with the pelvis suitably elevated by adequate support. The tissues over the sacral hiatus are anesthetized, using a 2-cm. hypodermic needle and the minimal amount of 2-per-cent local anesthetic, in order not to blur the defined contours of the hiatus. A 20-gauge, 5-cm. needle is then attached to a 25-ml. syringe, preferably of the ringed type. The needle is introduced through the hiatus at an angle of 45 degrees to the skin. It is lowered as it is advanced in the mid-line. The bevel should face upward, to prevent the cutting edge piercing the bony cortex and the fluid entering the spongy bone. The needle is rotated several times and the plunger continually withdrawn.

Should cerebrospinal fluid appear in the syringe, the injection should be aban-doned, since the dura has been pierced. If blood appears, the needle may be withdrawn slightly and then advanced again. Some 5 ml. of the fluid are injected, with the palm of the free hand placed over the sacrum, to detect ballooning of the tissues due to the presence of misdirected fluid. The remaining fluid is then injected slowly and firmly.

Injection Material. The common local anesthetics are 0.5-per-cent lignocaine or 0.25-per-cent bupivacaine (plain solutions), and 25 ml. is used. Steroid of personal choice may be added. Its antiinflammatory properties are of value in this type of injection.

Complications. The most serious complication is perforation of the dura, with consequent spinal anesthesia. Headache and episodes of hypotension occur but are unusual.

Injection is commonly accompanied by a short exacerbation of pain, which disappears within a few minutes, and the patient becomes either completely or partially relieved of low back and peripheral pain, so that manipulation or traction may be carried out.

Dural Puncture. Minimization of this danger is assisted by attention to the length of the needle introduced, by continuous rotation of the needle, and by repeated aspiration tests. If spinal anesthesia results, ventilation with oxygen must be used and the circulation assisted with dextran or other suitable blood substitutes. Treatment must be continued until the normal respiratory and cardiovascular state is restored.

Hypotension. This is more likely to occur if the block is extensive and may be prevented by the intramuscular injection of a vasopressor drug.

Intravascular Injection. When the central nervous system is involved, with evidence of toxicity, pentothal may be given intravenously.

Penetration of the Rectum. This has been known to occur during injection of the epidural space. Antibiotics should be administered prophylactically.

Lumbar Epidural Block

The indication for lumbar epidural block is persistent pain of sciatic type which has failed to improve with conservative treatment, or because of the severity of the pain itself. The technique consists essentially of the introduction of a needle into the epidural space at a selected lumbar intervertebral level. The patient is placed in the lateral position, lying on the painful side.

Dawkins, quoted by Mehta, emphasizes that, in this type of block, none of the mechanical safeguards to prevent the piercing of the dura are completely efficient, and experience and familiarity with the procedure are to be preferred.[20]

The lateral position is chosen, since the injected material may sink and encompass the affected nerve root. The skin over the selected level is infiltrated with 2 per cent local anesthetic, using a hypodermic needle. A spinal needle with a short bevel, to minimize the risk of entering the dura, is then introduced through the interspinous ligament and the resistant ligamentum flavum at the selected level. At this stage, 5 ml. of normal saline are contained in the syringe and consistent pressure is maintained on the plunger: a sudden loss of resistance indicates that the epidural space has been entered. Further loss of resistance to the plunger will accompany this sensation. The needle is rotated a number of times and aspiration is carried out on several occasions.

If cerebrospinal fluid appears in the syringe, it is wise to change the intervertebral level. If blood appears, the needle is withdrawn slightly and saline is used to clear it. Further aspiration should then be carried out. If the barrel of the syringe remains clear of cerebrospinal fluid and blood, the syringe is changed for one containing 8 ml. of 1 per cent plain lidocaine and 2 ml. of suitable steroid. The contents are slowly injected, with intervals for aspiration.

If there is doubt as to the presence of cerebrospinal fluid in the syringe barrel, the needle should be disconnected and the drops of fluid issuing from the needle permitted to fall upon the dorsum of the bare hand. If the fluid is warm it is probably cerebrospinal fluid, and the procedure should be halted.

During injection, the patient may complain of increased pain in the back or leg, and the injection should then be slowed. The patient is left for 10 minutes on his side and then moved to a supine position for 30 minutes, after which he may return home. The injection may be repeated within a week. The complications of this procedure are the same as those described for caudal block and are treated in the same manner.

Paravertebral Root Block

The most common nerve roots affected by lumbar intervertebral disc herniation are the L5 and S1: less commonly the L4 root may be involved. This type of block may be used, diagnostically if other neurological signs are not present, or therapeutically, as part of conservative treatment. It has proved a useful aid in the relief of root pain.

If the nerve root has been trapped the benefits are short-lived, but when pressure is exerted on the root by a sequestrum, straight leg raising of 40 degrees may be converted to 90 degrees, with relief of the root incarceration. This depends, naturally, upon the mobility of the material holding the root captive.

Technique. The block should be carried out under direct roentgenographic guidance, but this is not always convenient or possible. Roentgenographs of the lower lumbar spine (particularly an anteroposterior view) should, however, be available. The patient is positioned prone across a suitable abdominal support, to diminish lumbar lordosis. A 22-gauge needle, 6 to

10 cm. long (depending upon the patient's obesity and somatic type) is used, with a 3 cm. skin marker.

The 5th Lumbar Root. The roentgenographs are inspected to preclude a sacralized 5th lumbar transverse process. The transverse process lies tangential to the superior border of the spinous process. The site of entry is sprayed with ethyl chloride and the needle directed at the transverse process or passed over the superior border of the sacrum. The needle is inserted painlessly through the skin and either "walked" inferiorly off the transverse process or superiorly from the superior border of the sacrum. The needle is withdrawn slightly and redirected medially toward the intervertebral foramen. When paresthesia is elicited, the needle is withdrawn slightly, and careful aspiration is performed for cerebrospinal fluid or blood. A mixture of 6 ml. of 1 per cent lignocaine or other suitable anesthetic mixed with steroid is injected slowly; aspiration being attempted several times during the procedure.

The first sacral root may be reached through the first sacral foramen, which lies 4 to 5 cm. inferior and slightly medial to the entrance route for the 5th lumbar root. The same precautions are observed and the same amount of fluid used.

The complications of this type of block are similar to those of caudal block but are less common.

"PHYSICAL THERAPY"

With the increased understanding of the pathology of low back pain there has been a reorientation of many of the concepts of physiotherapy and a reassessment of the value of the modalities which, for many years, have been used empirically in this area. The advent of steroids, the potent antiinflammatory analgesics and the electromyograph have produced a greater interest in kinesiology, exercise, and postural reeducation, with consequent elimination of many of the traditional but unproved modalities.

Heat

Heat, in its moist and dry forms, has been prescribed since time immemorial. The same types of backache are treated in the same Roman spas in Europe today with the same temporary benefit but no permanent effect. Diathermy, radiant heat, and infrared radiation have little place in the treatment of deep seated pain, other than as preliminaries to more sqecific therapy.

Massage

Superficial or sedative massage in its many varieties is largely without specific benefit other than its placebo effect and the pleasant sensation of relaxation that it induces. Deep cross-friction, on the other hand, given firmly and vigorously to defined and palpable structures such as the long and short posterior sacroiliac ligaments, permits minor adhesions to be broken down and local vascularity to be increased. This type of massage should not be given vigorously enough to cause bruising.

Percussion, given rhythmically and lightly up and down the lumbar spine with the ulnar border of the fists, is of value as a preliminary to passive movements such as extension thrusts.

Electrical Stimulation

Electrical stimulation may be used with some benefit in psychological backache. It is otherwise worthless in the treatment of low back pain.

Counterirritation

Judging from the large number of "healing" unctions, ointments, and rubrifacient creams sold all over the world counterirritation still enjoys a vogue. There is little doubt that the vigorous rubbing and sense of local warmth reassures and comforts the patient for a period.

Ultrasound

Ultrasound is a high frequency wave form generated by the oscillation of a crystal in a field of rapidly alternating polarity. Frequencies vary from 3 megaherz (MHz). It may be applied in a pulsed form, using a stationary head, or as a continuous form of energy from a mobile head, in order to avoid overheating of the tissues. Dyson and Bond described the generation of heat, micromassage and alteration of membrane permeability, and experimental stimulation of tissue regeneration, and the reversible effect of blood cell flow.

Ultrasound is primarily thermal in its effect, but has not been shown to be superior to other varieties of deep heat. It is most effective in the treatment of indolent, uninfected, superficial ulcers, where its stimulus to epithelialization is unparalleled by any other modality; in the presence of superficial scarring and fibrous tissue; for the breakdown and resolution of superficial hematomas, and in the treatment of sprained ligaments and tendons.

Contraindications. Ultrasound must not be used in the presence of neoplasm, since metastases may be caused. It should be used with discretion over the epiphyses in young patients. The uterine area should be avoided in pregnancy. Acute infections should be treated with circumspection. The eyes and gonads should not be irradiated.

Dosage. The common superficial dosage is 0.5 watts per square centimeter. A high dose will not necessarily increase the therapeutic effect and may be painful and resented by the patient. Treatment may last for 8 minutes at the first session and build up gradually to 15 minutes, increasing by 2-minute intervals.

THE USE OF SCLEROSANT INJECTIONS IN LIGAMENTOUS PAIN

Kellgren noticed that when deep periosteum was briefly stimulated, the patient could correctly localize the pain, but if the duration of the stimulus was increased, the pain spread and was poorly localized.[13] Kellgren injected muscles, interspinous ligaments, subcutaneous ligaments, and other deep structures with 0.1 to 0.3 ml. of 6-per-cent saline solution. He found that the introduction of the needle produced a pain of too short a duration to be accurately localized, but found the introduction of 6-per-cent saline resulted in local, and then referred, pain which lasted several minutes.[14,15,16] The areas of somatic reference of the pelvic ligaments have been mapped out by Hackett, who largely pioneered the treatment of damaged and relaxed ligaments by the injection of sclerosing solutions.[10] The area of segmental pain arising from the lumbar interspinous and capsular ligaments resemble, but are not congruent with, the dermatomes, and some confusion may arise in distinguishing areas of reference.

Hackett stated that when ligamentous tissues weaken at the fibro-osseous junction as the result of a strain, tear, or degeneration, the stability of the joint is impaired, with consequent painful disability due to ligamentous incompetence (relaxation). Where the ligament is not robust and is subjected to forces in two planes, a tear may take place in the ligamentous integument itself, for example the rent in the interspinous ligament. The vulnerability of the interspinous ligament to the combined forces of flexion and rotation has been described before. Gross flexion and extension alone commonly do not rupture the interspinous ligaments. Instead, compression fractures of the vertebral bodies and arches result, but if a torsional force is exerted with the spine in slight flexion, the interspinous ligaments may suffer damage, with or without dislocation or fracture-dislocation of the spine. One may deduce, therefore, that a combination of these forces insufficient to produce fracture or dislocation may result in deformity and tears of these ligaments.

Indications

Trauma to the ligamentous structures of the lumbosacral spine may present as an acute or chronic episode. Since the lumbosacral ligaments form a closely interrelated mechanical structure, the symptoms and signs arising from them present rather as a symptom complex than as evidence of isolated ligamentous damage. This is the common pattern, but individual ligaments may present as a single source of pain. The history and clinical picture are familiar. The patient presents what is commonly and correctly diagnosed as acute or chronic lumbar intervertebral strain; acute or chronic lumbosacral strain, or chronic sacroiliac strain. These conditions are strains in one form or another of joints and, therefore, of the supporting structures of the joints, mainly the ligaments and joint capsules.

The treatment of the acute phase follows traditional conservative patterns: rest on a firm surface, heat and massage, and splintage in the form of a well-fitting corset when required.

It has been emphasized before that the interspinous ligament is so frequently damaged in acute lumbosacral strain and that the injection of 3 ml. of local anesthetic and 1 ml. of steroid into this ligament as the diagnosis is made, produces substantial amelioration of the pain. By this means the diagnosis is confirmed and treatment is materially assisted. It is, however, when the condition enters the chronic phase that treatment and relief become problematic.

Local pain in the lumbar spine, of ligamentous origin, like local pain of disc origin, is poorly localized by the patient and is described as a fairly diffuse backache. Pain originating in the sacroiliac ligaments is more easily identified, and, in my experience, the commonest locus of pain in the back is at the level of one or the other posterior superior iliac spines.

Deep somatic referred pain in the lower limbs may be distinguished without great difficulty from pain of root origin. While the actual areas of reference are close enough to cause some confusion, deep somatic pain is never accompanied by any neurologic deficit. While superficial sensation may demonstrate some hyperalgesia, intact superficial reflexes and motor power, absence of tender muscle bellies, or anesthesia and paresthesias indicate that the pain is not of root origin.

It is in no way proposed that the syndrome of ligamentous pain is a distinct and separate entity from pain and disability originating from lumbar disc herniation, but rather that both are components of intervertebral joint inefficiency, ligamentous incompetence in most cases being the final product of lumbar intervertebral disc breakdown. This becomes evident when the chronic ligamentous strain and inefficiency emerge as a clinical pattern once disorganization of the intervertebral disc has taken place.

It is well known that during pregnancy the corpus luteum secretes a hormone called relaxin, which causes relaxation of the ligamentous structure of the pelvis, thus permitting a certain resiliency of the otherwise rigid, bony birth canal. Relaxation of these ligaments may be followed by postpartum failure of involution, and they may become a source of disabling local and referred pain. This type of backache is a fairly common complication of childbirth and, in resistant cases, the patient is passed through the whole gamut of conservative treatments, only to find impermanent relief in the form of a corset. The prospect of additional pregnancies is regarded with trepidation.

Because of the mechanical relationship of the lumbosacral and sacroiliac joints, it is usual to find one or more of the long, posterior sacroiliac ligaments involved in primary strain of the lumbosacral joint. The upper fibers of the long posterior sacroiliac ligament refer pain over the posterolateral aspect of thigh to the lateral aspect of the calf. The lower fibers refer pain down the posterior aspect of the thigh and along the lateral aspect of the foot. The short posterior sacroiliac or interosseous ligament refers pain down the posterior aspect of the thigh as far as the lower border of the popliteal fossa. The iliolumbar ligament, particularly in its lateral extent, refers pain to the iliac fossa and testis in the male and to the labium majorum in the female. The only ligaments that can be palpated effectively are the supraspinous and long posterior sacroiliac ligaments and, when affected, the latter will exhibit marked tenderness, particularly at the posterior superior iliac spine.

Methods

Apart from the mechanical maneuvers which can be used to elicit pain from injured ligaments, Hackett stated that the introduction of a needle, together with initial pressure of a few millilitres of local anesthetic into the tender fibers, is sufficient to produce local and referred pain before local anesthesia takes place. This has not been my experience, and I have used an 8-per-cent solution of saline for the purpose of eliciting and reproducing referred pain. Saline (0.5 ml.) is introduced into the ligament under suspicion. Within 30 seconds the patient complains of local pain at the injection site, which rapidly assumes the character of deep somatic pain and which is referred into a fairly well-defined area. The patient is asked to compare and contrast the quality, intensity, and distribution of pain with the pain of which he complains. Careful explanation of the purpose of the

test usually renders the patient both cooperative and helpful. The needle is left *in situ*, and if the characteristics of the pain are identified by the patient, the evidence may be accepted as part confirmation of the diagnosis. Two milliliters of local anesthetic are then run in through the same needle, which is left *in situ*, and the pain of the test injection is abolished. Sclerosis of the affected ligaments is then carried out.

Pathology

The introduction of a suitable sclerosant into the fibers of a ligament results in an aseptic local inflammatory reaction within 48 hours, which is followed by the presence of rapidly maturing fibroblasts. One month later, fibrous tissue is present, and the inflammatory reaction diminishes, until, some 40 days after injection, only healthy fibrous tissue remains.

The patient is instructed to return home to bed as soon after the injection as possible. Local heat, in the form of an electric pad or hot water bottle, is of value. Simple analgesics are prescribed 4-hourly for 48 hours. The sclerosing injections are conveniently given on a Friday afternoon, so that, if necessary, the patient may have complete rest over the weekend and return to work at the commencement of the week, without loss of employment. (Nervous patients may be given the first injection in a nursing home, with the use of preliminary sedation.)

Material

The material which I have used on this series is Sylnasol (G.D. Searle), which is a 5 per cent solution of the sodium salt of a vegetable fatty acid. I have carried out well over 1,000 injections with this material and can report no complications or side-effects, either local or general. I have used a 25 per cent solution of Sylnasol in normal saline, and local anesthetic. The amount of solution injected depends, of course, upon the number and size of the ligaments to be treated. The usual quantity injected at one session is 16 ml., but I have employed as much as 25 ml. without ill effects. In view of the rather painful inflammatory reaction following injection, I have sought other agents which are as efficacious in their sclerosing action and yet not so violent in their immediate local reaction. Hackett has recommended the following mixture: phenol (25%), dextrose (25%), Glycerine (25%), water (add to make 100%). This is diluted with a 1 per cent solution of lignocaine hydrochloride (Leostesin) into a solution of one part of sclerosing agent to 2 parts of local anesthetic. It is my practice to give 20 ml. at one session. I have carried out over 4000 injections with this material, and the local reaction is substantially less painful than with Sylnasol, the immediate symptomatic inflammatory reaction terminating within some 12 to 24 hours.

Technique of Injection

Iliolumbar Ligament. The patient lies prone on a pillow or prop, to decrease lumbar lordosis. The transverse processes of L4 and L5 are identified and contacted by use of a vertical 5-cm., 23-gauge needle. When the tips of the transverse processes have been located, the injection is commenced at the fibro-osseous junction of the ligament, and then the needle is redirected laterally and the injection continued through the length of the ligament to its iliac attachment. Here again, the deposition of fluid should be made when the needle contacts bone. The needle is then withdrawn slightly, so as to deposit fluid within the ligament itself. Ten milliliters of the solution may be used in the treatment of this ligament, 1 ml. being injected at each contact of the needle. Two insertions of the needle through the skin should be sufficient; the needle is then maneuvered in the subcutaneous tissues without being withdrawn. (Fig. 10-16).

Interspinous Ligament. The patient lies prone on two pillows and a 3-cm., 23-gauge needle is inserted through the supraspinous, into the interspinous, ligament. Four milliliters of fluid are deposited, and great care is taken to avoid entry into the epidural space. If the ligament is lax or has suffered injury, the flow of fluid

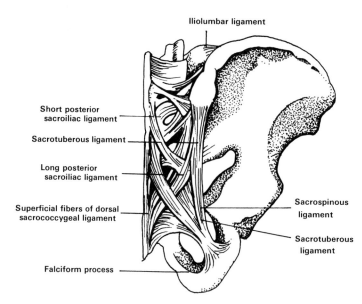

Iliolumbar ligament

Short posterior sacroiliac ligament

Sacrotuberous ligament

Long posterior sacroiliac ligament

Superficial fibers of dorsal sacrococcygeal ligament

Falciform process

Sacrospinous ligament

Sacrotuberous ligament

Fig. 10-16. Posterior pelvic ligaments.

is unimpeded, and very little pressure is required to depress the plunger of the syringe. The needle should contact the fibro-osseous junction at the spinous process: deposition of fluid is made here and then throughout the length of the ligament. Occasionally, the tip of the needle may escape from the interspinous ligament and be directed laterally and may accidentally enter the dural root sleeve. If cerebrospinal fluid is seen to enter the syringe, the needle should be withdrawn and redirected. As an additional safety measure, injection is carried out as the needle is withdrawn. Care must be taken to avoid piercing the ligament flava and thus effecting entry into the dural space.

After three injections at 2 week intervals, an increased resistance is experienced to the entry of the needle, and it becomes increasingly difficult to inject the fluid into the ligament.

Long Posterior Sacroiliac Ligament. The patient lies prone and the lumbosacral depression is located with the thumb. A 5-cm. needle is inserted 3 cm. lateral to this at an angle of 45 degrees. The needle contacts the attachments of the ligaments to the ilium. One milliliter of fluid is deposited at each contact, some 6 milliliters in all. The needle is then withdrawn and inserted inferior and lateral to the posterior superior spine, and an additional 4 ml. is deposited at each contact as the needle is moved medially toward the sacrum. Care must be taken to contact bone here, because of the immediate proximity of the sciatic trunk. The needle is again withdrawn and reinserted 3 cm. medial to, but at the same level as, the posterior superior spine. An additional 7 ml. is deposited into the ligamentous attachment over the dorsum of the sacrum. The sacral foramina must be carefully avoided. Finally, the needle is turned anterolaterally at an angle of 45 degrees and 1 ml. is deposited into the short sacroiliac and interosseous ligaments. It is advisable to use a syringe with a needle-locking device, since considerable resistance to the injection material is experienced as sclerosis takes place.

Injections are tolerated extremely well by patients of varying ages and both sexes. The injections are given at intervals of 2 weeks, and each patient receives an average of five to six injections. Three injections are usually sufficient to produce an effective sclerosis of the interspinous ligaments. Over a period of 20 years, 5000 injections have been carried out with satisfactory results and no complications of any kind. Hackett claimed a relief rate of 82 per cent, and my results, in carefully selected patients, have approximated this figure. The impression gained is that relief is experienced, commonly, for 2 years or longer in some 80 per cent of patients. When patients return complaining of recurrence of pain and are anxious to continue the injections, they insist that following sclerosis they experienced a sensation of security in the low back.

Patients suffering from lumbar intervertebral ligamentous strain or lumbosacral ligamentous strain are provided with a well-fitting Freeman-type corset to wear for the first 6 weeks of treatment. Patients suffering from sacroiliac ligamentous strain are provided with the same type of corset, to which a supratrochanteric strap has been added. While under treatment, patients are instructed not to carry out any heavy lifting and to avoid bending and working in the flexed position.

Postlaminectomy Pain. A number of patients fail to find relief from low back pain following laminectomy, with or without fusion, for intervertebral disc herniation, despite clear indications for surgery, competent technique, and suitable postoperative treatment.

Following decompression of the affected root, the patient experiences relief from referred pain in the leg, while motor weakness and neurologic deficit improve. Many of these patients, however, complain of failure to obtain relief from low back pain itself. The residual pain described is of a lesser degree than the preoperative low back pain and is of a more diffuse and aching quality. This type of pain is not an uncommon sequel in patients who have suffered chronic disc herniation and who finally come to operation after a long period of disability. Examination may reveal that, while patients have been relieved of the pain and disability of intervertebral disc origin, the secondary involvement of the lumbosacral and sacroiliac ligaments is the cause of residual pain. In the small series of patients seen by me, sclerosis of these ligaments has given substantial relief.

EXERCISE

Opinions differed widely in the past about the place of active excercise in the treatment of low back pain, particularly of disc origin. Vigorous active exercises have no place in the treatment of the acute phase of lumbar disc derangement or other acute conditions involving the lumbar spine.

Exercises are prescribed to increase the power of the back musculature, to increase the mobility of the spinal joints, to stretch remote, contracted structures such as the hamstring muscles, and to improve and maintain posture.

Nachemson, in his studies of exercise and its effect on intradiscal pressure, stressed that many of these exercises increased the load in the lumbar spine greatly, and quoted Kendall and Jenkins and Lindström and Zachrisson, that isometric exercises, alone or combined with traction, give better results than the commonly prescribed flexion-extension patterns of exercise.[17,19] At the same time he emphasized that passive motion has its own risks (Fig. 10-17).

Except after prolonged bed rest or a long period of incarceration in a brace, the massive extensors of the lower lumbar spine rarely require strengthening exercises. Those designed to mobilize the lumbar spine, to mold and hold its contour in the optimal postural attitude, and to permit it to carry out its multiplicity of functions with maximum efficiency, are necessary. They should be directed at those muscles that control the shape and position of the lumbar spine relative to the gravitational forces and stress with which it has to contend.

Lewer Allen demonstrated electromyographically that the rectus abdominis muscle does not contract when the trunk

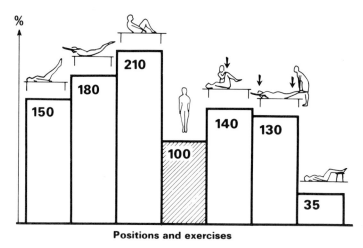

Positions and exercises

Fig. 10-17. Relative change in pressure (or load) in the third lumbar disc with various muscle-strengthening exercises in living subjects. Traditional exercises and their effect on discal pressure are analyzed in this table. The dangers of resisted and antigravity exercises in the early stages of low back pain are illustrated. (Nachemson, A. L.: Spine. 1:59, 1976. © 1976 Harper & Row Publishers, Inc. Hagerstown, Md.)

Fig. 10-18. Lumbar isometric exercises: crook lying.

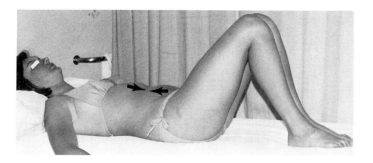

is flexed from the erect position, except to force flexion to its ultimate stage.[1] Floyd and Silver analyzed the interactivity of the component muscles of the anterior abdominal wall by the use of multiple electromyographic electrodes.[8] They pointed out that the head-raising type of exercise against gravity benefits significantly only the rectus abdominis, while bilateral straight-leg raising, with its fixation effect upon the pelvis, caused activity in the whole abdominal wall.

Campbell emphasized the importance of the oblique and transverse muscles in the act of expiration.[3] The patient should, therefore, strongly contract the abdominal wall and couple this with strong voluntary exhalation.

Failure to accentuate the important part synchronized respiration plays in association with abdominal-strengthening exercises has diminished the effect of this form of therapy in the past.

TYPES OF EXERCISE

The program of exercise may be drawn up once the patient is free from pain and gravity-free mobility is satisfactorily demonstrated. Exercises clearly will vary in load, frequency, and goal in different patients. Age, sex, local conditions of the bony and ligamentous apparatus of the lumbar spine must be assessed, as well as the state of the patient's musculature. Exercise load is carefully graded to the patient's ability and power.

Lumbar Isometric Exercises

"Crook-Lying." This exercise may be carried out while the patient is still bedfast. The patient lies supine with one pillow under the head and with the hips and knees comfortably flexed (Fig. 10-18).

The exercise begins by the patient taking a deep inspiration. The patient is then asked to contract the abdominal muscles by pulling the umbilicus toward the spine. At the same time he exhales as forcibly as possible. Since the abdominal muscles are the most powerful of the expiratory muscles, the action of abdominal contraction is increased substantially.

At the same time as the expiratory phase, he carries out isometric contraction of the abdominal muscles. The importance of the expiratory phase cannot be overstated, and the synchrony of the two groups must be achieved.

Gluteal Contractions. The patient is taught to contract the gluteal muscles. The action is gentle at first and is gradually increased to maximum contractions.

A Combination of Abdominal and Gluteal Contraction. The two exercises described above are now carried out simultaneously.

"Pelvic Tucking." The patient is asked to flatten his back against the supporting surface and to carry out Exercise 3, combining it with upward tilting of the pelvis, while holding the lumbar spine flat against the supporting surface in order to abolish lordosis (Fig. 10-19).

Initially, the patient may find difficulty

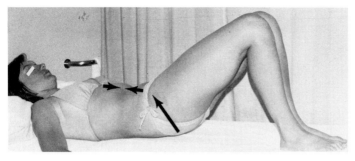

FIG. 10-19. Pelvic "tucking."

in combining these movements, but rapid progress from five to 15 combined movements is possible. Suitable rest intervals should be given.

The same exercise is taught in the *standing* position, but postural faults are not corrected at this stage. The patient is encouraged to carry out the exercise until he is proficient. When proficiency has been attained, the patient carries out his exercises as often as his activities permit, for example while walking.

The above exercises primarily increase the efficiency of the abdominal muscles, the rectus abdominis in particular. The use of powerful expiration will tend to activate the oblique and transverse muscle as well. The exercises are primarily designed as an early stage of activity and rehabilitation after intervertebral breakdown. It is doubtful whether patients who have suffered "disc" episodes will benefit from heavy, resisted exercises, because of the consequent rise in intradiscal pressure.

Resisted Exercises

The patient lies supine on a firm surface. The legs are extended and the arms lie by the sides. Respiratory synchrony is essential for all exercises involving the abdominal wall. The exercise begins with deep inspiration. The patient, keeping the hips and knees extended, sits up to an angle of 90 degrees, expiring deeply. It is important that no assistance be given to the patient by holding down the feet, since this will permit the flexors of the hips to assist the movement of sitting erect. If the extended legs are voluntarily pressed against the supporting surface, inhibition of the hip flexors takes place. Again, this exercise primarily contracts the rectus abdominis.

The patient lies supine with the pronated hands beneath the buttocks, in order to help abolish lordosis. (Fig. 10-20, 10-21). The exercise again commences with deep inspiration. The extended legs are flexed at the hip joints to 45 degrees, simultaneously with deep expiration.

Both exercises are commenced in groups of five and increased as needed.

Quadriceps Exercises. The quadriceps muscles are exercised in order to increase their power, this being essential for weight lifting with a straight lumbar spine (Fig. 10-22).

The patient who has suffered low back breakdown is taught at all times to lift weights by holding the weight close to the trunk and flexing and then extending the knees with the lumbar spine straight. The limit of lifting in this manner is the ultimate weight of the object.

Stretching Exercises

Hamstrings. Short hamstrings are a common cause of increased lordosis, and stretching exercises for these muscles are part of a program to diminish the exaggerated lumbar curve (Fig. 10-23). The muscles are tested by instructing the patient to touch the toes with the knees ex-

FIG. 10-20. Resisted exercises.

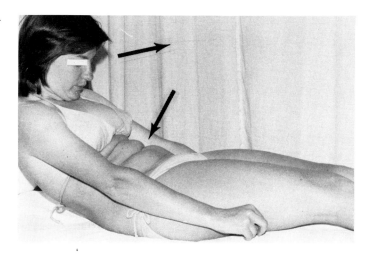

tended. The degree of failure will give an indication of muscle shortage.

The hamstrings may be stretched by asking the patient to carry out repetitive "sit-ups," with assistance being given by holding the feet, or by tilting the supporting surface to assist spinal flexion. Touching the toes in the erect position should be discouraged because of the increased intradiscal pressure it causes.

BRACING

The purpose of bracing is, in the main, to permit ambulation while allowing local rest of the low back. Unfortunately, the lower the lesion, the greater the problem of splintage becomes. The lowest level of the brace must allow mobility of the hip joints and permit the patient to sit. It is, nevertheless, essential that the inferior border of the brace extend as far below the lumbosacral joint as possible, so that the paravertebral supports do not produce adverse leverage on this key joint.

Corsets

The muscles of the lower spine, including the abdominal wall, play a significant part in its support. The trunk musculature, by increasing the pressure within the thoracic and abdominal cavities, effectively decreases the stress on the lower

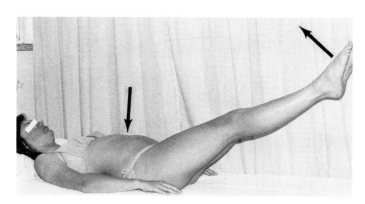

FIG. 10-21. Resisted exercises.

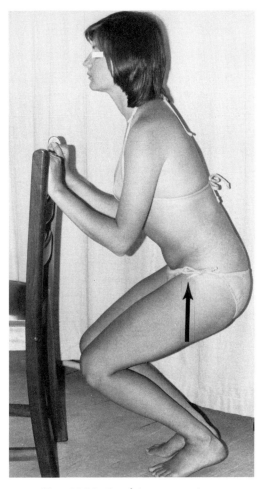

FIG. 10-22. Quadriceps exercises.

intervertebral discs and lumbar vertebrae. A strong anterior abdominal wall is one of the most efficient agents in this mechanism, and weakness, whatever the cause, increases the vulnerability of the lower spine to stress.

The operative principle of the corset is to increase the pressure in the abdominal cavity. It is essentially a tube of strong material, usually of canvas or man-made fiber, which is reinforced posteriorly by paravertebral steels. It should be molded accurately to the lumbar curve and its effect controlled by lateral lacing. It is commonly lighter than a brace and more cosmetically acceptable; but, unlike the brace, it is not rigid. It is warmer in hot weather, but more comfortable to sleep in.

Braces

Despite its greater rigidity a well-fitting brace, by virtue of its resistance to change of shape on movement, may be more comfortable than a corset and, because of its open framework, cooler in hot countries. It should produce less friction, since there is less surface area in contact with the skin. The brace limits spinal movement in the vertical planes, and when a supratrochanteric band and iliac crest

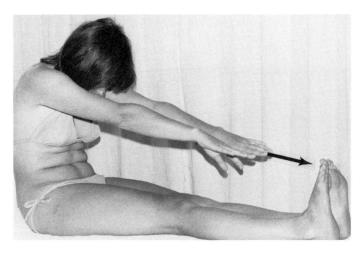

FIG. 10-23. Hamstring stretching exercises.

steels are added, rotation is limited to a reasonable extent. It should be noted that the classical braces were not designed to diminish axial stress. No brace, however well designed, is able to control the lower segments of the lumbar spine as well as it can the lumbodorsal spine.

Norton and Brown, in a review of back supports, believed that the longer braces have a lever action. In forward flexion of the trunk the main force is concentrated at the lumbodorsal junction, too high to control the important lower levels, so that flexion at the lumbosacral and adjacent joint was greater when this type of brace was worn than without it. They also commented upon the possibility that specific patterns of flexion exist that may be clinically significant and that patients vary in their lumbar flexion; those with the most action probably being the most vulnerable.

The origin of low back bracing and splinting is as old as ancient Egyptian medicine and progressed from simple materials, such as tree bark, used to form a malleable support, to the highly sophisticated braces and splints of the medieval armorers. Today, although we recognize the difficulties, we are still at a stage of mechanical compromise. C. P. Taylor, in the middle of the last century, designed a brace which utilized the classical three-point method of support, using a force at the pelvis and shoulders to produce extension of the back and a forward force in the midspinal region. Jordan, in his authoritative treatise on orthopedic appliances, classified spinal braces into two main types: the positive supporting spinal brace and the active correcting brace.[11] He proceeded to discuss the three-point method of fixation.

Most patients resent the idea of incarceration within a brace, with its attendant mechanical and cosmetic disadvantages, and it is important to explain the specific purpose and value of the appliance in lay terms. Modern braces use light metals

and materials; one of their few advantages.

Braces are at their best in patients of moderate weight, since the brace must be close-fitting. Obese patients should be advised to diet before fitting and their reduced weight must be maintained.

Leather has remained the covering of choice, despite the discovery of plastic materials, since it produces little friction to the skin and is absorbent. The brace must be well-fitting, to prevent unnecessary movement. Its fastenings should be within easy reach of the patient and of simple design (self-retaining buckles or Velcro), and pressure points must be noted and carefully prepared.

The same three-point principle is largely used today, and braces consist of minor variations of the long Taylor brace and the various shorter types. The most effective and comfortable is the Amsterdam.

The Taylor brace consists of a rigid posterior framework extending from a supratrochanteric band with two further superior straps, which are attached to a free abdominal pad extending from pubis to xiphisternum. It is held in place by two shoulder straps. It is designed to prevent flexion and is least effective in the lower lumbar spine (Fig. 10-24).

The dynamic extension brace was devised by Coplans and Helfet some 20 years ago (Fig. 10-25) and has been used consistently since. It consists of a padded plate fitted to the small of the back, from which extends three twisted springs: one around the pelvis to fix the brace; the second along the crest of the ilium, which takes pressure on the anterior superior spine, and the third twisted upward to form pectoral pads. The brace is effective.

The back-plate is stable and remains applied to the countour of the patient's back during all movements. Its efficiency is tested by asking the patient to sit down and to stand up from a chair. The plate

(Text continues on p. 178)

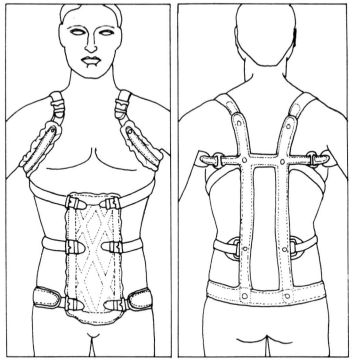

FIG. 10-24. The Taylor brace.

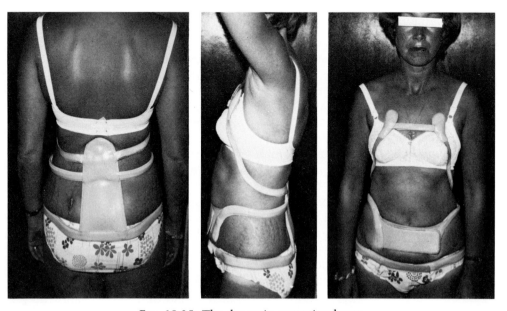

FIG. 10-25. The dynamic extension brace.

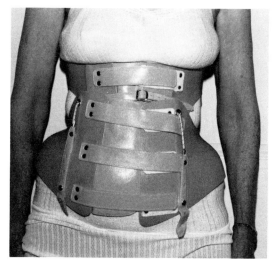
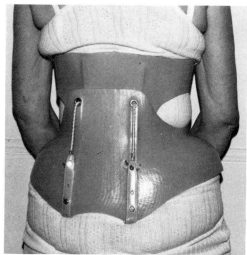

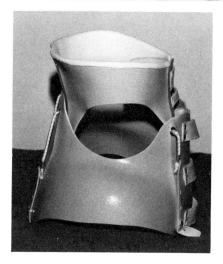

FIG. 10-26. The Coplans brace.

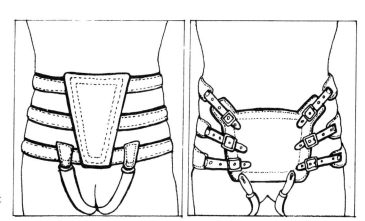

FIG. 10-27. The Goldthwait brace.

should not move away from the patient. No rigid brace can do this (i.e., remain firmly applied during all movements).

The Coplans Brace. None of the braces described effectively prevent axial stress, except in terms of movement from the vertical position. The fundamental purpose of this brace is to produce an upward lift or, rather, diminish the axial weight on the lower lumbar spine. It is of light, molded fiber and consists of two parts: a thoracic corset which lies within a molded pelvic base, both of these closed anteriorly by a simple corset device with lacing. Four elastic cords are attached in pairs anteriorly and posteriorly to the lower, free margin of the thoracic component and are then threaded through eyelets on the upper, free margin of the pelvic support, and act as pulleys. The elastics may be tightened suitably to pull the thoracic corset upward, producing a supporting or traction effect on the lumbar spine. It is astonishing how little force is required to produce such an effect (Fig. 10-26).

This type of brace weighs a little less than 2 pounds and has been used for 20 years in conditions such as acute episodes of spondylolysis, spondylolisthesis, chronic lumbosacral strain, and peripheral root pain, requiring reduction of the load on the lumbar spine. It is comfortable, and its materials ensure that it is easy to keep clean.

The Amsterdam brace is a short, comfortable brace, based on a supratrochanteric band and short paravertebral steels ascending as high as D10. It has hooped steels, taking purchase over the iliac crests, and is fastened anteriorly by a short corset. It prevents hyperextension and permits the patient to lean back upon the paravertebral steels.

The Goldthwait brace, sometimes called the Osgood sacroiliac brace, is a short brace consisting of two paravertebral steels covered with leather and forming a lumbar pad and, anteriorly, a rigid abdominal pad. The anterior and posterior pads are joined together by three adjustable lateral straps (Fig. 10-27). The brace reinforces the pelvic ring with its lower strap and produces intraabdominal pressure with the anterior pad. It is a compromise lumbosacroiliac device.

POSTURE

Exercise has, as its primary goal, an efficiently operating back, which implies a satisfactory posture. Since man's unique mechanical design demands a life-long, unrelenting battle against gravity and its associated stresses, his ideal posture must necessarily be that which he can maintain most effortlessly throughout the activities of daily living. Most prescriptions of correct posture depict man in the "stand-easy" position. The "standing erect" posture is, unfortunately, of little practical use in the machine-dominated Western world. The inhabitants of less sophisticated societies, particularly in Africa, do not suffer either the same degree of low back disability or postural imbalance. Posture must, therefore, be considered in relation to activities and not to Man as a standing, motionless pillar. Mechanically satisfactory posture must not be confused with appearance.

The effects of common pathological conditions, such as myopia, flat feet, adolescent kyphosis, even when minimal, are important. It is evident that there exists a correct posture which is a suitable and personal compromise for each patient.

The inability of man to stand still for lengthy periods is well known but will bear reemphasis. Shifting from one leg to another; rest against any support which may offer itself; the many variations of standing and sitting which occur naturally; all indicate that a satisfactory, motionless posture is neither practical or possible. No statue or other work of art exists depicting motionless, vertical Man.

It is not a naturally occurring phenomenon, and too much time is spent in teaching patients to assume static and unnatural attitudes.

Joseph stated that the use of the adjective "postural" when applied to muscles such as the soleus, gluteus maximus, quadriceps, and erectores spinae, is unwarranted.[12] It should be reserved for muscles that are required to achieve or maintain correct posture. Since the ankle is stabilized by the calf muscles, the knee and hip joints by their ligaments, and the vertebral joints by parts of the erectores spinae, these muscles will exhibit electrical activity only when the subject sways from the vertical "stand easy" position, and are otherwise silent.

Opinions vary as to the ideal postural attitude. Tucker described an attitude which he called, "active, alerted posture." This consists of standing erect, with feet slightly apart and the toes slightly flexed. The knees are slightly flexed. The buttocks are contracted in what Tucker described as a "pinch proof" manner. The umbilicus is "buttoned" to the spine. The shoulders are slightly elevated and flexed. The head is extended as if reaching for the ceiling and attempting to touch it with the vertex (Figs. 10-28, 10-29). The impression this posture gives is one of alertness and readiness for action; but it is a preparation for movement and does not utilize the principles of relaxed standing posture with minimal muscle contracture as discussed earlier in the chapter.

Posture and exercise are parts of the same mechanism by which man maintains his body in an optimal attitude against gravity. Efficient posture connotes the achievement of a desired and comfortable stance embodying minimal muscular expenditure. The advent of electromyography and the ability to measure intradiscal pressure, have largely eliminated traditional and anachronistic concepts. Correct posture is of maximal importance during three decades of life,

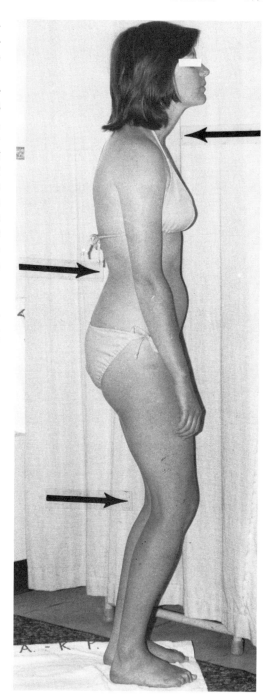

FIG. 10-28. The model demonstrates what is traditionally accepted as poor posture: everted feet, slight genu valgum with femoral rotation, pelvic tilting. The abdominal wall is slack, and lordosis is evident. Shoulders are flexed; the upper dorsal spine is kyphotic; and the head is "cantilevered."

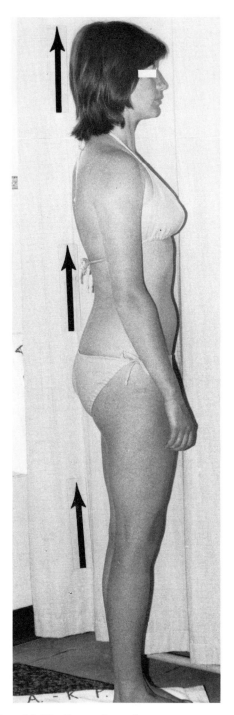

FIG. 10-29. Correction of poor posture, accomplished in the main by gluteal "tucking," abdominal wall contraction, and revision of the position of the head, so that the vertex reaches vertically upward. The lordosis is corrected.

since by this time bone has been shaped and molded and ligaments contracted into patterns that are no longer truly malleable. While further deterioration may be prevented, dynamic correction is difficult to achieve.

Postural faults may be resolved broadly under two headings: (1) mobile imbalance which is imposed upon a normal locomotor system and normally oriented psychological attitude, and (2) deformity, which is the result of symmetrical imbalance or pathological causes. The first group is easily treated by individual therapy, which is continued on a group basis as soon as adequate improvement is demonstrated. Compromise must always be accepted for the wide variations of the norm which occur in the different somatic types encountered. However, it is the second group that constitutes the therapeutic problem, and here treatment must be handled on an individual level, the program and goal having been carefully ventilated by the physician and the therapist. Where compromise is accepted, a precisely limited goal should be defined, otherwise loss of patient cooperation and interest results. The author has treated the problem of posture thematically in the section on Exercise, and has employed the evidence of electromyography and the mensuration of intradiscal pressure as material evidence.

The shape of the body, with its multiplicity of spinal and costal joints, is molded and prepared in youth for the ultimate form that it must assume for its final struggle against gravity, when elasticity has diminished and musculature becomes feeble. Each skill, from the crouching stance of the boxer, to the fluent perfection of the ballet dancer, makes its lasting imprint on the individual. Similarly, pathological conditions, ranging from asthma to congenital variations of the spine, must have the same effect. A superficial rigid uniformity exists only in the serried ranks of soldiers,

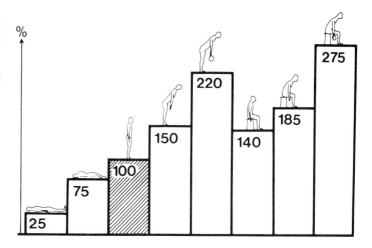

FIG. 10-30. Relative change in pressure (or load) in the third lumbar disc in various positions in living subjects. This graphic evaluation clarifies the importance of both correct posture and intermittent rest. (Nachemson, A. L.: Spine. 1:59, 1976. © 1976, Harper & Row Publishers, Inc., Hagerstown, Md.)

and our attention should be engaged by the posture of motion, rather than the static motionless stance of tradition.

It is beyond the scope of this chapter to attempt the description of correct posture in motion and in the numerous attitudes which the body assumes sequentially. However, the fundamental rule remains immutable: optimal function with minimal expenditure of energy; or in precise terms, good posture requires minimal electromyographic activity and intradiscal pressure (Fig. 10-30).

Where, then, do the problems of posture commence? It is not possible for a depressed and troubled patient to exhibit good posture, and psychogenic causes therefore require consideration and solution. Posture is fluid, since it is the response to the input of multiple impulses into the sensorium and the constantly changing motor patterns which result. The teaching of correct postural attitudes, usually begins with placement of the head in its proper relationship to the trunk. The reverse should be true, since the feet are the base upon which true posture is built, stage by stage (see Fig. 10-29).

The Feet. The foundation of all standing posture derives from the use of the correct weight-bearing areas of the feet, in order to avoid the lateral and torsional stresses on the legs and their joints, which finally must affect the inclination of the pelvis.

A firm anterior abdominal wall is essential to sustain intraabdominal pressure and to prevent exaggerated lordosis and abnormal pelvic tilting. Strong gluteal muscles assist this action. Costal cage function depends largely on correct spinal alignment.

Satisfactory posture of the head demands a correct lordotic curve of the cervical spine, which in its turn must be influenced by the inferior curves of which it is a continuum.

The shoulders are permitted to hang freely and the arms to mold themselves naturally to the sides.

The head is balanced on the delicate mobile cervical spine by the cervical musculature, in the main the posterior muscles, while the vertex is thrust upward in Tucker's "alerted" attitude.

Because of his evolutionary sacrifice of "field" vision for stereoscopic vision, man requires a monitoring attitude of his head for the enlargement of his visual input, and the posture of his head is, therefore, an important part of his defense mechanism.

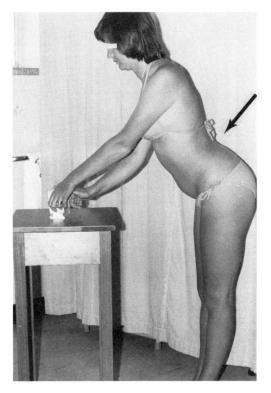
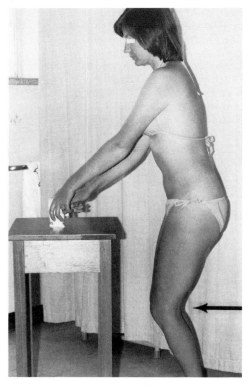

A   **B**

FIG. 10-31. *(A)* The inherent danger of a slack abdominal wall, increased lordosis, and angle of tilt of the hips, making the lumbar spine vulnerable. *(B)* Correction of these faults: the pelvic angle has been straightened by flexing the knees, the abdominal wall is contracted, and lordosis is abolished.

CORRECT WEIGHT LIFTING

It is evident that correct posture can be monitored accurately by electrical means, without delving into the mechanics of the spinal bones. When flexion takes place in a standing position, electrical activity ceases in the extensors of the spine as soon as full flexion is reached, with consequent lengthening and relaxation of the erector spinae muscles. Floyd and Silver reported that in extension from this position, with the subject's hand loaded with a weight of 56 pounds, initial lifting commences at the hip joints, while the extensor muscles of the spine continue electrically silent.[9] There exists, therefore, a critical angle when weight is supported by inert tissues only, and it seems reasonable to assume that this is the angle of maximal vulnerability of the spine, which is momentarily bereft of the control of the powerful extensors. A good deal of low back pain could be avoided if a brief but succinct explanation of the mechanism of the lumbar spine were taught to senior Secondary School students during their gymnastic instruction, and the handling of common, heavy objects by ergo-dynamic methods demonstrated to them. These consist essentially of maintaining the spine in its least vulnerable attitude, while thrusting, pulling, and lifting is carried out, using the weight of the body. From a prophylactic and rehabilitative point of view, this type of handling exercises should be introduced to pupils at High School level, to reduce low back injuries in an industrial society (Fig. 10-31).

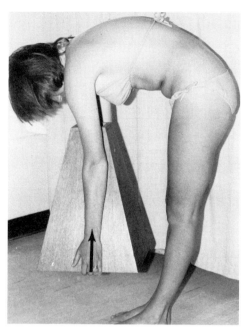

C

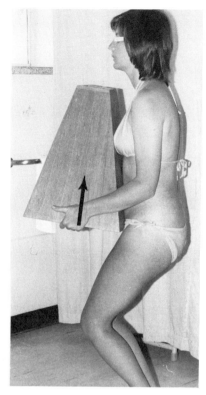

D

FIG. 10-31 *Continued.* *(C)* The "vulnerable angle" described by Floyd and Silver, demonstrates loss of control by the spinal extensors. *(D)* The correct method of lifting, holding weight close to the trunk and using the quadriceps to lift.

REFERENCES

1. Allen, C. E. L.: Muscle action potentials used in the study of dynamic anatomy. Brit. J. Phys. Med., *11*:66, 1948.
2. Barry, P. J. C., and Hume-Kendall, P.: Corticosterioid infiltration of the extradural space. Ann. Phys. Med., *6*:267, 1962.
3. Campbell, E. J. M.: The functions of the abdominal muscles in relation to the intra-abdominal pressure and the respiration. Arch. Middlesex Hosp., *5*:87, 1955.
4. Coplans, C. W.: Lumbar disc herniation. South African Med. J., *25*:881, 1951.
5. ———: Lumbar Intervertebral disc herniation. South African Med. J., *27*:182, 1953.
6. Cyriax, J.: Text Book of Orthopaedic Medicine. vol. 2. London, Cassel & Co., 1959.
7. Dawkins, M.: The identification of the epidural space; a critical analysis of various methods employed. Anesthesia, *18*:66, 1963.
8. Floyd, W. F., and Silver, P. H. S.; Electromyographic patterns of activity of the anterior abdominal wall patterns in man. J. Anat., *84*:132, 1950.
9. ———: The function of erectores spinae in certain movements and postures in man. J.Physiol., *129*:184, 1955.
10. Hackett, G. S.: Joint Ligament Relaxation Treated by Fibro-osseus Proliferation. Springfield, Charles C Thomas, 1956.
11. Jordan, H. H.: Orthopaedic Appliances. New York, Oxford University Press, 1939.
12. Joseph, J.: Man's Posture, Electromyographic Studies. Springfield, Charles C Thomas, 1960.
13. Kellgren, J. H.: Observations on referred pain arising from muscle. Clin. Sci. *3*:175, 1938.
14. ———: On the distribution of pain arising from deep somatic structures with charts of segmental pain areas. Clin. Sci., *4*:35, 1939.
15. ———: Some painful joint conditions and their relation to osteoarthritis. Clin. Sci., *4*:193, 1939.
16. ———: Somatic stimulating visceral pain. Clin. Sci., *4*:303, 1939.
18. Kohler, R.: Contrast examination of lumbar interspinous ligaments. Acta Radiol., *52*:21, 1959.
19. Lindström, A., and Zachrisson, M.: Physical Therapy on Low Back Pain and Sciatica. Scand. J. Rehabil. Med., *2*:37, 1970.
20. Mehta, M.: Intractable Pain. Philadelphia, W. B. Saunders, 1973.
21. Nachemson, A.: Toward a better understanding of low-back pain: a review of the mechanics of the lumbar disc. Rheum. Rehabil., *14*:129, 1975.
22. Norton, P. L., and Brown, T.: The immobilizing efficiency of back braces. J. Bone Joint Surg., *39A*:111, 1957.
23. Steindler, A.: Kinesiology of the Human Body. Springfield, Charles C Thomas, 1955.
24. Trevor-Jones, R.: Osteoarthritis of the paravertebral joints of the 2nd and 3rd cervical vertebrae as a cause of occipital headache. South African Med. J., *38*:392, 1964.
25. Tucker, W. E.: Home Treatment and Posture. Edinburg, Churchill Livingstone, 1973.

11 The Radiology of Backache

Pieter D. de Villiers

Pain-producing diseases of the spine include infections, metabolic disease, and primary and secondary tumors of the vertebrae or neural elements. The complex intervertebral joints are prone to degenerative arthrosis and to arthritis of a multitude of forms (including ankylosing spondylitis, rheumatoid arthritis, and the "variants" associated with ulcerative colitis and psoriasis), Reiter's syndrome and gout, pyrophosphate arthropathy, and brucellosis. In a major proportion of cases pain is due to disease of the intervertebral discs and ligaments. Peripheral pain may be caused by spinal disease or peripheral neuritis. In addition, the symptoms of diseases of the spine and nervous system may be complicated or mimicked by psychological stress backache.

INDICATIONS

The golden rules of radiology are to avoid all unnecessary examinations and to make every examination that is essential thorough and complete. The requirements of an orthopaedic surgeon's request for roentgenographic examination of a painful back differ from those of the family doctor. Presumably preliminary examinations would have been completed and simple forms of treatment applied, and the patient's complaint is already serious enough or chronic enough to warrant, among other forms of treatment, at least consideration of an operation.

ROENTGENOGRAPHY

The Radiology Department will do five or six routine views of the lumbar spine. Every spine exposure should be made on a long film (17 x 7 ins.), so as to include the sacroiliac region as well as the lower thoracic vertebrae (Fig. 11-1).* It is an advantage to perform anteroposterior and lateral examinations with the patient standing erect, to insure a natural stance, and the operator should not correct curvatures or impose false curvatures to accommodate the film or technique. When lateral views fail to show the intervertebral disc spaces "open," it is impossible to distinguish between a tilted disc space and a narrowed space. When erect, contralateral, and tilt views fail, tomography may provide the most accurate assessment. Similarly, the oblique views should ideally "open" all the paravertebral joints, including the sacroiliac joints. It is advis-

---

*In all myelograms illustrated in this chapter the letter or letters always indicate, in addition to the right or left side of the patient, the side(s) of symptoms, and a small ball-bearing on the patient's back marks the site of the lumbar puncture, for future reference by the radiologist and the surgeon.

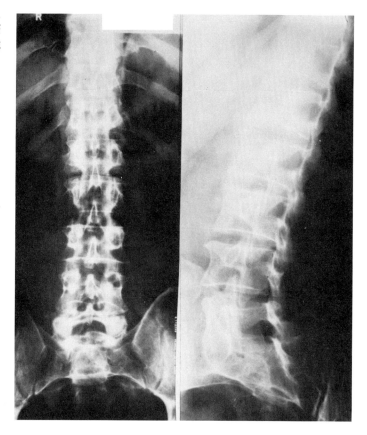

FIG. 11-1. Routine anteroposterior and oblique views of the lumbar spine, including the sacroiliac joint.

able to add lateral stress views of the lumbar spine, erect, in full flexion, and in extension. Cinematography and observation on the fluoroscopic screen have been less informative than simple large films on which details can be studied and measured.

The whole pelvis, being part of the structural and functional unit of the back, is included in every examination of the lumbar spine. In the experience of many orthopaedic surgeons are examples of disastrous maldirection of investigation and treatment of backache, subsequently found to have been due to disease of the pelvic bones or joints. Clinical or roentgenographic information may lead to additional special examinations of the sacroiliac joints, including tomography. Sometimes examination of the thoracic spine is similarly indicated. The routine lateral film of the thoracic spine is a midline thick-layer tomograph or zonograph, because it is impossible to see the necessary details of the thoracic spine on lateral views through the ribs, lungs, diaphragm, and shoulder girdle (Fig. 11-2).

The interpretation of baffling signs in the bones and joints of the back is sometimes simplified by the examination of other parts of the skeleton. Occasionally a chest film will serve as a "mirror of systemic disease," apart from its possible value for the anesthetist.

INTERPRETATION

Mistakes are less often due to faulty interpretation than to inadequate roentgenography, but a few remarks may be appropriate.

Incredibly, an anatomically narrow

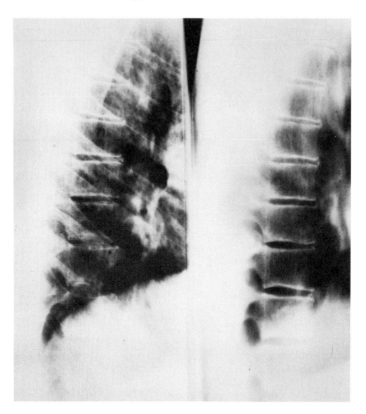

FIG. 11-2. Plain lateral film of the thoracic spine compared with routine zonography. In the ordinary film the view is obscured by ribs, lung vessels, the diaphragm, and the shoulder girdle.

lumbosacral disc space is still often regarded as "narrowed" when, in fact, partial sacralization, present in nearly half the population, is perhaps more often a sign of strength than of weakness at that level: a rudimentary disc is not prone to herniation, degeneration, or instability.

The interpretation of the roentgenographic appearance of paravertebral joints is notoriously unreliable: paravertebral joints which appear to be normal may be a cause of severe disability. Spondylolisthesis may even develop as a result of degenerative disease of paravertebral joints which appear normal on oblique views. On the other hand, loss of space in these joints is much more difficult to assess than narrowing of a disc space. "Sclerosis" is commonly diagnosed in patients with an anatomically well developed subarticular cortical layer. Tomog-

raphy only occasionally helps to clear up some of the various misinterpretations.

Tropism, or assymmetry in the interpretation of paravertebral joints is seen too often in painless backs to be taken really seriously. On the other hand, malaligned lower lumbar and lumbosacral paravertebral joints (i.e., joints which are not parallel to those at the higher levels on oblique views), are commonly seen to develop early and cause severe degenerative disease with advancing years.

The more complicated paravertebral sacroiliac joints are equally difficult to interpret. The subarticular cortical layer varies even more than in the lumbar facet joints. The wide and ill-defined appearance of normal young joints account, for many miraculous cures of "early Marie-Strumpell spondylitis." Conversely, patients may be in discomfort, and possibly incapacitated, from undoubted sacroiliac strain which defies demonstation by roentgenographs.

The value of roentgen assessment of instability (Chap. 6) is liable to be overestimated—on the one hand, because slight rotation is easily mistaken for a sliding movement, and on the other hand, because important rotational instability cannot be demonstrated at all.

Many of the true roentgenographic abnormalities demonstrated may be incidental or not directly related to the patient's symptoms, and care should be taken lest an unexpected roentgenographic finding such as spondylolisthesis becomes an indication for operation in a patient whose symptoms in themselves would not have called for operation. Roentgen findings which are often clinically irrelevant include Schmorl's nodes, large osteophytes, and signs of disc degeneration such as narrowing, a vacuum sign, and calcification in a disc or annulus, all of which are seen in a large percentage of the population, many of whom have no symptoms referable to the back.

Arterial calcification may be noted in roentgenographs of the spine and pelvis, but circulatory insufficiency, occasionally mistaken for spinal disease, is not always so obvious.

MYELOGRAPHY

Plain films of the bony walls of the spinal canal do not allow accurate assessment of the state of its contents. For instance, it is common to find the symptomatic prolapsed disc at a different level from the narrow disc space.

Myelography first became acceptable as a regular diagnostic method with the development of Myodil (ethyl iodophenylundecylate) in 1944. Myodil shares with all other oily contrast media the triple disadvantages of impenetrable density, immiscibility with body fluids, and "reluctance" to enter narrow spaces. More-

over, and particularly because it is almost completely nonabsorbable, Myodil, unless it is completely removed, leads to progressive subarachnoid fibrosis.

Since 1970 relatively safe water-soluble contrast media have been developed in the place of oily Myodil and watersoluble but highly irritating Abrodil, which required anesthesia. In 1970 Ahlgren reported the use of Dimer-X (dimeglumine iocarmate) in lumbar radiculography.[1] Gonsette's report of 1971 on the use of Dimer-X covered much of what was later confirmed by others in larger series.[2] He even attempted thoracic and cervical myelography with this medium.

We have performed myelograms with Dimer-X in 3000 patients in the last 3½ years. Although the manufacturers' original instructions advised against the use of Dimer-X above the level of the L2, our cases include examination of the lumbar segment, usually with the lower thoracic segment (in 2661; full thoracic segment in 512; and cervical canal in 444 instances). The incidence of reactions with examinations at higher levels is not significantly greater than for lumbar radiculography.[3,4] More recently a non-ionic water-soluble medium, Metrizamide (Amipaque) has been used successfully for lumbar radiculography and then for thoracic and cervical myelography.[6,7] The regular use of water-soluble contrast media for myelography has strongly influenced the investigation of disc disease and backache generally. It is no longer true to say that the objective of myelography is merely to localize clinical disc prolapse. For surgeons who have experienced its diagnostic accuracy, water-soluble myelography has become routine before any spinal operation and plays a part in the decision to operate as well as in the choice of operation.

Technique

We introduce Dimer-X by lumbar puncture in all examinations of the lumbar, thoracic, and cervical regions and have found in practice that proper diffusion of contrast is obtained by injection with the patient sitting, rather than lying on the side. The dose is 10 ml. for nearly all adults: the previously recommended dose of 5 ml. is usually too small for diagnostic accuracy. The large dose allows adequate examination of the whole lumbar segment (Figs. 11-3—11-6) and routine inclusion of the lower thoracic segment. The extension into the lower thoracic region occasionally reveals unsuspected disease in patients with known lower lumbar disease (Fig. 11-7). The large dose also makes it possible to do successful stress views in the erect position in flexion and extension in selected patients (Figs. 11-8, 11-9). An anterior pressure effect on the spinal sac may be increased or decreased in flexion, depending,

presumably, on the state of the disc, the integrity of the posterior ligament, and the degree of stability at the particular level. Tomography may clarify an uncertain appearance (Fig. 11-10).

Contrast medium may be withdrawn after lumbar myelography in patients with arachnoiditis, a very narrow canal or where there is any other reason for fearing undue reaction, but withdrawal of a large volume of cerebrospinal fluid is likely to increase the incidence and severity of postmyelography headache. After full thoracic and cervical myelography, diffusion of contrast medium makes its withdrawal impractical and probably unnecessary.

Diagnostic Reliability

The diagnostic accuracy of water-soluble myelography in disc herniation

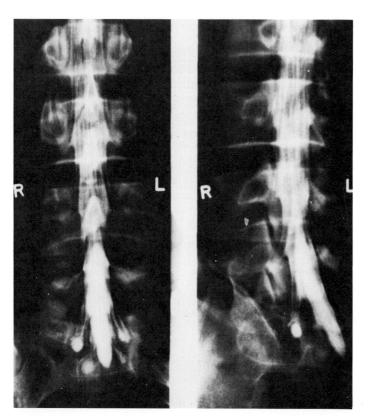

FIG. 11-3. Routine frontal and oblique views of lumbar water-soluble myelography, with filling of nerve root sheaths and, incidentally, of a root sheath diverticulum (so-called arachnoid cyst).

FIG. 11-4. Three of the routine views on lumbar myelography: disc prolapse with a large right anterolateral pressure effect.

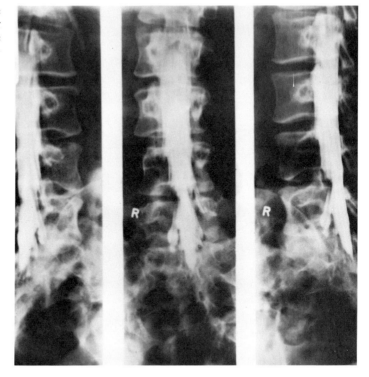

FIG. 11-5. Disc prolapse with more subtle right anterolateral pressure effect: three of the routine views.

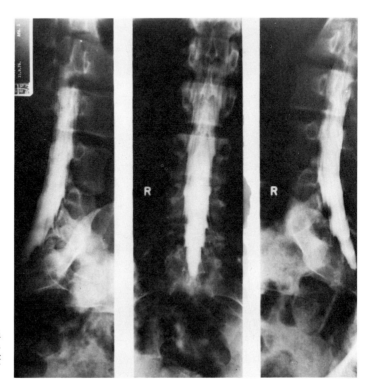

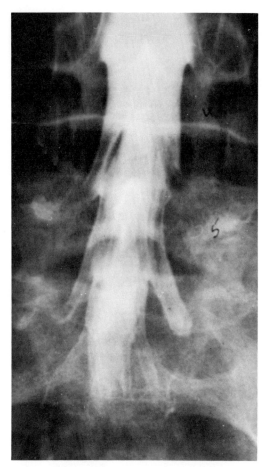

Fig. 11-6. Disc prolapse with lateral pressure effect confined to the nerve root: single anteroposterior view.

gives the surgeon confidence to avoid unnecessary operations and to limit the extent of necessary operations. In our series, the demonstration of prolapsed discs has been constantly confirmed in those patients who underwent surgery. In very rare instances even water-soluble myelography may fail to reveal a lateral disc prolapse, but on the whole a negative examination is reassuring when referred pain arises from the discs and other intervertebral joints and is not caused by nerve root compression. A false-negative result with protrusion at the level of the lumbosacral junction is possible when an anatomically large space is present between the disc and the dural sac, but this kind of disc protrusion is not a likely cause of nerve root compression.

Some years ago a review of 5 years' experience at the Nuffield Orthopaedic Centre at Oxford revealed the clinical localization of disc prolapse to be correct in only 39.2 per cent, whereas myelography achieved an accuracy of 75 per cent with Myodil and 90 per cent with a water-soluble medium (Abrodil).[10]

Water-soluble myelography with an adequate dose and proper diffusion makes it possible to determine the diameters of the canal accurately, but not its cross-sectional shape. It does serve to demonstrate other pathology which may simulate disc protrusions and to reveal the occasional occurrence of disc prolapse at more than one level.

Regarding false-positive findings, water-soluble media are not prone to the artifacts that are so common with Myodil and other oily materials. On the other hand, no experienced surgeon should be induced by dramatic myelographic demonstrations to operate on abnormalities that are indeed present but which may not be causing the patient's symptoms, or to operate without due regard for the known natural history of the disease or consideration of associated psychological factors. We have occasionally been impressed by the persistence of large pressure effects in patients whose symptoms had resolved on conservative treatment.

Advanced age is not a contraindication to myelography, except when it prevents operation. Contrary to our previous belief, disc herniation appears to be as common in old as in young people.

Reactions

Myelography should never be undertaken lightly or for any but really serious indications. It is never an out-patient pro-

FIG. 11-7. *(A)* The routine lateral views on lumbar myelography at three levels confirming the presence of suspected lower lumbar disc disease but also revealing the presence of a more serious lesion in the lower thoracic region with obstruction of the canal. *(B)* Two further oblique views of the lower thoracic region again demonstrate the obstruction by an extradural lesion.

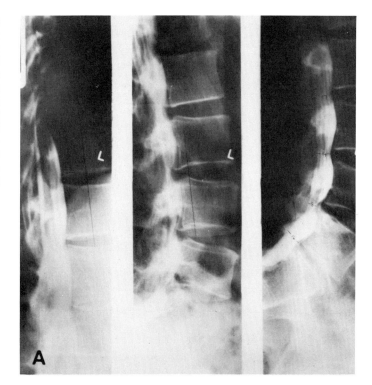

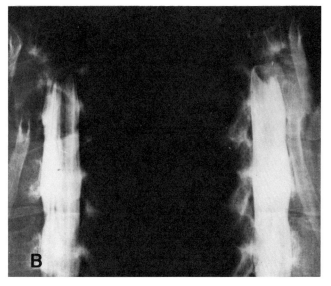

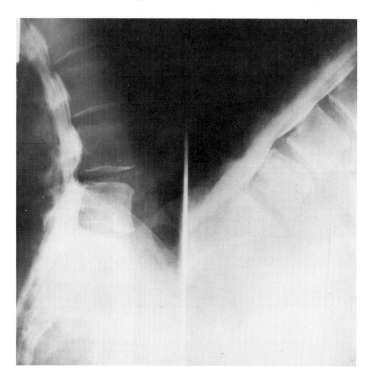

FIG. 11-8. Routine lateral stress views: anterior pressure effects at the levels of disc degeneration tend to decrease in flexion. Instability of L4 on L5, with tilt and shift.

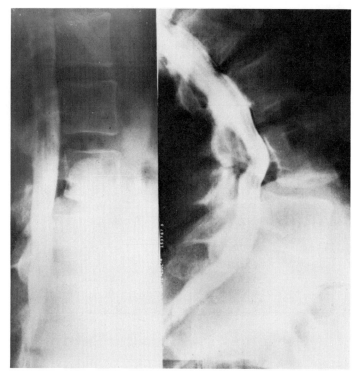

FIG. 11-9. Stress views: spondylolisthesis and instability of L4. In extension, the nerves are pinched between two pressure effects: anteriorly, at the level of disc degeneration at L4–5; posteriorly, produced by the posterior arch at and above the body of L4. Both defects are relieved on flexion.

cedure. Dimer-X is absorbed and excreted in up to 24 hours, during which time the patient must be nursed with the head raised and under strict supervision. We elevate the head of the bed by 20 cm. and raise the patient's head on two or three firm pillows.

Apart from the well-known early complications of headache and clonic muscle spasms and the unlikely possibility of convulsions, nearly 10 per cent of patients suffer from a "hangover" for a week afterward, and occasionally headache muscle pains, and general malaise may persist for up to 3 weeks. Patients must certainly be warned of the possibility of some degree of temporary disability after the examination, and, as a general rule, surgeons would be well advised to postpone nonurgent operations on the spine for a week or two after myelography.

Headache Before and After Myelography. It is generally accepted that one third of patients will develop headache after myelography or after lumbar puncture with any contrast medium, that the headache is sometimes severe, may be delayed for a day or two after examination and that it may persist for up to 3 weeks. Apart from this, however, any radiologist who does many myelograms and is concerned with the recording and management of reactions, cannot escape being impressed by the common association of headache with backache. Of all our patients referred for myelography, some 40 per cent gave a history of headache, which was severe in nearly half, judged by the fact that their headaches were accompanied by nausea at least, or necessitated periods of bed rest. Of all our patients undergoing Dimer-X myelography 30 per cent complained of headache of varying degrees of intensity and persistence after examination, but 80 per cent of these gave a history of being prone to headaches of similar degree, anyway. In only 6 per cent of the total number of myelograms was the headache or its severity "unexpected."

It is not surprising that headache and backache occur together, considering that the head and spine are parts of the same system, that the cranial cavity and the spinal canal are continuous and share a common subarachnoid space. However, psychological stress may be another common factor, which appears to be borne out by the fact that the incidence of results described as "normal or unimportant" in our myelograms, being 24 per cent overall, was twice as high in headache sufferers as in patients without a history of headache. Surgeons are well aware of the occurrence of stress backache. They may be well advised to take the headache history of their patients, as well as the nature and severity of their reactions after myelography, into account when they decide on investigation and treatment.

Spasm. Dimer-X causes clonic spasm of the muscles of the back and lower limbs in 3 per cent or more of patients within 24 hours of myelography, usually not amounting to more than momentary discomfort, but occasionally severe and even with the risk of causing compression fractures of vertebral bodies. Spasms are controlled by diazepam. We now give patients 10 mg. of diazepam by intramuscular injection before examination and repeat the same dose afterward. At any sign of muscle spasm diazepam is repeated, intravenously if necessary, and then 6-hourly or as often as may be required during the rest of the 24 hours. It should be pointed out that 94 to 97 per cent of patients do not have spasms.

Convulsions. Dimer-X is an irritant which must not be allowed to flow over the brain surface. If a patient is overtilted during examination or allowed to lie flat after examination it will certainly cause convulsions. Indeed, convulsions may be expected to occur once in 500 examinations in spite of due care: epilepsy is regarded as a relative contraindication, and occasionally convulsions after Dimer-X will uncover previously unrecognized epilepsy.

ARACHNOIDITIS, SUBARACHNOID ADHESIONS, AND FIBROUS SPINAL STENOSIS

After Dimer-X myelography 10 per cent of patients suffer from general malaise, headache, nausea, pain, and stiffness for a week or longer, and the symptoms are strikingly aggravated by the erect position and activity. Are these signs of arachnoiditis?

We have found evidence of subarachnoid fibrosis in 105 of 1500 consecutive myelograms (Figs. 11-10—11-19). Of these, 103 occurred in the 369 patients who had had previous procedures, and only two in the 1131 patients who had not

Table 11-1. Incidence of Fibrosis in 1500 Myelographic Examinations

	Number of Cases	Fibrosis Number of Cases	%
	1500	105	7
Virgin (canal)	1131	2	0.17
Previous Procedure(s)	369	103	28
Myodil Myelography	41	31	76
Dimer-X Myelography	67	6	9
Operation	123	24	20
Operation + Myodil	90	81	90
Operation + Dimer-X	40	12	30
Operation + Myodil + Dimer-X	8	4	–

had previous myelography or posterior spinal operation (Table 11-1).

Subarachnoid fibrosis typically affects the lowermost segment of the thecal sac. It starts with obliteration of the narrow spaces in emergent nerve root sheaths, followed by adhesion of nerves within the sac, together and to the sac walls, and eventually by fibrous stenosis of the sac

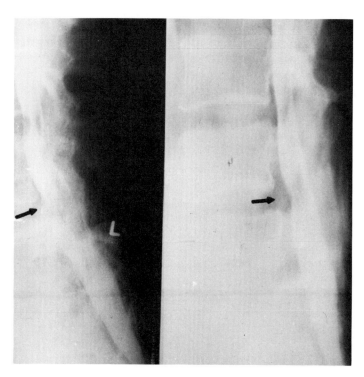

FIG. 11-10. Comparison of lateral plain film and tomogram of a lumbar myelogram: posterolateral fusion tends to obscure the detail of the canal on the ordinary film.

FIG. 11-11. Fibrous obliteration of nerve root sheaths after Myodil myelography and laminectomy, with only slight narrowing of the thecal sac.

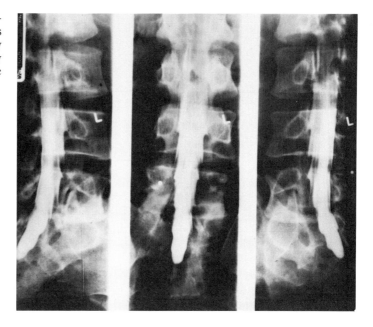

itself. The disappearance of visible nerves from the center of the sac, noted by many observers but not explained, is due simply to their adherence to the sac walls. Fibrous spinal stenosis is common com-

pared to the rare condition, bony stenosis.

Arachnoid adhesions are practically never seen in patients who have not been subjected to myelography or posterior

(Text continues on p. 198)

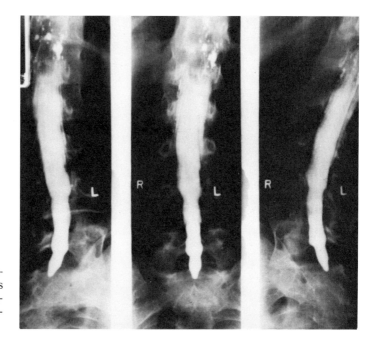

FIG. 11-12. Moderately severe fibrous spinal stenosis after myelography and laminectomy, with visible droplets of retained Myodil.

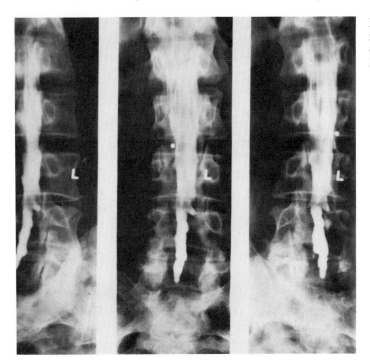

FIG. 11-13. Fairly severe fibrous spinal stenosis secondary to laminectomy and Myodil retention.

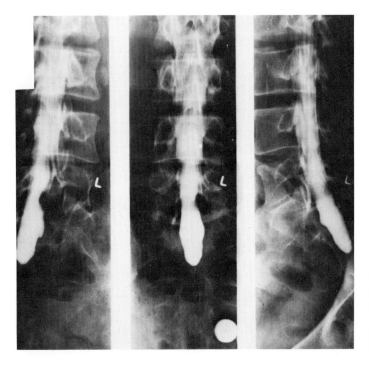

FIG. 11-14. Fibrous spinal stenosis after myelography and laminectomy, without relief of symptoms. The impression of a disc prolapse is seen on the left side.

FIG. 11-15. Subarachnoid fibrosis with fibrous stenosis and adherence of nerves in bundles and to the sac walls.

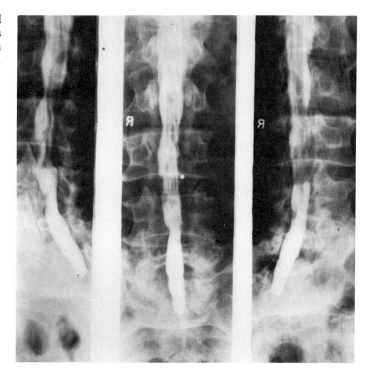

FIG. 11-16. Fibrosis is present following myelography and surgery, with a posterior fibrous tissue defect in relation to the laminectomy, as well as fibrous occlusion of nerve root sheaths and fibrous stenosis of the lower part of the sac.

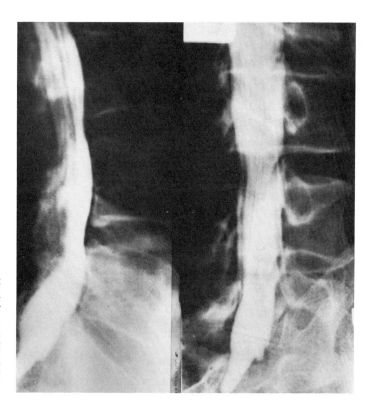

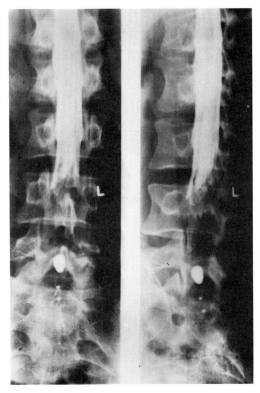

FIG. 11-17. Fibrous obliteration of the thecal sac. Myodil remains.

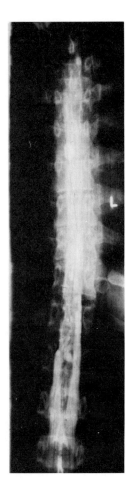

FIG. 11-18. Fibrosis in the thoracic region, with Myodil droplets and lateral filling defects. Demonstration of the cone of the spinal cord on routine thoracic myelography with Dimer-X.

spinal operations. We have seen roentgenographic evidence of spinal fibrosis in two patients with open wounds of the spinal canal (in another series) but never after vertebral compression fractures or anterior fusions. It has been absent in a few patients with a history of meningitis, and also in the larger number who had had previous lumbar punctures. We recently did a myelogram on a patient who had been subjected to 17 lumbar punctures in the course of management of resistant meningitis, and found no sign of subarachnoid fibrosis. We have not seen the condition in bilharzia sufferers, except those who had also been subjected to myelography and open operations on the spinal canal.

Dimer-X myelography produces visible evidence of subarachnoid fibrosis in 9 to 10 per cent of cases, usually mild and limited to the lowermost segment of the thecal sac. The use of a larger dose probably increases the incidence of fibrosis, but the risk may be minimized by diluting the Dimer-X with the total volume of cerebrospinal fluid available in the spinal canal. It is unsafe to let patients lie completely supine after Dimer-X myelography, nor should they be permitted to sit upright. If the Dimer-X is confined to the bottom of the thecal sac, a concentration of nearly 100 per cent results. If 10 ml. of Dimer-X is dispersed through the whole

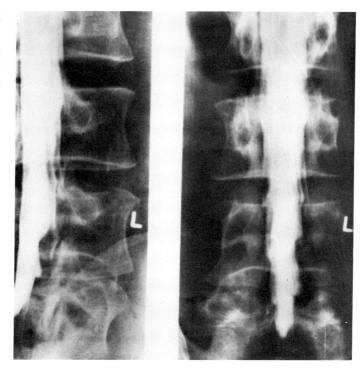

FIG. 11-19. Disc prolapse and localized fibrosis after laminectomy: Left anterolateral pressure effect; distortion of the root sheath above; elevation and obliteration of the root sheath below, and fibrosis of the lowermost extremity of the thecal sac.

length of the spinal canal it may be diluted to 10 to 20 per cent.

Although a symptomless control series is not feasible, from the observation of symptomatic patients with spinal fibrosis and from the changes and progression of their symptoms, we believe that severe fibrosis causes symptoms, including backache, pain in the lower limbs, sensory and motor impairment, and that symptoms may be severe and progressive after Myodil retention. We know of no effective treatment for established subarachnoid fibrosis, but we do routinely administer long-acting systemic cortisone after myelography, in the hope of preventing it. Intrathecal Depo-Medrol, however, has apparently been the cause of some of the most severe cases of fibrous spinal stenosis we have ever seen.

Fibrosis should be preventable to some extent. The only causes of arachnoid adhesions and fibrous spinal stenosis of practical importance are myelography and posterior spinal operations. The incidence

of fibrosis after Dimer-X myelography is 10 per cent; after all Myodil myelograms, 76 per cent; after Myodil retention, probably 100 per cent, and after posterior spinal operations, 20 per cent.

With combined and repeat procedures the incidence of fibrosis becomes very high.

Any operation on the back should be planned, with the help of adequate investigation, to be the last. A myelogram should be done once only, and performed so as to provide all the information possible. The greatest risk of myelography is not muscle spasm, nor headache, nor even fibrosis, but diagnostic inaccuracy.

Air Myelography

Because of its complete safety from permanent side effects some experienced investigators still favor air myelography. However, it requires replacement of a very large volume of cerebrospinal fluid, with corresponding discomfort, and introduces the danger of diagnostic inaccuracy, especially when used only occasionally.

Discography

We have used discography rarely in the past and not again since Dimer-X became available. It may serve to demonstrate abnormality in a disc which has not protruded. This may be an advantage or a disadvantage for the patient, depending on the interpretation. Discography carries risks of its own and can perhaps contribute little that is not more simply achieved by "water-soluble" myelography.[3]

Venography

Venography provides an indirect method of demonstrating abnormalities in the spinal canal which may be interpreted as causing pressure on the cord or nerves, although these neural structures are not visualized.[5] We have no personal experience with the technique, but have been impressed by demonstrated results. However, whether by painful intraosseous injection or time-consuming selective catheterization, the investigation is unlikely to gain wide appeal in the face of the simple and effective alternative examination by "water-soluble myelography."

Computerized Axial Tomography

This new noninvasive form of examination of various body levels may occasionally be of value in disease of the spine.[4] It would certainly provide for the first time a simple and effective, if expensive, method of demonstrating clearly the shape of the spinal canal in cross-section. The thin transverse sections would necessarily have to be limited to highly selective levels.

POSTOPERATIVE EXAMINATION

Not all cases in which pain persists, recurs or is aggravated after spinal operations are hopeless. In more than half of these patients a roentgenographically demonstrable lesion is present which may explain the symptoms, and many of these can be treated. Among these abnormalities are those of persistent disease, recurrent disease, conditions which are secondary to the previous abnormality or to corrective surgery, and further entirely new abnormalities unrelated to the previous history. The lesions include the following: disc prolapse, persistent or recurrent, at the same or different level; disc degeneration, preexisting or following previous disease or operation, at the same or a different level; fibrosis; instability, preexisting or secondary; nonunion of fusion, or pseudarthrosis; infections; disease in the lower thoracic region.

Combinations and multiple abnormalities are particularly common in postoperative cases of backache. Even more than in preoperative examinations, abnormalities may be demonstrated which have no bearing on the symptoms of a particular patient. It should be noted especially that a spinal fusion which shows no roentgenographic bony union is often stable and that even a pseudarthrosis with instability may be painless.

An unsuccessful surgical result is commonly followed by failure to respond to other forms of treatment. Similarly, the cause of postoperative pain is not often roentgenographically demonstrable, particularly in the case of pain-neurosis, whether preexisting or caused by previous procedures. A negative examination conscientiously performed nonetheless has a positive value.

Instability may be particularly difficult to assess roentgenographically at this stage, and it bears repeating that we have no technique that demonstrates all rotational instability (see Chap. 5).

In roentgenographic reinvestigation after failed surgery, review of previous examination and comparison with previous films is of prime importance. The roentgen reexamination does not differ in any essential detail from the routine examination for backache. The examination should, if possible, be more meticulous than before. Stress views and tomography should not be omitted, and myelography should be properly performed, and the lower thoracic region included in the examination.

REFERENCES

1. Ahlgren, P.: IX Symposium Neuroradiologicum. Goteberg, Aug. 1970, Book of Abstracts, p. 135.

2. Gonsette, R.: 1971, Clinical Radiology, 22:44, 1971.
3. Holt, E., 1968, J. Bone and Joint Surg., 50, 720.
4. Sagel, Stuart, S., Stanley, Robert, J., and Evens, Ronald, G., 1976 Radiology 119, 321–330.
5. Schobinger, R. A., Krueger, E. G. and Sobel, G. L. 1961, Radiology, 77:376.
6. Skalpe, Ingar, O., and Amundsen, Per, 1975, Radiology 115, 91–95.
7. Skalpe, Ingar, O., and Amundsen, Per, 1975, Radiology 116, 101–106.
8. de Villiers, P. D., 1974, S. Afr. Med. J., 48, 2629–2633.
9. de Villiers, P. D., Lombaard, M., Nel., 1976: S. Afr. Med. J., 47, 2461–2464.
10. Wright, F. W., Sanders, R. C., Steel, W. M., and O'Connor, B. T., 1971. Clin. Radiol., 22, 33–43.

12 The Failures of Surgery for Lumbar Disc Disorders

George F. Dommisse and R. P. Gräbe

"The last part of surgery, namely operations, is a reflection on the healing art. . . . No surgeon should approach . . . operation without . . . reluctance"; so wrote John Hunter in 1749.

Classic contributions by Schmorl,[16] Beadle,[4] Keyes and Compere,[11] and especially by Mixter and Barr,[14] established the "pathological disc" as a clinical entity and its surgical removal as a justifiable means to an end. Nothing since that time has evolved to alter these two concepts, but a degree of disillusionment has undoubtedly crept in, and a first-class procedure has acquired a measure of disrepute.

During the period 1937 to 1970, no fewer than 22,888 "laminectomy" operations for lumbar disc were reported in 53 publications which Spangfort reviewed.[17] To these, Spangfort added a further series of 2,504 operations performed in two major clinics in Sweden, and submitted the data to a computer-assisted analysis. The conclusions of this major investigation are significant.

The mortality in the collected series was negligible, varying from 0.1 to 0.3 per cent. The morbidity was high, with recurrence of symptoms (backache, sciatica,

or both), within the year in 48 per cent of 7,391 patients, operated by 71 surgeons, and reported in 23 publications. When the reasons for failure were sought, it became clear that ". . . patients with complete herniations . . . [had] the best results, and negative exploration the poorest." Clearly, accuracy of diagnosis is mandatory if improved results of operation are to be had.

There are other reasons for failure, and there are shibboleths which must be dispelled. First among them is the postulate that laminectomy may do some good and it can do no harm. Kennedy and Elsburg[10] considered the introduction of air might bring some local relief, while others thought that by removal of part of the wall of the spinal canal spatial compromise was relieved. The modern concept is more acceptable, namely that preoperative diagnosis determines treatment, whether surgical or conservative. The "surprise factor," which may or may not be uncovered by surgery, is justified only when all reasonable aids to diagnosis have been enlisted, including observation over a reasonable period of time.

The second shibboleth is that persistent subjective complaints, without positive physical signs, constitute an indication for operation. The contrary is, however, the case for the diagnosis is *ipso facto* in

This work was supported, in part, by The Medical Research Council of South Africa, by the University of Pretoria, and by the Department of Hospital Services of the Transvaal Provincial Administration.

202

doubt, and operation may prove a "negative exploration." Aggravation of the psychological component will then ensue.

Thirdly, operation undertaken early rather than late will ensure the quickest and the best result. Delay, on the other hand, may have irreversible neural effects. The facts are inconsistent with the hypothesis, for a favorable result will follow nonoperative measures, and a conservative regime alone will generally suffice. One of us (RPG) conducted a retrospective review of 1590 patients with lumbar backache, examined and treated over a period of 12 years. In 1536 patients (96.6%) conservative measures alone yielded a satisfactory end-result, and operation was performed in only 3.4 per cent of the series. In no single instance was the quality of the end-result adversely influenced by delay, nor was the complication of sphincter disturbance (attributable to ischemic neuropathy of the roots of the cauda equina) observed.

The fourth shibboleth is that laminectomy for disc is a procedure which can be undertaken effectively by the occasional surgeon in the general operating theater and without the routine cooperation of a team of multidisciplined specialists. If the low incidence of fatalities has contributed to this view, then the awesome morbidity revealed by Spangfort should deter. When the first operation has failed, then the spectre of "second-hand surgery" rears its head. If the number of failures is to be reduced, then the principle of the specialized unit must be applied. This is the modern trend: results in numerous other fields testify to its worth. A spinal surgeon rather than an orthopaedic or a neurosurgeon is the appropriate leader of the team; he should have medical, laboratory, and paramedical services at this command.

There is a fifth shibboleth, that the psyche dominates and that the result of surgery is determined by the psychological status preoperatively, rather than by objective physical signs. We subscribe to the opposite view; namely, that organic (somatic) factors dominate and dictate the nature of the psychological response. To attribute a surgical failure to a preexisting mental flaw is to diminish the quality of the service. It offers a dubious explanation and contributes little, if anything, toward success.

The shibboleths referred to here are controversial, negative factors which serve as a measure of the varying standards currently being applied. In the pages which follow we shall limit comment to some of the more positive and objective fields. They include accuracy of diagnosis, the anatomy and the microanatomy of the part, refinements of surgical technique, and some causes of surgical failure.

ACCURACY OF DIAGNOSIS

For treatment to have a chance of success, the diagnosis of a herniated disc must be recognized as a tri-phasic exercise: First, the *presence* of a herniated disc, which is determined by the history and the physical signs including plain roentgenograms; second, *the degree and severity* of the herniation, as judged by the response to conservative treatment. In this phase, time is a valuable diagnostic aid. Third (and only when it has been decided to operate), the *precise localization* of the lesion must be made so that the surgical procedure which follows is definitive, not exploratory. In the latter, myelography with a water-soluble contrast medium is our method of choice (see p. 187). There are other valid methods of special investigation, which in some hands have proved satisfactory.

Important in the history are the onset, response to rest and activity, the nature and location of pain, the degree of disability in varying situations, and the nature of previous treatment. A complete general examination to exclude other factors is mandatory.

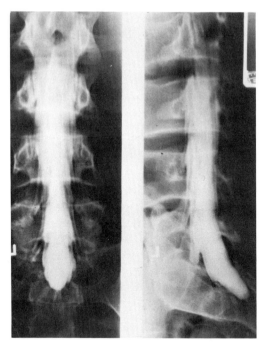

FIG. 12-1. A normal myelogram using a water-soluble contrast medium. The cauda equina, the sheaths of the spinal nerves, and the outline of the normal dural sac are well displayed. (Courtesy P. D. de Villiers)

Physical Signs

Spinal Signs. Limitation of movements, especially of flexion, with pain and increasing spasm of the extensor muscles on forcing movements, are of particular significance. In severe cases, a rigid back during ambulation is diagnostic of an irritable spinal lesion.

Tension Signs are based on the normal amplitude of movement which the 4th and 5th lumbar and the 1st sacral spinal nerves enjoy, permitting straight-leg raising to about 90 degrees. Spangfort found: "In the total material, the [straight-leg raising] sign was positive before operation in 95.7 per cent of the patients. In 2,157 patients with verified herniations it was positive in 96.8 per cent."[17] This was the single most important sign, but a high percentage of false-positives was also noted. The "crossed Lasègue sign" was positive in only 21.6 per cent, but when present was associated with a "high degree of significance" and proved to be less sensitive but more specific than ipsilateral limitation.

Neurological signs involve essentially the 5th lumbar and 1st sacral spinal nerves, less often the 4th lumbar and occasionally the 2nd and 3rd sacral spinal nerves.

Impairment of the ankle reflex was reported in 50 per cent of patients by Barr[2] and "in other reports during the following 3 decades . . . [in] an average of 50 to 60 per cent."[17] In his own series, Spangfort reported that the total incidence of this sign was 29.7 per cent. Paresis of ankle extensors was noted by the same author in 30.2 per cent. It had specific reference to herniation at the L4–5 intervertebral level.

By contrast, impairment of the ankle jerk indicated herniation at the lumbosacral level. In a retrospective review of verified complete herniations, either or both of these neurologic deficits has been recorded in 87 per cent during preoperative examination. Spangfort concluded, "The rate of negative explorations was significantly higher in patients without neurologic signs than in other subgroups."

Myelography, using a water-soluble contrast medium, has brought a new clarity to the field and has proved almost, if not completely, accurate (Fig. 12-1). When employed for the corroboration of clinical diagnosis it has proved completely reliable in hitherto unoperated cases. Special points in technique are described elsewhere in this volume. When observed, they enhance the accuracy of diagnosis and reduce the number of false-positive readings to an effective minimum.

Three aspects of myelographic diagnosis are the positive identification of the individual elements of the cauda equina, the complete filling of the sheaths of each

FIG. 12-2. The roots of the cauda equina within the dural sac. The spinal canal is capacious, and the spinal nerves are loosely disposed. (Dommisse, G. F.: Morphological aspects of the lumbar spine and lumbosacral region. Orthop. Clin. North Am., 6:163, 1975)

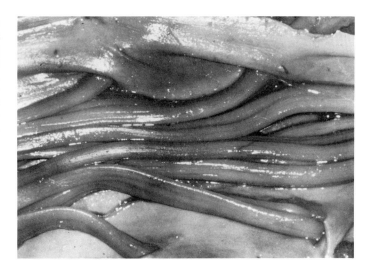

of the spinal nerves, and the well-filled, generously rounded curves of the dural sac. The pathological features are discussed in Chapter 4.

Anatomy and Microanatomy

The lumbar spinal canal is centrally placed, while the paired canals or tunnels for the escaping spinal nerves (nerve roots) are directed laterally. In each instance, the available space may be compromised under abnormal conditions.

The average anteroposterior diameter of the central lumbar canal is 15 to 16 mm., while the transverse diameter is much greater, being 22 to 25 mm. between the L1 and L5 vertebral levels. The canal becomes wider and flatter and is admirably adapted to accommodate the cauda equina (Fig. 12-2).

The canal or tunnel for the spinal nerve is directed obliquely outward at an angle of 30 to 40 degrees (Fig. 12-3). It has an inner, entrance foramen, which is defined rostrally by the notch below the vertebral pedicle, and an outer orifice commonly known as the intervertebral foramen. The tunnel between the inner and outer

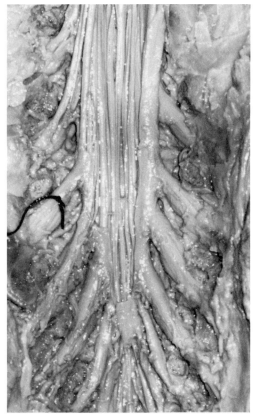

FIG. 12-3. The lumbar spinal nerves are directed outward at an angle of 30 to 40 degrees.

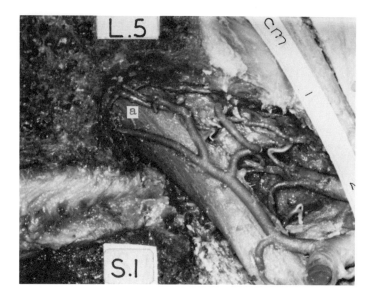

FIG. 12-4. The fifth lumbar spinal nerve, ventral view. The length of the canal is indicated. The posterior spinal ganglion is marked *a*. The veins have been excised. (Dommisse, G. F.: Morphological aspects of the lumbar spine and lumbosacral region. Orthop. Clin. North Am., 6:163, 1975)

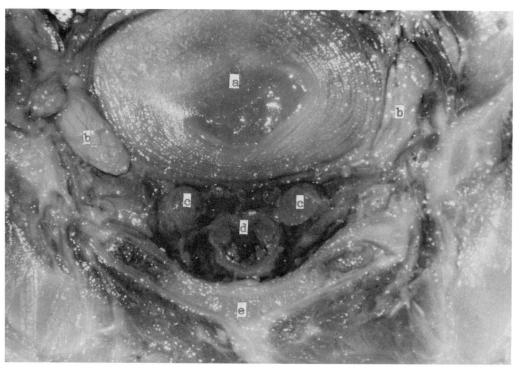

FIG. 12-5. Cross-section of the spinal canal at lower lumbar level. *(a)* Nucleus pulposus, *(b)* segmental spinal nerve in tunnel, *(c)* segmental spinal nerve of next succeeding level, *(d)* dural sac with distal spinal nerves of the cauda equina.

foramina (Fig. 12-4) varies in length at different levels, and in the adult male measures 2.5 to 3.0 cm. at the L5–S1 level.

In the healthy person the canal provides ample accommodation for the posterior spinal ganglion (Fig. 12-4), the spinal nerve, the segmental arteries, and the regional veins. The significance of the segmental arteries has been emphasized elsewhere.[6,7] Numerous radicular arteries for the supply of the spinal nerve and radicles occur at every level. Medullary feeder branches of the segmental arteries occur at occasional, irregular levels only. The artery of Adamkiewicz has been found to enter the canal as far caudad as the L4 level, where it may be involved in disc lesions and in disc surgery.

The most common site of herniation of the nucleus pulposus is directly apposed to the spinal nerve of the next succeeding level (Fig. 12-5C). Compression of the nerve is between the herniated disc and the neural arch or the superior articular facet of the vertebra. The emerging spinal nerve is proximal to and immune from compression, except only when the herniated material is projected laterally into the tunnel.

The posterior spinal ganglion enjoys a protected position under cover of the vertebral pedicle and is not implicated in the more common type of herniation of the disc (Fig. 12-6). The same applies to the emerging segmental nerve of that level. By contrast, the next most caudad nerve crosses the disc space and is displaced medially or laterally by a herniated disc; alternately it is compressed between the prolapse and the ligamentum flavum or the anterior surface of the superior facet of the vertebra below. Narrowing or stenosis of the canal for the spinal nerve occurs under several conditions, and the presence of narrowing may be suspected when the sheath of the spinal nerve fails to fill with contrast medium during myelography (see Fig. 12-1).[12] Inevitable

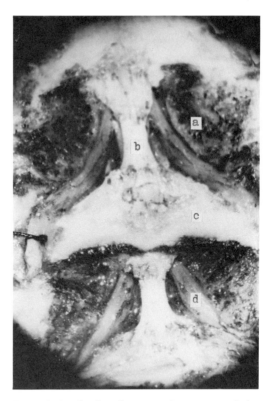

FIG. 12-6. The lumbar spinal nerves and the posterior spinal ganglia, ventral view. The vertebral bodies have been totally removed to display the posterior longitudinal ligament and the posterior rim of the annulus fibrosus. The vertebral pedicle *(a)*, the posterior longitudinal ligament *(b)*, the annulus fibrosus *(c)* and the posterior spinal ganglion *(d)*.

stenosis of the canal takes place in the presence of lumbar spondylosis with degenerative narrowing of the disc space and with retrospondylolisthesis (Fig. 12-7).

The Dura Mater

The dura mater is a complex membrane with a rich intrinsic blood supply (Fig. 12-8). It responds to noxious stimuli by means of the reactions of inflammation, with hyperemia and swelling, which may resolve or which may terminate in chronic fibrosis and thickening, or arachnoiditis. Thickening of the dura

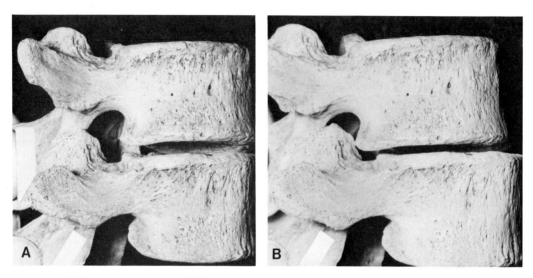

FIG. 12-7 *(A)* Degenerative spondylosis at L4–5 level, with severe narrowing of the disc space. The tunnel for the emerging spinal nerve is unimpeded. *(B)* Degenerative spondylosis at L4–5 level, with retrospondylolisthesis. The tunnel for the emerging spinal nerve is severely obstructed.

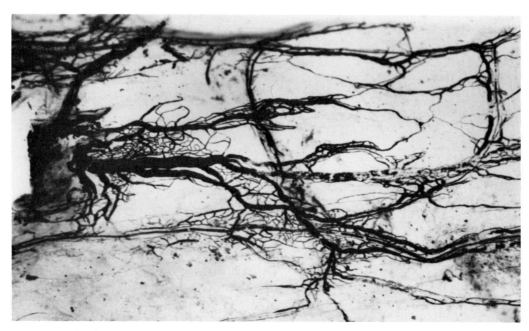

FIG. 12-8. The dura mater. The intrinsic blood vessels have been filled with India ink, and the specimen rendered transparent by the Spalteholz technique.

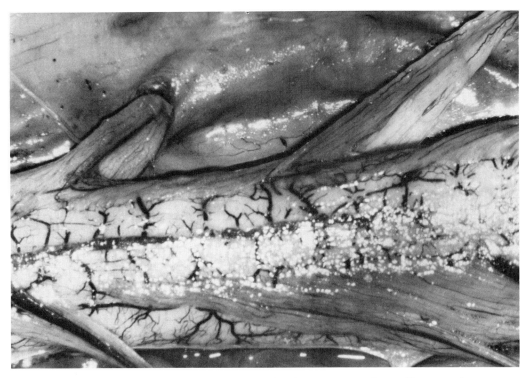

FIG. 12-9. The spinal nerve penetrates the dura mater at the axillary pouch.

mater may result in obliteration of the sheath and in compression of the spinal nerve (Figs. 12-9, 12-11). The spinal nerve and the posterior spinal ganglion enjoy a rich blood supply (Fig. 12-10). These structures are sensitive to the effects of ischemia and respond by means of ischemic radiculopathy (Fig. 12-11). Intraneural fibrosis with interference of the conduction potential of sensory and

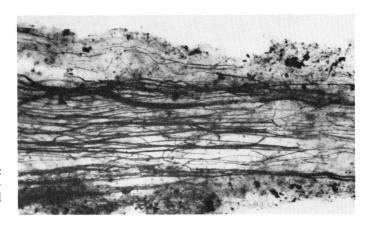

FIG. 12-10. The intrinsic microcirculation of the posterior spinal ganglion and spinal nerve.

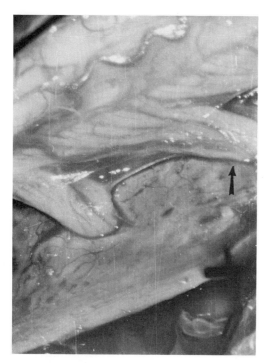

Fig. 12-11. Ischemic radiculopathy of a cervical spinal nerve as seen at operation is clearly visible on this marred photo. The arrow points to the unhealthy, shrunken nerve. (Courtesy Professor R. Lipchitz)

motor axons follows, a condition described elsewhere as "the battered root syndrome."[5]

Artery of Adamkiewicz

The artery of Adamkiewicz is the largest of the anterior medullary feeder arteries in the lumbar segments of the spinal cord (Fig. 12-12). It occurs commonly at the T10 and T11 vertebral levels, but is occasionally found as far caudad as the L4 spinal nerve. It can suffer damage by compression, ligation, or cautery during surgery for disc, with paraplegia as an occasional result. The exact levels at which medullary feeder arteries may be encountered vary; spinal angiography is a rarely used, esoteric procedure. Reasonable care

during operation will preserve the medullary feeder arteries. An awareness of the risk associated with their loss is mandatory.

Batson's Vertebral Venous Plexus

The intraspinal, extradural component of Batson's plexus (Fig. 12-13a) is of primary concern in the surgery of the lumbar disc. The communicating channels between the extradural and the extravertebral veins (Figs. 12-13B and 12-14) accompany the spinal nerves in the tunnels and are of equal surgical significance. Congestion of the vertebral veins may be of a general nature, as in asphyxia and when pressure is exerted on the inferior vena cava. This latter factor is to be avoided during surgical procedures.

Congestion of the veins of the pelvis is a factor in backache and menorrhagia. Congestion of the extradural veins is an unlikely factor in the production of backache and root pain—compression results in collapse, not congestion, of the veins, and this collapse is the basis of venography.[9] It is readily accounted for by the richness of the plexus and by the reversibility of blood flow in this low-pressure, valveless venous system.

THE FAILURES OF SURGERY

Failures are due to incorrect diagnosis, to the wrong operative procedure, and to faulty technique. Incorrect diagnosis is sometimes attributable to incomplete examination, particularly inadequate roentgen examination. Two common pitfalls in diagnosis are postpartum sacroiliitis and scoliosis.

Postpartum Sacroiliitis

Diastasis of the symphysis pubis occurs commonly in the late months of pregnancy, reaching maximum deformity during parturition. The sacroiliac joint or joints are inevitably implicated, and there

FIG. 12-12. The artery of Ademkiewicz, at T11 level on the left side in this human neonatal cadaver specimen. (Dommisse, G. F.: J. Bone Joint Surg., *56B*:225, 1974)

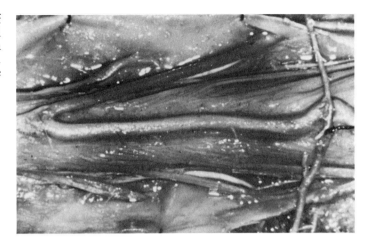

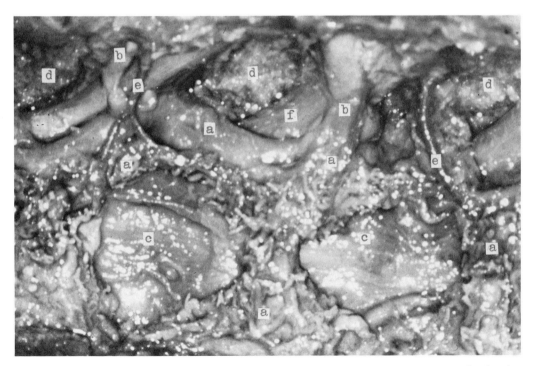

FIG. 12-13. The intraspinal, extradural component of Batson's venous plexus, in the lumbar spine: *(a)* the plexiform and cavernous venous channels; *(b)* the communicating veins between the extradural and the extravertebral components of the plexus; *(c)* the dura mater, ventral aspect; *(d)* the vertebral pedicle; *(e)* intraspinal extradural arterial branches; *(f)* the segmental spinal nerve.

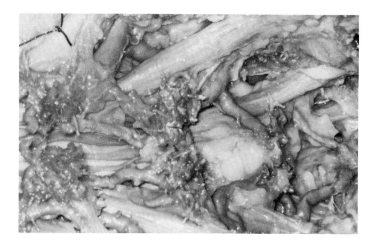

FIG. 12-14. Lumbosacral spinal nerves (ventral view). Large veins connect the extradural venous plexus with the lumbar and azygos veins. The lumbosacral spinal nerves are accompanied in their course through the nerve tunnel by large venous channels.

is failure of complete restitution, with permanent sacroiliac instability and with the reactive changes of osteitis condensans ilii (Fig. 12-15). The inclusion of the entire pelvis in the roentgenographic examination of the backache sufferer is mandatory. "Osteitis pubis" in the male is usually associated with prostatitis and with backache.

Lumbar Scoliosis

Lumbar scoliosis is associated with lumbar backache; sometimes also with spinal nerve pain. The patient is unaware of the deformity because it is not a cosmetic problem. Roentgenographic examination of the spine with the patient erect is essential, in order that the deformity may be detected during the early stages (Fig. 12-16).

The rotational element of the lordosis-scoliosis deformity is responsible for disruption of the fibers of the annulus fibrosus, and for the vertebral instability which is inevitable. There is disruption of the intervertebral disc, with clinical signs and symptoms resembling those of herniation of the nucleus pulposus. Roent-

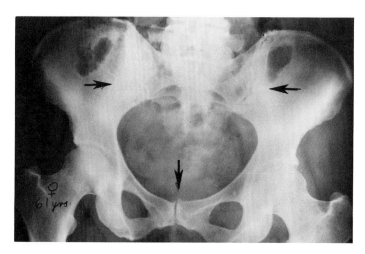

FIG. 12-15. Postpartum sacroiliitis with "osteitis condensans ilii" of severe degree, in an elderly, multiparous female. Instability with sclerotic changes, narrowing, and displacement at the symphysis pubis provide the key to diagnosis.

FIG. 12-16. *(A)* Lumbar scoliosis of moderate degree in a 39-year-old female who suffered backache. *(B)* The same patient, 14 years later. The scoliosis and accompanying changes are obvious. Intractable pain compelled extensive surgery.

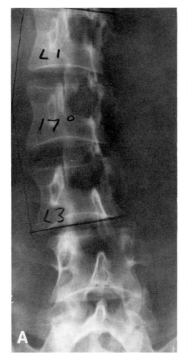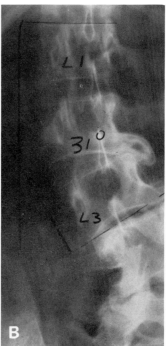

genographic examination of the erect spine is mandatory if diagnostic errors are to be avoided.

Arteriovenous Malformation

Yasargil has shown that vascular malformations of the spinal cord are not rare (Fig. 12-17).[19] The incidence in the experience of Krayenbühl and Yasargil was 4.35 per cent of 961 spinal tumors.[19] The symptoms and signs reported by Yasargil included "lumbar ischalgia," "dysesthesia" of the legs, "lumbalgia," weakness of the legs, bladder weakness and in-

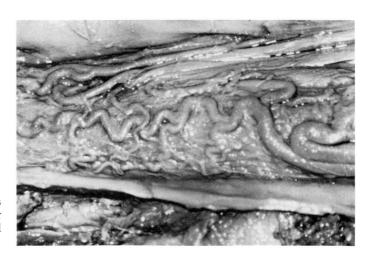

FIG. 12-17. Arteriovenous malformation in the lumbar spinal canal of a 4-week-old infant (cadaveric dissection).

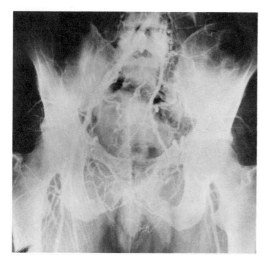

FIG. 12-18. Aortic angiogram of a male of 40 years. Left iliac artery occlusion is total. A myelogram done elsewhere proved negative and was an unjustified procedure. (Courtesy of P. D. de Villiers)

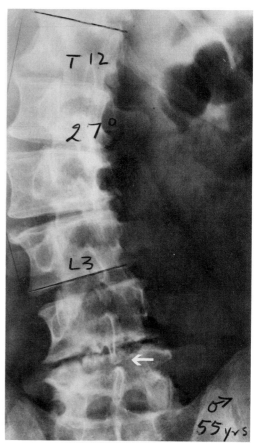

FIG. 12-19. Lumbar scoliosis in a male, age 55 years. Operation for lumbar disc removal and interbody grafting 17 years earlier relieved pain but failed to arrest the progressive deformity of lumbar scoliosis.

continence, girdle pains, and sexual disability, generally of a slowly progressive nature. Recognition of the condition is essential, and the response to timely surgery is gratifying. Myelography, especially with the use of a water-soluble contrast medium will reflect the possible diagnosis. Special methods of examination, including selective angiography and venography, will provide confirmatory evidence (Fig. 12-18).

Occlusion of the Aorta or Iliac Artery

The symptoms of abdominal and pelvic aneurysms resemble closely those of herniation of the lumbar disc, and also of spinal stenosis. The correct diagnosis is confirmed by the presence of a pulsating abdominopelvic tumor and the absence of the arterial pulses in the affected leg. The routine inclusion of aortic or iliac aneurysm in the differential diagnosis is mandatory.

The Wrong Operation

Failure to arrive at the correct diagnosis may result in the wrong procedure (Fig. 12-19). Lumbar scoliosis, unlike thoracic curvatures, leads to progressive degenerative spondylosis, paravertebral osteoarthritis, and painful instability. Timely recognition of the scoliotic background of the complaints may be secured by the routine adoption of roentgenographic examination of the erect spine. Degenerative spondylosis of the lumbar spine is associated with spinal stenosis. Extensive fusion procedures (Fig. 12-20) fail to relieve the symptoms of stenosis and are associated with a high incidence of pseudarthrosis.

The presence and extent of stenosis of

FIG. 12-20. *(A)* Anteroposterior view of the lumbar spine of a 54-year-old male with degenerative spondylosis and with bilateral posterolateral fusion L1–L5 vertebrae. *(B)* Same patient, lateral view with retrospondylolisthesis and stenosis clearly seen at L4–5 vertebral level.

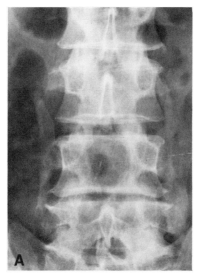
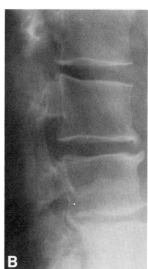

the central canal of the spine and of the nerve root tunnel or tunnels may be confirmed myelographically. The relief of stenosis by means of a posterior decompression procedure may be anticipated, with relief of symptoms and with restoration of function.

Three reasons for failure merit special consideration; they are postoperative arachnoiditis (Fig. 12-21), ischemic degeneration of the spinal nerve and posterior spinal ganglion, and recurrent prolapse of the disc. The frequent occurrence of postoperative arachnoiditis with thickening of the dural membrane and with constriction of the dural sac is attributable to trauma and has been observed also following fractures and open injuries. It is reasonable to assume that it follows upon hematoma formation in the extradural space, with subsequent organization and the formation of excessive connective tissue—a feature of the appearances encountered at so-called second hand surgery. In seeking an explanation for the obliteration of the sheath of the spinal nerve, the same pathological process of arachnoid thickening and extradural scar tissue formation may provide a solution. Degenerative radiculopathy (See Fig.

12-11) has been described as the "battered root problem" in which there are irreversible changes of intraneural fibrosis.[5] The matter requires further investigation. Degenerative radiculopathy may precede operation and be due to trauma or nerve root compression. Clearly, the persistence of nerve root symptoms cannot, under these circumstances, be ascribed to the operation and equally clearly, a meticulous neurologic examination conducted preoperatively is in the best interests of patient and surgeon.

Herniation of disc material may recur at the site of an earlier operation, or elsewhere, no matter how complete the removal has been. The elimination of this complication may be facilitated by the use of a temporary postoperative brace which firstly assures the prevention of postural hyperlordosis of the lumbar spine and, secondly, provides support for the back through the medium of the abdominal cavity. At the same time, vigorous postoperative exercises conducted in the supine position and aimed more particularly at the muscles of the anterior abdominal wall and at the gluteus maximus are advised for an adequate period. In this manner, posture is cor-

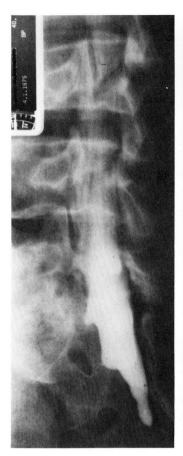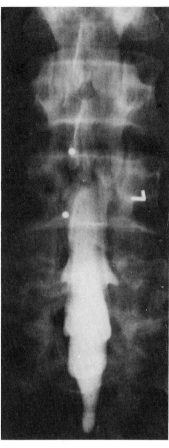

FIG. 12-21. Myelogram with a water-soluble medium demonstrates late postoperative arachnoiditis with fibrous stenosis of the dural sac and with obliteration of the sheath for the spinal nerves at several levels on both sides. (Courtesy P. D. de Villiers)

rected and hyperlordosis, with the attendant risk of reinjury of the posterior part of the annulus fibrosus, may be avoided.

TECHNICAL AIDS TO SURGERY

Three technical aids to the surgery of the spine and to lumbar disc procedures offer advantages: microsurgery, bipolar cautery, and hypotension anesthesia.

Microsurgery is not new. It has been used by the otologist for more than 50 years, and for many years also by the ophthalmic surgeon, the neurosurgeon, and vascular and plastic surgeons. In recent years it has attracted the attention of orthopaedists. A full range of surgical instruments is available, without which the use of the operating microscope is impracticable. Yasargil has traced the history and described the neurosurgical techniques adopted in his clinic.[19] The method can readily be acquired and the advantages, which are many, can be briefly summarized: It enhances the quality of surgical technique and it enables the gentlest handling of tissues (Fig. 12-22). When combined with bipolar cautery and with hypotensive anesthesia it enables perfect visualization of important microanatomical features and permits accurate, effective hemostasis.

Bipolar cautery offers considerable advantages over the more commonly used unipolar variety.[13] It is effective in coagulating fine vessels without spread of the coagulum beyond the immediate

FIG. 12-22. Microsurgical technique allows a clear view of the operative site. *(A)* Herniation of the nucleus pulposus at L5–S1 level on the right side. The swollen spinal nerve is displaced medially, and the sheath of the nerve has been punctured during access. *(B)* After removal of the herniated disc, the punctured sheath with a cerebrospinal fluid leak is clearly visible and easily repaired. (× 10)

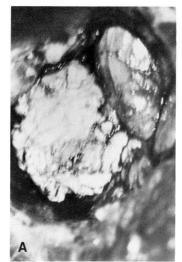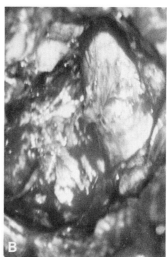

point of cautery and without damage to surrounding tissues.

Hypotension anesthesia is controversial but has proved its value in a series of more than 200 procedures for scoliosis by the senior author during the past 5 years. There have been no complications attributable to the method. Enderby declared: "Deliberate hypotension remains today an ill defined and often poorly understood technique . . . The practical advantages . . . become obvious when attempting an extensive and hemorrhagic surgical dissection. The ability to reduce bleeding to insignificant proportions is an outstanding procedure. . . . By its aid, intricate operations . . . can be made easier, more exact."[8]

Our thanks are recorded to: Dr. H. A. Grové, Director of Hospital Services; Professor H. W. Snyman, Dean of the Faculty of Medicine at the University of Pretoria; Dr. E. van Wyngaard, Superintendent of the H. F. Verwoerd Hospital, Pretoria; Professor I. S. de Wet, Head of the Department of Orthopaedics; Professor D. P. Knobel, Head of the Department of Anatomy; Mrs. L. Watson, for typing and secretarial services; and Mrs. C. Vermeulen, for photographic reproductions.

REFERENCES

1. Adamkiewicz, A. A.: Die Blutgefässe des Menslichen Rückenmarkes: 11. die Gefässe der Rückernmarksoberfläche. Sitzungsbericht Kön. Akad.Wissensch. Math.-naturw., *85*:101, 1882.
2. Barr, J. S.: Sciatica caused by intervertebral-disc lesions. J. Bone and Joint Surg., *19*:323, 1937.
3. Batson, O. V.: The function of the vertebral veins and their role in the spread of metastases. Ann. Surg., *112*:138, 1940.
4. Beadle, O. A.: The Intervertebral Disc. Medical Research Council, Special Report Series 161. London, His Majesty's Stationery Office, 1931.
5. Bertrand, G.: The battered root problem. Orthop. Clin. North Amer. *6*:1305, 1975.
6. Dommisse, G. F.: The blood supply of the spinal cord. A critical vascular zone in spinal surgery. J. Bone Joint Surg., *56B*:225, 1974.
7. ———: The Arteries and Veins of the Human Spinal Cord from Birth. Edinburgh, Churchill Livingstone, 1975.
8. Enderby, G. E. H.: Guest Editorial: Some observations on the practice of deliberate hypotension. Brit. J. Anaesth., *47*:743, 1975.
9. Helander, C. G., and Lindbom, A.: Sacrolumbar Venography. Acta Radiol., *44*:410, 1955.
10. Kennedy, F. and Elsburg, C. A.: A peculiar and undescribed disease of nerves of the cauda equina. Amer. J. Med. Sci., *147*:645, 1914.
11. Keys, D. C., and Comprere, E. L.: The normal and pathological physiology of the nucleus pulposus and experimental study. J. Bone Joint Surg., *14*:897, 1932.
12. Kirkaldy-Willis, W. H., Paine, K. W. E., Jean Cauchoix, J., and McIvor, G.: Lumbar spinal stenosis. Clin. Orth., *99*:30, 1974.
13. Malis, L. I.: Bipolar coagulation in microsurgery. Donaghy, R. M. P. and Yasargil, M. G. (eds):

Microvascular Surgery. St. Louis, C. V. Mosbey, 1967.

14. Mixter, W. J., and Barr, J. S.: Rupture of the intervertebral disc with involvement of the spinal canal. N. Engl. J. Med., *211*:210, 1934.

15. Percy-Lancaster, R.: Backache in pregnancy and pelvic arthropathy. J. Bone and Joint Surg., *49B*:199, 1967.

16. Schmorl, G.: Die pathologische Anatomie der Wirbel-saüle. Verh. Dtsch.Orthop. Ges., *21*:3, 1926.

17. Spangfort, E. V.: The lumbar disc herniation. A computer-aided analysis of 2,504 operations. Acta Orthop. Scand., Suppl. 142, 1972.

18. De Villiers, P. D. and Booysen, E. L.: Fibrous spinal stenosis. A report on 850 myelograms with a water-soluble contrast medium. Clin. Orth., *115*:140,1976.

19. Yasargil, M. G.: Microsurgery applied to neurosurgery. Stuttgart, Georg Thieme, 1969.

13 Rheumatic Disorders of the Lumbar Spine

Louis Solomon and Louis Berman

THE JOINTS OF THE LUMBAR SPINE

There are two types of joint in the adult lumbar spine—the true synovial joints or diarthroses formed by the posterolateral articular processes, and the nonsynovial fibrous or fibrocartilaginous amphiarthroses, the intervertebral discs and ligaments (Fig. 13-1). The sacroiliac joint has both components: the caudal two thirds of the joint has a true synovial articulation, while the most cephalad third, embraced by the sacroiliac ligaments, is an amphiarthrosis. Both types of joint may be affected by inflammatory disorders, but a polysynovitis will involve only the posterior intervertebral joints and the distal part of the sacroiliac joint.

The Posterolateral Intervertebral Joints

These small synovial joints are formed by the superior and inferior articular facets of adjacent vertebrae. Their bony facets are covered by a thin (1 mm.) layer of hyaline cartilage; the joints are enclosed by a loose and rather flimsy capsule, which is lined by synovial membrane. Movement is limited to a gliding and rotating action between the facets, allowing flexion, extension, lateral bending, and rotation of varying degrees at each intervertebral level. The cumulative effect of these small degrees of movement at a number of levels accounts for the extraordinary ranges of movement in the spine as a whole; conversely, true stiffness of the spine implies some restriction at multiple levels.

The Intervertebral Discs and Ligaments

The fibrocartilaginous intervertebral discs are firmly attached to the vertebral bodies between which they lie, lending stability to the vertebral column as a whole. The superior and inferior surfaces of the vertebral body are slightly concave, the perimeter being thickened and strengthened by a ring of compact bone; it is to this that the annulus fibrosus and the adjacent intervertebral ligaments are attached.[6]

The anterior and posterior longitudinal ligaments extend along the ventral and dorsal surfaces of the vertebral bodies throughout the length of the spine, blending with the outer fibers of the annulus fibrosus at the disc spaces. The anterior ligament blends also with the underlying periosteum, but the posterior ligament is bow-strung across the slightly concave vertebral body. Between the pedicles at the waist of the body, the vertebral vessels pass beneath the posterior longitudinal ligament, entering and leaving through the medullary sinus.

The other important syndesmoses of

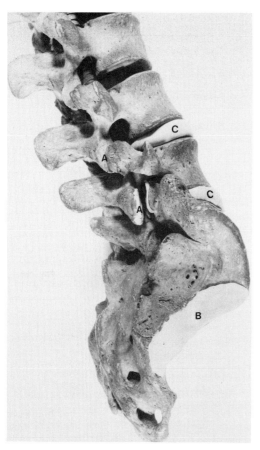

FIG. 13-1. Anatomy of the lumbosacral spine, showing the diarthrodial zygapophyseal joints *(A)*, the sacroiliac joint *(B)* and the fibrocartilaginous intervertebral discs *(C)*.

the spine are the supraspinous ligaments, the interspinous ligaments, the intertransverse ligaments, and the ligamenta flava.

MOVEMENTS OF THE LUMBAR SPINE

The direction and range of motion at any level of the spine are determined by the size and configuration of the adjacent vertebrae, the shape of the intervertebral disc, the plane of the zygapophyseal joints, and the strength of the intervertebral ligaments. Generally speaking, flexion occurs equally well throughout the spinal column, while extension is freer in the cervical and lumbar regions than elsewhere, and any restriction of this movement is noticed at a comparatively early stage. Not surprisingly, therefore, a loss of extension is the earliest physical sign of inflammatory disorders of the lumbar spine. Rotation, on the other hand, is almost completely prevented in the lumbar spine because of the anatomical plane of the zygapophyseal joints. Obviously, therefore, the range of rotation is no guide whatever to the state of the lumbar spine; more important, limited rotation in a patient complaining of "lumbar" backache should alert one to the fact that the dorsal spine may be affected as well.

PATHOLOGY

Rheumatic disorders of the spine are characterized by two basic pathological lesions: synovitis of the diarthrodial intervertebral joints and inflammation at the fibro-osseous junctions of the syndesmotic joints. The progress of these lesions, and the bony reactions which they evoke, account for all the changes observed.

It should be said at the outset that detailed descriptions of vertebral pathology in rheumatoid arthritis and similar disorders are limited by the difficulties of obtaining suitable material for study, especially in the important early stages of disease. Schemata which have been worked out are, therefore, based on relatively small numbers of specimens and are, to some extent, theoretical.

Synovitis of the Diarthrodial Joints

As in other synovial joints, inflammatory arthritis of the zygapophyseal and sacroiliac joints commences as a synovitis. Round-cell infiltration of the subsynovial layers is accompanied by vascular congestion and inflammatory exudate. In the later stages periarticular erosion occurs; the articular cartilage is ultimately lost, and the supporting bony structure crumbles under normal load. That these changes do not occur with equal frequency throughout the spine has been a matter of comment and speculation. Only the cervical spine is severely affected in rheumatoid arthritis, and here zygapophyseal erosion, ligamentous attenuation, and bone destruction frequently lead to intervertebral subluxation. The dorsolumbar spine is seldom, if ever, affected to this extent, and clinical problems related to lumbar arthritis are uncommon in rheumatoid disease.

Rheumatoid synovitis, in general, affects the more mobile joints more severely than it does those with a limited range of movement; indeed, one of the most effective ways of counteracting the synovitis is by immobilizing the affected joint. It is likely, therefore, that in a disease such as rheumatoid arthritis, which manifests as a synovitis, the restrained joints of the lumbar spine will be affected only slightly while the freely mobile cervical joints will be more severely involved. Certainly in those inflammatory disorders in which the spine becomes stiff due to ankylosis of the vertebral bodies, the zygapophyseal joints will show no evidence of synovitis. Zygapophyseal erosion and ankylosis in those cases is due to primary involvement of the periarticular ligaments.

Inflammation of the Fibrous and Fibrocartilaginous Joints

Rheumatoid arthritis does not affect the fibrous joints directly, and changes in the intervertebral discs and ligaments are therefore not seen. Our knowledge of the pathological features of the synchondroses in ankylosing spondylitis is derived largely from the work of Cruickshank[12] and Ball.[2] The initial changes are localized to the fibro-osseous junctions, where ligaments and fibrocartilaginous discs attach to the bone. Common sites are, therefore, the inter-vertebral discs, the ligamentous parts of the sacroiliac joint, the symphysis pubis, and the manubrium sterni. These fibro-osseous junctions, as well as those formed by tendon insertions into bone, are known as "entheses," and it has been proposed that the inflammatory disorder should be termed "enthesopathy." It is a clumsy term which has not found general acceptance, but it does serve to focus attention on this long-neglected entity and offers a unified explanation for the widespread features of the ankylosing arthropathies.

The basic sequence of change proceeds through four stages: (1) an inflammatory reaction with round-cell infiltration at the fibro-osseous junction and osteoporosis or osteoclastic resorption of the adjacent bone; (2) granulation tissue formation and erosion of bone at the enthesis; (3) replacement of granulation tissue by fibrous tissue; (4) and ossification of the fibrous tissue leading to ankylosis of the joint.

The characteristic results of this sequence of change are determined, to some extent, by the anatomical characteristics of the particular joint. Thus, in the manubrium sterni and symphysis pubis, both fairly flimsy synchondroses, the fibrocartilaginous disc is totally replaced by bone, resulting in solid ankylosis. The sacroiliac jonts, although diarthrodial, still suffer the same effects due to inflammation of the extremely dense periarticular ligaments. When the joint is encased in bone, segments of articular cartilage may still remain within, but eventually solid ankylosis occurs.

Most interesting of all are the changes around the intervertebral disc. Ossification of the perivertebral connective tissue across the surface of the disc gives rise to small bony bridges or syndesmophytes linking adjacent vertebral bodies. Two types are discernible.

The marginal syndesmophyte, which is characteristic of ankylosing spondylitis, replaces the superficial layers of the intervertebral disc and appears to lie deep to the longitudinal ligament. The origin of the new bone formation is still uncertain, but the commonly held view is that ossification occurs directly in the superficial layers of the annulus fibrosus.[13,28] Schilling and Schacherl, however, have demonstrated ossification within the layers of the delicate intervertebral ligament that joins the margins of the vertebral bodies superficial to the disc itself.[22] Whatever the case, the longitudinal ligament itself is not necessarily involved, for syndesmophyte formation occurs laterally as well as anteriorly and posteriorly. Intervertebral bridging over several adjacent levels gives rise to the "bamboo spine" which characterizes long-standing ankylosing spondylitis.

Nonmarginal syndesmophytes are usually larger than the marginal type and span a greater distance across the intervertebral space. Though occasionally seen in idiopathic ankylosing spondylitis, they are more characteristic of the spondylitis associated with psoriasis and Reiter's disease.[17]

Involvement of the anterior longitudinal ligament, which is closely applied to the anterior surface of the vertebral body, results in new bone formation in the anterior concavity of the body. This, together with marginal erosion of the vertebral body, produces the roentgenographic effect of squaring of the vertebra. The fact that this does not occur on the posterior surface may be because the posterior longitudinal ligament is not applied to the underlying bone but is bow strung across the posterior concavity (see p. 219). Around the zygapophyseal joints the capsules and periarticular ligaments undergo similar changes, resulting in bony ankylosis with articular cartilage still intact within the osseous casing.

Occasionally, the central part of the disc is involved in the inflammatory process, producing more extensive erosion of the adjacent vertebral bodies and the roentgenographic appearance of a "spondylodiscitis."

Changes in Paravertebral Muscles

Standard histologic techniques have in the past failed to reveal any change in paravertebral muscles related to inflammatory disorders of the spine. Recently, however, histochemical methods and electron microscopy have shown that structural and biochemical alterations do occur.[5] There is a generalized loss of Type 2 muscle fibers as well as cytoarchitectural changes in Type 1 fibers, including moth-eaten appearance and target or targetoid formation. Electron microscopy shows multiple defects, including loss of myofilamentous alignment, Z-line streaming, and abnormal folding of the basement membrane. Tubular aggregates, lipid bodies, and membranous bodies are also present to varying degrees.

RHEUMATOID ARTHRITIS OF THE SPINE

Rheumatoid disease is characterized by polysynovitis affecting the peripheral joints and tendon sheaths, including those of the hands and feet. Theoretically, the synovial joints of the spine could be involved as well. In actuality, it is only the cervical spine which is commonly affected, roentgenographic changes occurring in about 30 per cent of all patients with long-standing disease.

Patients with rheumatoid arthritis seldom complain specifically of backache, and even when questioned, they admit to lumbosacral pain no more frequently than a similar segment of the general population. It is surprising, then, to find that roentgenographic changes in the sacroiliac joints have been reported by several authors.[25] Repeated attempts in our own clinic to show similar changes in the lumbar zygapophyseal joints have been unrewarding.

Localized erosive lesions of the vertebral bodies have been described but are rare.[16] They have been attributed to granulation-tissue proliferation, extending from the marrow spaces of the vertebral body into the end-plate. Clinically these patients complain of intense pain on spinal movement or straining, and the roentgenographic changes closely resemble those of disc space- or vertebral infection.

Treatment. The treatment of rheumatoid spondylitis is that of the underlying disease. Instability does not occur in the lumbar region, and local measures are seldom called for.

ANKYLOSING SPONDYLITIS

For many years, ankylosing spondylitis was regarded as an atypical form of rheumatoid arthritis, and it was only after 1963 that it appeared in the American Rheumatism Association classification as a distinct entity. Nevertheless, the clinical features were described as long ago as the 17th century,[11] and the classic papers of Von Bechterew,[4] Strümpell,[27] and Marie[19] had established it as a well-recognized disorder some time before the advent of roentgenography. It is a chronic, inflammatory, polyarthritic disease affecting mainly the vertebral and sacroiliac joints and leading, ultimately, to bony ankylosis and rigidity of the spine.

The incidence of ankylosing spondylitis is estimated at about 1 per cent in western European populations, but it is thought to be much less common in American blacks and African Negroes.[3,26] It is a disease of young people, the symptoms usually commencing before the age of 30 and not infrequently in late adolescence. Males are affected much more frequently than females (ratios vary from 4:1 to 15:1). There is a definite familial aggregation, the incidence in proband relatives varying from 20 to 40 times that of the normal population.[15,20]

Clinical Features

The disease starts insidiously, with intermittent backache and stiffness recurring at intervals over a number of years. About 25 per cent of patients in our series admitted to at least one episode of severe backache before the age of 15, and several years prior to the appearance of lumbosacral stiffness. Many of these patients were found to have undergone physiotherapy, manipulation, and myelography before the true diagnosis emerged.

A more revealing symptom, though usually not the earliest, is stiffness. This is initially limited to the lumbosacral region and, to the observant patient, manifests as an inability to extend the spine as well as before. It is usually most severe during the early morning and late afternoon. Sometimes it is the cervical spine which is more noticeably affected and, when associated with pain, this may be misdiagnosed as fibrositis. At other times the entire spine may be stiff and painful.[24]

In about 20 per cent of patients symptoms occur in the peripheral joints at the same time, or even before, the onset of backache. In children and adolescents especially, hips, knees, and shoulders may become painful and swollen before spinal symptoms occur, though roentgenographs in these cases usually show asymptomatic involvement of the sacroiliac joints. Other joints which may be affected are the temporomandibular, the manubria sterna, and the symphysis pubis.

Less common presenting symptoms are pain at the insertion of the Achilles tendon or on the plantar surface of the heel. Ocular inflammation occurs in about 17 per cent of patients at some stage, and in 2 per cent it is the presenting feature.[24]

The Spine. Ankylosing spondylitis may be detected early by careful examination of the spine; the late signs are so obvious as to require no more than an intelligent glance. The posture alone may be revealing; flattening of the lumbar lordosis, a slight forward thrust of the neck, and

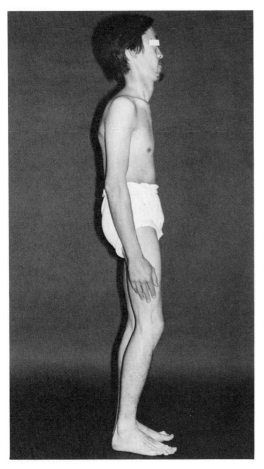

Fig. 13-2. Patient with ankylosing spondylitis. Note the typical posture with straight back, neck thrust forward, and hips and knees slightly flexed.

ried out by measuring the excursion of two points marked 15 cm. apart on the lumbosacral spine, from full extension to full flexion. Normally the distance between the two points should increase by at least 5 cm. during full flexion.

Pain on movement and tenderness of the paravertebral muscles are noted at the same time. The early loss of extension of the cervical spine may also be measured with accuracy. Normally, in the upright position, a young person should be capable of extending the head and neck, so that a line joining the occiput to the mentis forms an angle of at least 60 degrees with the horizontal. Anything below 45 degrees is abnormal.

Most difficult of all is clinical evaluation of the sacroiliac joints. Many ways of stressing these joints to elicit pain have been described; almost all are unreliable in that they fail to differentiate between sacroiliac and lumbosacral symptoms. The simple maneuver of placing the patient prone and forcibly extending the hip on each side, thus rocking the pelvis on the sacrum, is as good as any. Pain directly over the sacroiliac joint is suggestive of local disease.

Chest expansion is used as a measure of costovertebral stiffness, bearing in mind that this is normally diminished in the elderly, the obese, and those with pulmonary disease.[20,21] Expansion at the nipple line should be at least 5 cm. in normal young men.

In the most advanced stage of the disease the spine may be completely ankylosed from occiput to sacrum. Flexion contracture and ankylosis of the hip lends to these patients a characteristic gait, which, together with the rigid spine, gives an unequivocal picture. Sometimes ankylosis occurs in a position of deformity (dorsolumbar flexion and cervical flexion and rotation), so that the patient has difficulty directing his gaze ahead of his feet (Fig. 13-3).

slight flexion of the hips and knees are tell-tale signs of spinal stiffness (Fig. 13-2). The patient is then asked to flex and extend the spine. Inability to reach within 20 cm. of the floor is a sign of lumbar stiffness. An earlier sign, however, is the restriction of lumbar extension. This is often missed, as the patient "cheats" by slightly flexing the hips and knees. If the knees are grasped from behind and pulled into full extension, the true range of lumbosacral extension is revealed. A quantitative estimate of lumbar flexion is car-

The Paravertebral Muscles. Progressive

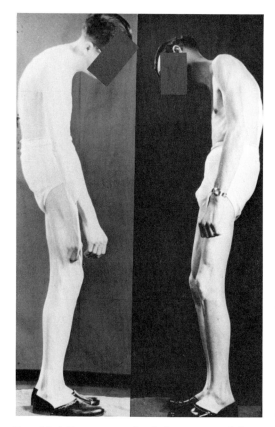

FIG. 13-3. Late stage of ankylosing spondylitis with rigid deformities of the spine.

wasting of paravertebral muscles leads to a characteristically flattened and atrophic appearance of the back in long-standing cases. These features, together with diffuse muscle pain and tenderness which extends well beyond the obviously involved segment, have led some people to believe that there may be neural involvement as well. Only recently, however, has it been shown by histochemical and electron microscopic techniques that the muscle fibers are abnormal in many of these patients.[5] The changes are described earlier in this chapter. Their precise relationship to the clinical features is still obscure.

Peripheral Joints. Involvement of peripheral joints is common in the later stages of ankylosing spondylitis and is present at the onset in about 20 per cent of cases. The hips, knees, and shoulders may show limitation of movement, and complete ankylosis of the hip was found in 12 per cent of one series of cases.[25] The metacarpophalangeal, metatarsophalangeal, and the temperomandibular joints may be painful and restricted in movement as well.

Extraskeletal manifestations include ocular inflammation, aortic valve disease, carditis, and, occasionally, pulmonary fibrosis. Cardiac conduction defects occur in about 8 per cent of patients.

Laboratory Investigations

Serologic tests for rheumatoid factor are negative in over 90 per cent of cases. This is one of the most characteristic findings of ankylosing spondylitis and certain other disorders which share many of the clinical features. It serves to emphasize the distinction from rheumatoid arthritis. The erythrocyte sedimentation rate is usually elevated in the active phase of the disease.

Roentgen Features

The cardinal sign—and also, in most cases, the earliest detectable feature—of ankylosing spondylitis is roentgenographic erosion of the sacroiliac joints (Fig. 13-4). Though usually bilateral and symmetrical, it need not necessarily be so. At an early stage one sacroiliac joint may be involved and the other not obviously so, or one may be more severely involved than the other. Sooner or later, however, the changes are bilateral. The ragged appearance of the sacroiliac joints, with periarticular osteoporosis, reflects the early pathological stage of fibro-osseous inflammation and osteoclastic bone resorption. With subsequent fibrous replacement of bone, the joint space appears to widen. This is usually most obvious in the middle third of the joint (Fig. 13-5). The final stage of ossification ap-

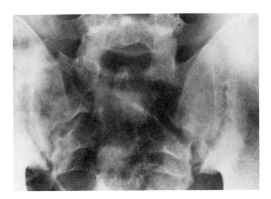

FIG. 13-4. Roentgenograph showing bilateral and symmetrical erosion of the sacroiliac joints. (See Fig. 13-5.)

pears as sclerosis, usually first on the iliac side of the joint, and proceeds to complete ankylosis (Fig. 13-6).

Next in diagnostic significance are the changes which accompany the formation of the marginal syndesmophytes. These usually commence at the dorsolumbar junction of the spine. The anterior corners of the vertebral bodies may show small areas of erosion at first; when this is accompanied by new bone formation an-

teriorly, with a reduction of the normal vertebral concavity, it results in the characteristic appearance of squaring of the vertebral bodies in the lateral films. (Fig. 13-7).[7] Later ossification of the surface layers of the disc leads to the delicate syndesmophyte which spans the gap between adjacent vertebrae (Fig. 13-8). Bridging of several adjacent intervertebral spaces gives the typical appearance of the "bamboo spine" (Fig. 13-9).

Early changes in the zygapophyseal joints are difficult to discern, yet joint space narrowing and even articular erosion may be demonstrated if sufficient care is taken to position the patient for the appropriate oblique projections. In the late stages, periarticular bone formation produces ankylosis of the posterior joints. When bilateral zygapophyseal ankylosis is accompanied by ossification of the interspinous ligaments over an extended segment, three longitudinal lines of sclerosis appear on the anteroposterior roentgenograph (Fig. 13-10).

Spinal changes, even at an early stage, may be accompanied by erosive arthritis of peripheral joints, especially the hips and knees (see Fig. 13-6). The roentgeno-

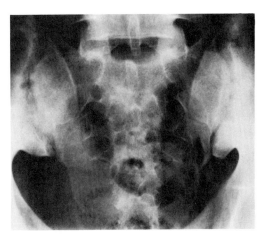

FIG. 13-5. Same patient as Fig. 13-4, 6 years later. The sacroiliac joints appear to be markedly widened, and there is dense periarticular sclerosis on the iliac side of the joints.

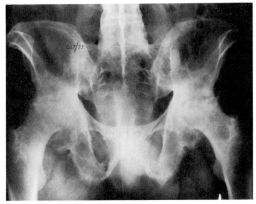

FIG. 13-6. Late stage of ankylosing spondylitis. The roentgenograph shows ankylosis of the sacroiliac joints and erosive arthritis of the hips.

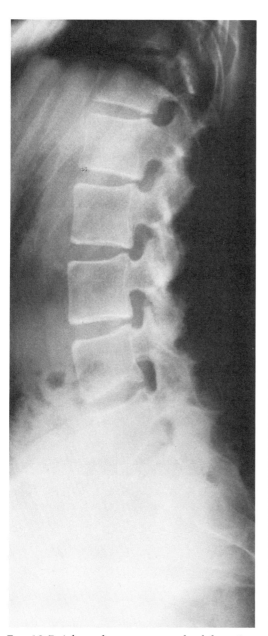

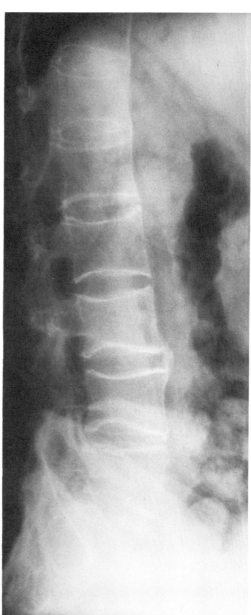

FIG. 13-7. A lateral roentgenograph of the spine shows erosion of the anterior margins and squaring of the vertebral bodies.

FIG. 13-8. Roentgenographic features in early ankylosing spondylitis. The anterior concavities of the lumbar vertebrae are flattened, and the intervertebral spaces are bridged by fine syndesmophytes.

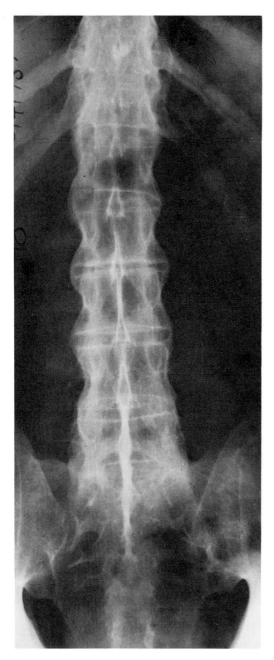

Fig. 13-9. Roentgenographic appearance of the "bamboo spine."

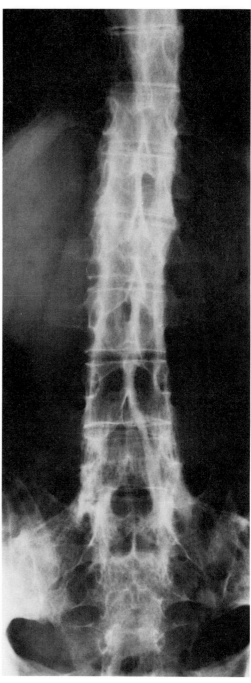

Fig. 13-10. A late case of ankylosing spondylitis. Ossification of the interspinous ligaments and the zygapophyseal joints produces three parallel lines of density running along the length of the lumbar spine. The sacroiliac joints are fused.

graphic features during the destructive phase are indistinguishable from those of rheumatoid arthritis. Unlike the latter, however, marked reactive new bone formation may lead to bony ankylosis of the synovial joints.

Extraspinal entheses which are often affected are the iliac apophyses, the ischial tuberosities (see Fig. 13-6), the femoral trochanters, and the ligamentous and tendinous insertions at the calcaneus (Fig. 13-11). Erosive changes or new bone formation extending into the soft tissues may occur.

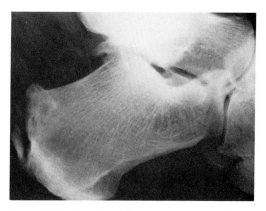

FIG. 13-11. Erosion, fragmentation, and new bone formation around the calcaneal apophysis.

Clinical Progress

The natural history of ankylosing spondylitis is one of recurrent acute or subacute episodes of pain, stiffness, and systemic activity. After some years the symptoms usually subside, but by then the patient may be left with permanent stiffness and deformity of the major joints. Sometimes these changes are limited to joints around the pelvis; more often the condition spreads up the spine to involve the dorsal and cervical segments, though this may take many years. The combination of spinal rigidity and ankylosis of the hips is particularly disabling, although in recent years the gloomy prognosis for these patients has been transformed by the advent of total joint replacement. Provided pain is adequately and safely controlled, patients with ankylosing spondylitis are surprisingly active, and their life span is said not to be shortened.[25]

Treatment

In the absence of a specific therapeutic agent, the treatment of ankylosing spondylitis consists of nonspecific antiinflammatory therapy, the control of pain, the preservation of movement, and the prevention of deformity.

Antiinflammatory Therapy. The most effective way of treating inflammatory joint disease is by rest and immobiliza-tion of the affected part. In the case of ankylosing spondylitis, however, complete rest and immobilization will increase the tendency to osteoporosis and ankylosis. The answer is a judicious compromise between rest and exercise, with adequate antiinflammatory drug therapy to combat pain and muscle spasm.

The most effective agents are indomethacin and phenylbutazone, which may have to be given in very large doses for months or years. Indeed, one of the striking things about patients with ankylosing spondylitis and the related disorders is their tolerance of large quantities of indomethacin, and doses of 200 mg. a day are not unusual during acute phases. Once the sedimentation rate has returned to normal and symptoms have subsided sufficiently to allow the patient to carry out his full exercise program, the dosage may be diminished progressively, and less harmful analgesics may be substituted for the more powerful antiinflammatory drugs.

Preservation of Movement. During the acute phases of the disease, pain and stiffness may be extreme. It is important, however, to encourage the patient always to think in terms of movement rather than rest, even if this has to be achieved

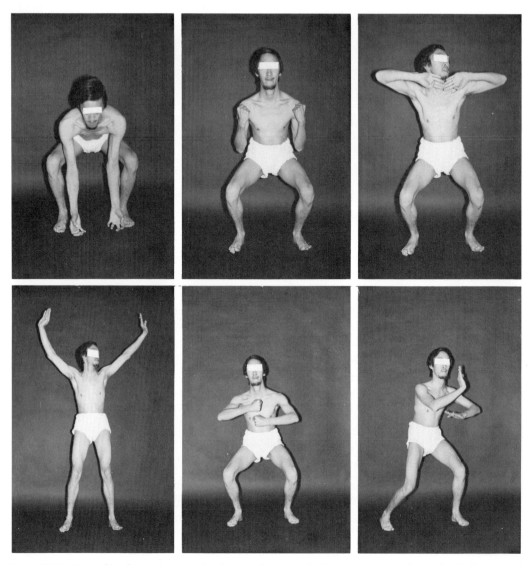

FIG. 13-12. Formalized exercises can be designed to put all the major joints through a full range of movement. The exercises shown here are based on traditional Chinese movements and include special breathing exercises as well.

by temporarily increasing antiinflammatory drugs. The patient should continue his normal pursuits as far as possible, avoiding only the more strenuous activities that involve lifting and straining. He should not sit in one position for long periods and, if desk work is essential, should get up, walk around, and exercise several times a day. He should be taught a series of exercises designed to mobilize shoulders, hips, spine, and costovertebral joints, to be carried out at least three times a day. This program is for life, and since simple, repetitive exercises are boring, they are soon abandoned. For this reason patients (and physiotherapists) should be encouraged to mold the exercises into games or dance rituals, the mastery of

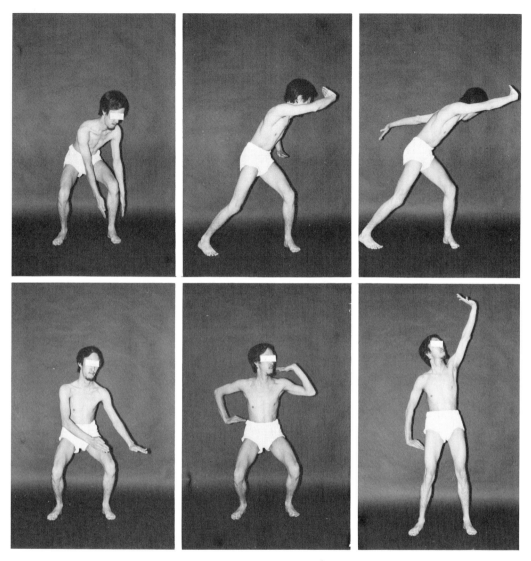

Fig. 13-12 *Continued.*

which will give a sense of pride and achievement (Fig. 13-12).

Prevention of Deformity. During the acute phase of the disease the patient tends to adopt those positions that are least painful: flexion of the spine, the hips, and the knees. With progressive stiffness and ankylosis, these deformities become fixed and produce a characteristic posture with flexion of the hips, a straight lumbar spine, and acute flexion and rota-

tion of the neck. At its worst this may make it impossible for him to lift his gaze more than a few paces ahead of his feet.

The prevention of these deformities is an important part of the physiotherapy program, and the liberal use of anti-inflammatory-analgesic preparations will make it possible to expand the mobilizing exercises into corrective therapy.

Correction of Deformity. Small degrees of fixed deformity in the spine and major peripheral joints can be corrected by controlled exercises and passive stretching before bony ankylosis supervenes. The opportunity of achieving even modest gains of this sort should never be neglected during the earlier and less disabling stages of the disease.

Ankylosis of one or both hip joints in unacceptable positions can be treated by total replacement arthroplasty. Certain modifications in the usual postoperative regime for these procedures should be adopted for patients with ankylosing spondylitis. Ankylosis of the cervical spine and limitation of chest expansion make anesthesia more hazardous than usual, and appropriate precautions should be taken in this regard. Provided the patient's general condition allows it, bilateral hip arthroplasty at one sitting is preferable, since postoperative rehabilitation of a single hip is often seriously impaired by the persistent deformity and ankylosis of the unoperated hip. Mobilization should begin immediately, as a certain amount of stiffening will take place during the months after operation.

Severe flexion deformity of the spine, which makes it impossible for the patient to lift his gaze more than ten paces ahead of his feet, is an indication for corrective surgery. In many cases adequate functional improvement may be achieved by ensuring full extension of the hip joints, if necessary by bilateral replacement arthroplasty. If the problem cannot be solved in this way, osteotomy of the spine should be considered.

The original operation of lumbar osteotomy was designed by Smith-Petersen in 1948. At the time it seemed an extremely hazardous procedure, but when the operation was carried out it was found to be easier than anticipated. Since then a large experience with this operation has been gained in various parts of the world and a reliable technique has been evolved. The need for the operation, however, has diminished, partly because it is now comparatively easy to mobilize the hip joints by low-friction arthroplasty, but mainly because the more severe deformities are being prevented by early, effective treatment. The operation is seldom carried out today.

SECONDARY ANKYLOSING SPONDYLOARTHROPATHY

For over a decade there has been an awareness that certain well-recognized disorders such as Reiter's disease and ulcerative colitis may be associated with features indistinguishable from those of uncomplicated ankylosing spondylitis. As more and more of these disorders have come to light, their common features have been delineated and they have been grouped under titles such as, "seronegative spondarthritides," and "ankylosing spondyloarthropathies."

The following criteria for inclusion in this group have been proposed by Moll and colleagues[20]:

1. The presence of an inflammatory peripheral arthritis
2. Negative serologic tests for rheumatoid factor
3. Absence of subcutaneous nodules
4. Roentgenographic sacroiliitis, with or without ankylosing spondylitis
5. Clinical overlap between members of the group
6. Familial aggregation

Disorders that satisfy all these criteria are idiopathic ankylosing spondylitis, Reiter's disease, psoriatic arthritis, ulcerative colitis, Crohn's disease, Whipple's disease, and Behçet's syndrome. If, however, one accepts the first four as major criteria which alone justify inclusion in the group, then conditions such as yersinia enterocolitis and the spondylitic form of Still's disease must qualify as well.

This is not to say that the spinal features of the specific diseases are indistinguishable from each other or that they resemble classical ankylosing spondylitis equally closely. Indeed, McEwen and co-workers have presented evidence that the spondyloarthropathies can be placed in two distinct categories[17]: (1) ulcerative colitis and Crohn's disease, which resemble idiopathic ankylosing spondylitis very closely and (2) Reiter's disease and psoriatic spondylitis, which resemble each other much more closely than they do the members of the other group. This, however, has been disputed by others, and it is undeniable that any large series of cases of idiopathic ankylosing spondylitis will include examples that resemble any of the secondary spondyloarthropathies.[20] Indeed, it is likely that all types of ankylosing spondylitis will ultimately be attributed to some underlying disorder, and the concept of "primary uncomplicated ankylosing spondylitis" will fall away eventually.

Clinical Features

As in idiopathic ankylosing spondylitis, backache and stiffness are the cardinal symptoms of secondary spondyloarthropathy. Complete rigidity of the spine, however, is less common in Reiter's disease, psoriatic arthritis, and yersinia enterocolitis than in idiopathic ankylosing spondylitis. Limitation of chest expansion is, likewise, less evident in these conditions than in ankylosing spondylitis.

Vertebral symptoms are accompanied, at some stage, by a peripheral arthritis in over 75 per cent of cases.[17,20] Whereas this is usually confined to the hips, shoulders, and knees in ankylosing spondylitis and ulcerative colitis, it frequently involves the smaller joints of the hands and feet in Reiter's disease, psoriatic arthritis, and yersinia arthritis.[17,29] In psoriasis destructive arthritis of the terminal interphalangeal joints is characteristic, though not inevitable. However, the findings of this particular feature in 100 per cent of their patients with psoriatic spondylitis

suggested to McEwen that this group might be more vulnerable than ever to terminal interphalangeal joint erosion.[17]

The clinical manifestations of the primary disease may not always be obvious. Any patient presenting with a seronegative spondyloarthropathy should be questioned carefully and examined for eidence of colitis, urethritis, conjunctivitis, psoriasis, and juvenile polyarthritis. Special investigations should include agglutination tests for yersinia enterocolitis and barium contrast roentgenography for ulcerative colitis and Crohn's disease.

Roentgen Features

Sacroiliac erosion is both the earliest and the most characteristic sign of secondary spondyloarthropathy. Its precise incidence, however, is difficult to determine and in any case depends largely on the duration of the underlying disease. In long-standing psoriatic arthritis it occurs in about 20 per cent of patients[20,29]; in Reiter's disease the frequency varies from 30 to over 50 per cent[20]; and in enterocolitis from 15 to 18 per cent.[20,32]

By the time the patient presents with backache and stiffness the roentgenographic sacroiliitis is usually bilateral and symmetrical, and in the more advanced cases (particularly those associated with ulcerative colitis and Crohn's disease) the changes are indistinguishable from those of ankylosing spondylitis.

Much has been made of the fact that the vertebral changes in secondary spondyloarthropathy differ significantly from those of classical ankylosing spondylitis, and MacEwen's group have divided their patients into two distinct types—those with classical ankylosing spondylitis, ulcerative colitis, or Crohn's disease, and those with Reiter's disease or psoriasis—largely on the basis that the former develop the typical marginal syndesmophytes already described, while the latter show a high proportion of "other

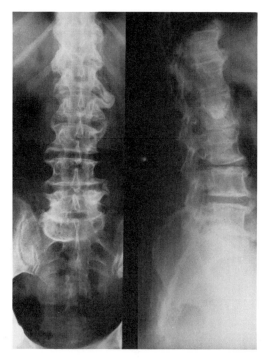

FIG. 13-13. Roentgenographs show "other than marginal" syndesmophytes in a patient with Reiter's disease.

than marginal" syndesmophytes (Fig. 13-13).[17] While it is true that patients with unequivocal Reiter's disease and psoriatic arthritis seldom manifest the full spectrum of roentgen changes seen in ankylosing spondylitis, or the tendency for these changes to spread relentlessly up the spine, the opposite does not hold, and many patients with classical ankylosing spondylitis develop large intervertebral spurs and bridges identical to those attributed to Reiter's disease.

Clinical Progress

In the secondary spondyloarthropathies the bowel or genitourinary disease usually precedes the vertebral involvement. Once the spondylitis is established, its severity bears little relation to the activity of the enterocolitis or urethritis, and it tends to persist even after the primary disorder has been successfully eradicated.

The peripheral arthritis, on the other hand, is often transient and may resolve completely once the primary disease is controlled.

ASSOCIATION BETWEEN THE SPONDYLOARTHROPATHIES

Numerous studies have shown close associations and overlap between the various ankylosing spondyloarthropathies. Psoriatic arthritis and Reiter's disease may, on occasion, be indistinguishable[30]; Reiter's disease also shares with ankylosing spondylitis, ulcerative colitis, Crohn's disease and Behcet's syndrome, certain common features, such as conjunctivitis, uveitis, and, occasionally, colitis.[14,20] Moreover, each of these disorders shows familial aggregation and a higher-than-usual prevalence in relatives of patients with any of the other disorders in the group.[18,20,31]

The Histocompatibility Antigen HL-A B27

The most convincing evidence of an association between the various ankylosing spondylo-arthropathies has been the recent discovery that they share a common histocompatibility antigen, HL-A B27, the presence of which is genetically determined (Table 13-1). The implications of this finding should be defined clearly. It is not suggested, for example, that HL-A B27 is in any way concerned with the etiology of the initial systemic disorder. Rather, it appears that of those individuals who contract the primary disease (ulcerative colitis, Reiter's disease, etc.) the ones who carry the appropriate histocompatibility gene will be predisposed to the development of sacroiliitis and spondylitis. Why they should be so predisposed is unknown. As a working hypothesis it has been postulated that a cluster of inherited immune responses may be associated with the same histocompatibility antigen (HL-A B27) as a

Table 13-1. Histocompatibility Antigen HL-A B27 in the Ankylosing Spondyloarthropathies

| Clinical Diagnosis | Patients | HL-A B27 Positive | | Reference |
		Patients (%)	Controls (%)	
Ankylosing spondylitis	75	96	4	Brewerton et al., 1973
	40	88	8	Schlostein et al., 1973
Reiter's syndrome	33	76	6	Brewterton et al., 1973
Psoriatic spondylitis	10	90	7	Brewerton et al., 1974
Ulcerative colitis with spondylitis	18	72.2	7.3	Brewerton et al., 1974
Yersinia arthritis	22	909	?	Aho et al., 1973

gene marker; those immune responses, operating in different combinations, may give rise to a number of different clinical syndromes which have in common a sacroiliitis and ankylosing spondylitis.

Treatment

Treatment with antiinflammatory drugs is usually sufficient to control the arthritis, but this may aggravate the enterocolitis. Progressive bowel disease may call for colectomy in its own right, and this will cure the peripheral arthritis as well. The spondylitis, howerver, is unaffected by colectomy and requires the same treatment as an idiopathic ankylosing spondylitis.

REFERENCES

1. Aho, K., Ahvonen, P., Lassus, A., Sievers, K., and Tillikainen, A.: HL-A antigen 27 and reactive arthritis. Lancet, *2*:157, 1973.
2. Ball, J.: Enthesopathy of rheumatoid and ankylosing spondylitis. Ann. Rheum. Dis., *30*:213, 1971.
3. Baum, J., and Ziff, M.: The rarity of ankylosing spondylitis in the black race. Arthritis Rheum., *14*:12, 1971.
4. von Bechterew, W.: Steifigkeit der Wirbelsäule und ihre Verkrümmung als besondere Erkrankungsform. Neurol. Zbl., *12*:633, 1893.
5. Berman, L., Isaacs, H., and Pickering, A.: Structural abnormalities of muscle tissue in ankylosing spondylitis. South Afr. Med. J., *50*:1238, 1976.
6. Bich, E. M.: The osteohistology of the normal human vertebra. J. Mount Sinai Hosp., *19*:490, 1952.
7. Boland, W. W., and Shebesta, E. M.: Rheumatoid spondylitis: Correlation of clinical and roentgenographic features. Radiology, *47*:551, 1946.
8. Brewerton, D. A., et al.: Ankylosing spondylitis and HL-A27. Lancet, *1*:904, 1973.
9. Brewerton, D. A., Caffrey, M., Nichl ., alters, D., Oates, J. K., and James, D. C. O.: Reiter's disease and HL-A27. Lancet, *ii*:996, 1973.
10. Brewerton, D. A., Caffrey, M., Nicholls, A., Walters, D., and James, D. C. O.: HL-A27 and arthropathies associated with ulcerative colitis and psoriasis. Lancet, *1*:956, 1974.
11. Connor, B.: The bones of a skeleton united without jointing or cartilage. Phil. Trans., B*29*:21, 1965.
12. Cruickshank, B.: Pathology of ankylosing spondylitis. Clin. Orthop., *74*:43, 1971.
13. Forestier, J., Jacqueline, F., and Rotes-Querol, J.: Ankylosing Spondylitis. Springfield, Charles C Thomas, 1956.
14. Jayson, M. I. V., and Bouchier, I.: Ulcerative colitis and ankylosing spondylitis. Ann. Rheum. Dis., *27*:219, 1968.
15. Kellgren, J. H.: The epidemiology of rheumatic diseases. Ann. Rheum. Dis., *23*:109, 1964.
16. Lorber, A., Pearson, C. M., and Rene, R. M.: Osteolytic vertebral lesions as a manifestation of rheumatoid arthritis and related disorders. Arthritis Rheum., *4*:514, 1961.
17. McEwen, C., et al.: Ankylosing spondylitis and spondylitis accompanying ulcerative colitis, regional enteritis, psoriasis and Reiter's disease. Arthritis Rheum., *14*:291, 1971.
18. Macrae, I., and Wright, V.: A family study of ulcerative colitis. Ann. Rheum. Dis., *32*:16, 1973.
19. Marie, P., and Astie, C.: Sur un cas de cyphose heredo-traumatique. Presse méd. 205.
20. Moll, J. M. H., Haslock, I., Macrae, I. F., and Wright, V.: Associations between ankylosing spondylitis, psoriatic arthritis, Reiter's disease, the intestinal arthropathies and Beçhet's syndrome. Medicine, *53*:343, 1974.
21. Moll, J. M. H., and Wright, V.: An objective clinical study of chest expansion. Ann. Rheum. Dis., *31*:1, 1972.
22. Schilling, F., and Schacherl, M.: Röntgen-

befunde an der Wirbelsäule bei Polyarthritis psoriatica und Reiter-dermatose: Spondylitis psoriatica. Z. Rheumaforsch., *26*:450, 1967.

23. Schlostein, L., Terasaki, P. I., Bluestone, R., and Pearson, C. M.: High association of an HL-A antigen W27 with ankylosing spondylitis. N. Engl. J. Med., *288*:704, 1973.

24. Sigler, J. W., Bluhm, G. B., Duncan, H., and Ensign, D. C.: Clinical features of ankylosing spondylitis. Clin. Orth., *74*:14, 1971.

25. Smukler, N.: Arthritis of the Spine. *In* Rothman, R. H. and Simeone, F. A. (eds.): The Spine. Philadelphia, W. B. Saunders, 1975.

24. Solomon, L., Beighton, P., Valkenburg, H. A., Robin, G., and Soskolne, C. L.: Rheumatic disorders in the South African Negro. Part I. Rheumatoid arthritis and ankylosing spondylitis. South Afr. Med. J., *49*:1292, 1975.

27. Strümpell, A.: Lehrbuch der spec. Pathologie und Therapie der inneren Krank leiten. ed. 8. Leipzig, Vogel, 1884.

28. Van Swaay, H.: Spondylosis ankylopoetica. Ein pathogenetische studie. Medical dissertation, Leiden, 1950.

29. Wright, V.: Psoriatic arthritis: a comparative study of rheumatoid arthritis and arthritis associated with psoriasis. Ann. Rheum. Dis., *20*:123, 1961.

30. Wright, V., and Reed, W. B.: The link between Reiter's syndrome and psoriatic arthritis. Ann. Rheum. Dis., *23*:12, 1964.

31. Wright, V., Sturrock, R. D., and Dick, W. C.: Seronegative spondarthritides. *In* Buchanan, W. W., and Dick, W. C. (eds.): Recent Advances in Rheumatology. Part 2. Edinburgh, Churchill Livingstone, 1976.

32. Wright, V., and Watkinson, G.: Sacro-iliitis and ulcerative colitis. Brit. Med. J., *2*:675, 1965.

14 Prolapsed Disc— From the Patient's Point of View

Michael Devas

I am an orthopaedic surgeon and at the time of my laminectomy I was 56 years old. At that time my wife had already had two spinal fusions for lumbar instability, and a son had also undergone a laminectomy for an adolescent disc protrusion. This is not a hard-luck story; I have learned much about backache and sciatica from the point of view of the patient since first taking an interest in the condition in 1956. Here I will emphasize certain aspects which, if dealt with at all, are often treated cursorily at best. For example, the patient who complains of "hot water pouring down the leg" need not be considered either neurotic or exaggerating. This is the best description available for a peculiar sensation which occurs in sciatica and which, once felt, will never be forgotten. Again, "I cannot keep my legs still" is not to be dismissed by thinking that the patient could keep them still if it was so wished. Once this has been experienced, sympathetic understanding takes the place of intolerant lack of interest.

HISTORY

The usual lumbago in early adult life was followed 15 years later by a routine sciatica with a lost ankle jerk. Treated conservatively, it improved to the extent that normal life was enjoyed; however, any hard exercise still produced a twinge behind the knee.

This "twinge," exacerbated at times, is probably more important than might be thought, because it stopped tennis and suchlike activities. The inevitable increase in weight took place; with increasing weight, life became even more sedentary, and even less activity would give the slight warning ache in the lateral hamstrings. Stress of any form would exacerbate the twinge; this was usually lack of rest from poor sleep at night, often because of anxiety or tension. Lack of sleep under happy conditions did not have the same effect. Deep, peaceful sleep is old-fashioned, but a benison without comparison.

Easter 1976 produced a severe second attack of sciatica; it came on during a period of extremely energetic work in organizing an international orthopaedic meeting in London with much extra travelling. I tried (foolishly) to continue to work until the sciatic scoliosis and my limp was noted by my colleague. Bed rest produced rapid improvement, and 2 weeks later I returned to work in a corset. Alas for advice! A heat wave made it too uncomfortable to do knee- or hip replacements in the corset, and it was discarded prematurely.

Sciatic Pain

Three months later, on holiday, pain began in the left leg. Slowly, over 3 days, it got more intense. It was at this stage that the hot water sensations occurred. These being new, I realized the root irritation was different and drove for 4 hours to get home. Sitting in a car had always been comfortable, even with sciatica (in contradistinction to many other sufferers), so much so that in the first attack I could get relief in the driving seat. However, once home, after the last journey, I could not leave the sitting position. How often have I not really believed graphic descriptions of being locked in position; unable to get upstairs, or forced to do this or that! Eventually I managed to get out of the car and onto my bed, but I had to put my legs on a chair, the affected knee and hip flexed as though in the sitting position. Any attempt to lower the leg produced a sharp searing pain into the buttock, thigh, and calf; "red-hot," "tearing," and many other lurid descriptive terms are not an exaggeration. It is this pain that can frighten a patient, and so the movement is not tried again. However, with the knowledge that the pain is just pressure on a nerve root, and after half an hour of rest, by moving with extreme slowness the problem of being locked in this position was overcome and the leg lowered to the bed in stages.

Lying in bed at home was comfortable. Drugs on demand from the bottle at the bedside (but moved at night) were the best method of controlling pain. The quality of the pain is very important, but despite the graphic descriptions, it is not a terrible pain in itself. Severe sciatica is a tiring pain, its very continuity causing frustration and irritability. The inability to move freely and having to sleep in the same position until some unguarded movement jerks one into wakefulness is both tiresome and tiring. It is not a fearful pain, but great care is taken to avoid it. It is remote, but nevertheless it prevents

walking. When it occurs it cannot be borne: one must get to the floor to lie. One cannot take one more step: yet even at the most severe it can seem absurd and be almost laughable. It is a stupid pain, but it cripples; it is an intense pain, but it is far down in the leg. Finally, it is a pain that is curiously difficult to remember.

It was impossible to walk from bed to toilet without aid. Crawling was easiest. Sitting on the toilet seat was a great problem because the back and leg would lock just as the sitting position was being achieved, so great care was needed to get down satisfactorily. A daily bowel action was helpful; without it pain was increased. After 10 days the straight-leg raising was not improving, and I was admitted for traction.

THE PAIN OF INSTABILITY

At the age of 30 during her third pregnancy my wife found that activities like stooping and lifting became difficult because of low backache. It was worse with the next pregnancy, and standing became difficult, necessitating a shooting stick when out and bed rest for the last 3 weeks. At no time was there severe pain but only the feeling of intense physical weakness that occurred when standing. After the child was born she returned to a normal life but could not manage heavy domestic work.

The fifth and sixth pregnancies were much the same but were helped by an orthopaedic maternity corset. Again the feeling of weakness of the low back was worse than the pain, which was not at first severe. The last 5 or 6 weeks of the pregnancies were spent in bed.

The important feature of the symptoms was the severe disability of not being able to stand. Although this is the classic feature of lumbar instability it is still difficult to describe, especially when the emphasis on low back pain is not present. Social events were curtailed if they necessitated standing; a cocktail party was quite unacceptable. Treatment, apart from the corset, made no difference, and physiotherapy was of little help.

Over the next few years the pain increased; it was like "being sawn in half" and "red-hot needles" in the back. Location was very difficult, but tenderness at the lumbosacral region, especially in the muscles, was present when the symptoms were severe. A manipulation was of no help. The only activity that was pleasant because it caused no pain was swimming, but neither did it help.

A screw fusion of L4 to the sacrum was done. The initial benefit was great, only to be followed by later deterioration. A normal myelograph was followed by 3 months in a rehabilitation center doing progressive exercises. After this, pain was much improved, but standing was still impossible for more than a few moments. Although daily exercises continued, after 6 years the pain had gradually come back. A radiculogram was normal. Exploration showed that the L3–4 level was unstable, and this was fused.

For a woman the frequent use of a bedpan after a fusion is very painful, particularly being lifted on to it. To overcome this, the patient should be rolled on to her side on top of several pillows; the bedpan is placed in position and the patient rolled back on to it. Before reversing the procedure, and after every micturition, the perineum must be cleansed. This is easiest—and best done—by douching with warm water. The bedpan is removed by rolling the patient and, while she is still on her side, the pressure points are dried and powered.

Describing the Symptoms

The difficulty of trying to explain what the problem is can be very great. The symptoms can be bizarre. When pain is severe, "burning rods" are descriptive and can be localized easily, but sometimes the pain is elusive and each muscle in the low back needs to be carefully palpated to find spasm; here is the source of the pain. The patient is embarrassed in having to admit that the pain, neither severe nor properly localized, nevertheless makes it impossible to stand without the feeling of being about to keel over, so it is not surprising that many similes should be used in the description of this absurd inability to do a simple normal activity such as standing. Thus a suitable comparison was found, in this case, with hunger. The surgeon was asked if he had ever been starving for several days. He was then asked if he could locate, at that time, the pangs of hunger. By this the very real problem, with its lack of precise or specific localization and detail, could be understood.

TREATMENT OF SCIATICA

Traction

Traction in itself is comfortable, but the top or proximal end of the strapping can irritate if it is not stuck down very firmly. Benzoic acid paint helped but smelled awful when present the whole time. Every part of the paint should be covered by the crepe bandage so that it does not stick to the sheets. The pull of the traction must not be chosen arbitrarily but adjusted to the weight of the patient, who will be lying in the head-down position; this makes the bottle troublesome to use and bedpans quite unacceptable. Constipation is certain unless a compromise is found, such as using a commode while the traction is maintained.

The symptoms in traction must be watched. Mine changed after a week. Whereas at first extended legs were most comfortable, overnight something happened, and from then on, despite the weights, the knees were flexed, especially at night. This was not the patient being difficult; it just occurred. Perhaps at this stage the disc had sequestrated completely.

Analgesics

Paracetamol with aspirin and codeine was the basic mixture augmented by two tablets of Diconal (dipipanone hydrochloride 10 mg., cyclizine hydrochloride 10 mg.) or pethidine, 100 mg. by mouth. While on traction the mixture alone by day was sufficient, but at night the stronger drugs were needed to ensure sleep and Phenergan (promethazine hydrochloride, 10 mg.) and butobarbitone were added. The ordinary methods of dosage for night sedation were completely inadequate. The routine of taking the night sedation at 10:00 p.m. meant waking at about 4:00 in the morning, thereafter to lie awake for some hours, perhaps drifting off into a fitful sleep just before being awakened for the morning nursing care. Therefore the Phenergan was taken at 8:00 o'clock, because it takes a long time to act for sleep, and the analgesics and barbiturate at 9:00. At the same time a dose of Piriton (chlorpheniramine 4 mg.) and a butobarbitone tablet with the basic paracetamol aspirin and codeine mixture was left by the bedside to be taken in the middle of the night on waking. This meant that each night, without having to summon aid, and as soon as pain awoke me, I could take the pills at my bedside and drift off to sleep. I awoke refreshed and not muzzy. I found throughout that the proper quantity of drugs to act as they should rarely caused any side effects. This was particularly true of Diconal and pethidine, which at no time did anything for me except relieve pain. There was certainly no well-being produced by either drug, despite their reputations, except the relief of the sciatica. It is said that Phenergan may exacerbate pain; but its excellent quality of promoting deep, prolonged sleep outweighs that aspect, which is easily overcome by taking analgesics at the same time.

Traction having failed and the orthopaedic meeting approaching, a plaster jacket was put on after a cast for a plastic jacket had been made. This was against the advice of my surgeon, who thought it would be too much standing. He was right; gradually the pain in the leg became more and more intense, despite adequate premedication. Eventually a vasovagal collapse put an end to standing, but fortunately the jacket was complete by then.

Awaking from the faint was the most comfortable interlude in the 3 months of this particular trouble. There was no pain, and I was completely at ease. I cannot explain this now, but at the time I believed that the plaster jacket was working. It did seem at first to help, but walking was still extremely difficult. Sticks, a walking frame, axillary crutches were all tried, but elbow crutches proved the best. Sitting was possible, which had been very painful before, so that lying or reclining in a comfortable chair was imperative except when hobbling from place to place. Thirty yards was about the limit of walking with the elbow crutches. Without them hardly a step could be taken. The plaster jacket did not work as a cure (it was not by now expected to) and it is probably unjustifiable for a patient to continue in it after 3 weeks if it has not started to give some improvement. For me it was procrastination to keep me about.

Personal hygiene is a freely used expression, but the problems are ill understood, especially when wearing a plaster jacket. The sciatica produced when trying to cleanse the perineum at toilet is great. Very careful positioning was necessary and often very sharp bouts of pain were produced. Further, proper washing of the perineum was almost impossible and help was often necessary. If the plaster jacket is cut away sufficiently to allow these functions to be done more easily by allowing more flexion of the hips, the jacket does not give sufficient immobilization of the spine. The proper jacket makes it almost impossible to do up a shoelace or to put on a sock, and this must be accepted. The plastic jacket was less good at immobilization but had many compensations. Particularly, it was possible to take a bath, and socks could be put on before the jacket was replaced. The plastic jacket and the elbow crutches kept me in much the same condition as the plaster jacket. This meant that to go around the orthopaedic meeting was impossible all at once and had to be done in stages. A wheelchair was the most comfortable seat I could find, both for its positioning of the body and for its mobility in the office.

The analgesic routine at this stage would be three codeine, three aspirin, and three paracetamol tablets and probably 100 mg. of pethidine. I am over 6 feet tall and weigh about 90 kg. Taken at 10:00 this would last until mid-afternoon, when a second dose would be taken, perhaps substituting Diconal for the pethidine. For special efforts, papaveratum would be substituted for the codeine, but no pethidine or Diconal was taken at the same time. The papaveratum (10 mg. per tablet) was prepared with soluble aspirin (500 mg.) in an effervescent mixture and was undoubtedly the best analgesic and left the mind clear without side effects or euphoria. Ten mg. of papaveratum is equivalent to 5 mg. of morphia. I found two tablets satisfactory, but this could be augmented with paracetamol. It was found important to take the drugs when pain was severe rather than at fixed times each day. If a weaker drug is being taken too often, then a stronger drug should be instituted. Thus, if the aspirin-codeine-paracetamol mixture lasted only for an hour, then it was important to add a stronger drug to the mixture, such as mentioned above.

Alcohol was certainly the best vehicle for taking tablets. Its analgesic effect was appreciable even if consumption did increase considerably at this time. No withdrawal symptoms were evident on returning to normal consumption after the operation.

Laminectomy

The symptoms were classical and I did not have a myelograph. I was frightened before the operation, of what I am not sure; perhaps vaguely of paralysis; even of not waking up. The fears were illogical and stupid, because I have had anesthetics before, but nevertheless were present. Being in "my own" hospital, dealt with by my own colleagues, and looked after by my own nurses, I could not admit to such vague fears. How much more may some timid patient suffer?

I woke, having had a sequestrated disc removed from the L5–S1 level on the left; the nerve root had been stretched very tightly against the ligamentum flavum. I awoke at about 5:00 o'clock that afternoon and I recall having three or four injections of Omnopon. Again, it was needed at 3½-hour intervals and not at the 4 hours that is so often prescribed. This is important, because when one wakes after an anesthetic and operation the pain locally is acute (but all the sciatica had gone), and adequate morphine dosage leaves the patient far happier the next day.

At 6:00 in the morning after the operation it was obvious I needed no more injections. Instead, having had a good night, a cup of coffee was the most desired drug. I could now appreciate properly the numbness of the first sacral distribution, conspicuous in the absence of pain.

I began to move at once, at first isometric calf exercises and rolling—with help—from side to side. At first painful, it was just possible if taken slowly. The quality of the nursing skill is all important. The pain was not so much from the operation wound itself but from a ridge of edema which formed on either side of the spine which was, as it were, squeezed out from the central part of the wound where pressure was maintained by body weight. After lying for a while on the side, the same thing occurred and was painful on returning to the supine. If the rolling continued to the opposite side, there was not a second ridge of edema and thus it was better to go from side to side rather than from side to back to side.

The pain from the operation rapidly decreased, and daytime drugs were withdrawn entirely at 3 days, but nocturnal sedation continued to obtain a good night. At the end of 1 week all night sedation was stopped. This was followed by a sleepless night (but what did it matter in hospital?) and the next night, 10 hours' sleep. It was at this time that drug withdrawal started the twitching in the leg and more knee movements and fidgeting. I believe this was caused by the large consumption of paracetamol, because on one occasion a small dose completely relieved the symptoms. After 4 days I started to walk. I was very wobbly, hardly having walked for over 3 months.

Rehabilitation

Walking was the important exercise. There was no need to do anything else, although, in bed, exercises using dumbbells had been done. Lying supine, both arms are lifted from the side to the perpendicular and each hand holding a 5-pound weight. This will exercise most of the spinal muscles isometrically and it was found to be a very helpful, tiring, and simple exercise.

At first the slightest hill was a problem, but after 4 weeks, 2 or 3 miles were possible and the hills seemed less steep. At 6 weeks it was possible to walk 5 miles. With each succeeding week exercise improved and distances were increased, and I was fitter 3 months after the laminectomy than I had been for some 15 years. Weight had been lost, exercise tolerance greatly improved, and even agility seemed better.

Sensibility

The lack of sensibility over the area supplied by the first sacral root has been mentioned; the absence of heat appreciation often gives rise to a cold feeling, and I know why a patient has "a cold foot" in sciatica, even if "warm water" is felt running down the leg.

CONCLUSION

The experience of a disc being removed after 3 months of severe sciatica has produced in me a firm conviction that most people who appear to complain of bizarre, odd, ludicrous, or even frankly impossible symptoms should be believed. With an increasing interest in lumbar stenosis, on which myelography or radiculography has to be done purely on the history and with no physical signs, I believe no symptom should be discarded lightly merely because it is difficult to appreciate or understand. Secondly, my prescription habits have altered, I hope for the better; no patient is standard or uniform, and analgesia should never be prescribed by rote; rather the merits of each individual should be assessed. Finally, I have always believed that my nursing staff were superb: having had practical experience of their skill my belief is now confirmed.

Index

Numerals in *italics* indicate a figure; "t" following a page number indicates a table.